Sex and Pregnancy

Sex and Pregnancy

From Evidence-Based Medicine to Dr Google

Edited by
Dan Farine
Mount Sinai Hospital, Toronto

Pablo Tobías González
Infanta Cristina University Hospital

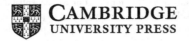

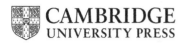

Shaftesbury Road, Cambridge CB2 8EA, United Kingdom

One Liberty Plaza, 20th Floor, New York, NY 10006, USA

477 Williamstown Road, Port Melbourne, VIC 3207, Australia

314–321, 3rd Floor, Plot 3, Splendor Forum, Jasola District Centre, New Delhi – 110025, India

103 Penang Road, #05–06/07, Visioncrest Commercial, Singapore 238467

Cambridge University Press is part of the University of Cambridge Press & Assessment.

It furthers the University's mission by disseminating knowledge in the pursuit of education, learning, and research at the highest international levels of excellence.

www.cambridge.org
Information on this title: www.cambridge.org/9781009015301

DOI: 10.1017/9781009025034

First published 2023

A catalogue record for this publication is available from the British Library.

Library of Congress Cataloging-in-Publication Data
Names: Farine, Dan, editor. | Tobías González, Pablo, editor.
Title: Sex and pregnancy : a guide for healthcare workers / edited by Dan Farine, Pablo Tobías González.
Description: Cambridge ; New York, NY : Cambridge University Press, 2022. | Includes bibliographical references and index.
Identifiers: LCCN 2022022830 (print) | LCCN 2022022831 (ebook) | ISBN 9781009015301 (paperback) | ISBN 9781009025034 (epub)
Subjects: MESH: Pregnancy | Coitus | Sexual Behavior | BISAC: MEDICAL / Gynecology & Obstetrics
Classification: LCC RG525 (print) | LCC RG525 (ebook) | NLM WQ 200.1 | DDC 618.2–dc23/eng/20220625
LC record available at https://lccn.loc.gov/2022022830
LC ebook record available at https://lccn.loc.gov/2022022831

ISBN 978-1-009-01530-1 Paperback

....

Dedicated to my sister and brother-in-law, Esther and Jacob Burstein.

Dan Farine

Manolo, Basilio, Carmen, Guillermo and Javier, thank you for your love and guidance.
Silvia, thank you for your strength and patience.
Manuel, thank you for your laughter and curiosity

Pablo Tobías González

Contents

Contributors

Duaa M. Bahkali
Department of Obstetrics and Gynecology, University of Ottawa, Ottawa, Ontario, Canada

Jon F. R. Barrett
Department of Obstetrics and Gynecology, McMaster University, Hamilton, Ontario, Canada

Giuseppe Benagiano
Department of Maternal and Child Health, Gynecology and Urology, "Sapienza" University of Rome, Rome, Italy

Cristina González Benítez
Department of Obstetrics and Gynecology, La Paz University Hospital, Madrid, Spain

Vincenzo Berghella
Department of Obstetrics and Gynecology and Division of Maternal Fetal Medicine, Thomas Jefferson University Hospital, Philadelphia, PA, USA

Silvia Barras Bermejo
Obstetrics and Gynaecology Department, Hospital Universitario Infanta Cristina, Parla, Spain

Hanane Bouchghoul
Department of Obstetrics and Gynecology, Bordeaux University Hospital, Bordeaux, France

Julia Burd
Department of Obstetrics and Gynecology and Division of Maternal Fetal Medicine, Thomas Jefferson University Hospital, Philadelphia, PA, USA

Francisco Marcelo Carvalho
Faculdade de Medicina Nova Esperança, João Pessoa, Paraíba, Brazil

Beatriz Maria Villar de Carvalho
Santa Casa University, São Paulo, Brazil

Yara Maia Villar de Carvalho
Faculdade de Medicina Nova Esperança, João Pessoa, Paraíba, Brazil

Crystal Chan
Mount Sinai Hospital, Sinai Health System, and Department of Obstetrics and Gynecology, University of Toronto, Toronto, Ontario, Canada

Jazleen Dada
Department of Obstetrics and Gynecology, Faculty of Medicine, University of Toronto, Toronto, Ontario, Canada

Ayelet Dangot
Department of Obstetrics and Gynecology, Lis Maternity Hospital, Tel Aviv Sourasky Medical Center, Tel Aviv University, Tel Aviv, Israel

E. Shirin Dason
Department of Obstetrics and Gynecology, Temerty Faculty of Medicine, University of Toronto, Toronto, Ontario, Canada

Karthika Devarajan
Department of Obstetrics and Gynecology, North York General Hospital, Toronto, Ontario, Canada

Trish Dinh
Department of Obstetrics and Gynecology, University of Ottawa, Ottawa, Ontario, Canada

Gian Carlo Di Renzo
Centre of Perinatal and Reproductive Medicine, University of Perugia; Department of Obsterics and Gynecology, IE Sechenov State University, Moscow,

Russia; and Wayne State University
Medical School, Detroit, USA

Yossef Ezra
Department of Obstetrics and Gynecology,
Hadassah Medical Center, and The Hebrew
University Medical School, Jerusalem,
Israel

Dan Farine
Mount Sinai Hospital, Maternal–Fetal
Medicine Division, Department of
Obstetrics and Gynecology, University of
Toronto, Toronto, Ontario, Canada

Eduardo Borges da Fonseca
Division of Obstetrics and Gynecology,
Federal University of Paraíba, João Pessoa,
Paraíba, Brazil

Marcos Luján Galán
Urology Department, Infanta
Cristina University Hospital, Parla,
Madrid, Spain

Noa Gilad
Mount Sinai Hospital, Toronto, Ontario,
Canada

Hanna R. Goldberg
Department of Obstetrics and Gynecology,
University of Toronto, Toronto, Ontario,
Canada

Pablo Tobías González
Obstetrics and Gynecology Department,
Infanta Cristina University Hospital, Parla,
Madrid, Spain

Gali Gordon
Department of Obstetrics and Gynecology,
Hadassah Medical Center, and The Hebrew
University Medical School, Jerusalem,
Israel

Ola Gutzeit
Rambam Health Care Campus, Haifa,
Israel

Doron Kabiri
Department of Obstetrics and Gynecology,
Hadassah Medical Center, and The Hebrew
University Medical School, Jerusalem,
Israel

Abi Kirubarajan
Department of Obstetrics and Gynecology,
Temerty Faculty of Medicine, University of
Toronto, Toronto, Ontario, Canada

**Evangelia Vlachodimitropoulou
Koumoutsea**
Division of Maternal–Fetal Medicine,
Department of Obstetrics and Gynecology,
Mount Sinai Hospital, University of
Toronto, Toronto, Ontario, Canada

Vered B. Lamhot
Rambam Health Care Campus, Haifa,
Israel

Michael Lavie
Lis Maternity Hospital, Tel Aviv Souraski
Medical Center, Tel-Aviv, Israel

Ángeles Leal García
Pelvic Floor Unit, Department of
Obstetrics and Gynecology, La Paz
University Hospital, Madrid, Spain

Hayley Lipworth
Division of Maternal–Fetal Medicine,
Department of Obstetrics and
Gynecology, Sunnybrook Health Sciences
Centre and Institute of Medical Sciences,
University of Toronto, Toronto, Ontario,
Canada

Hugo Madar
Department of Obstetrics and Gynecology,
Bordeaux University Hospital, Bordeaux,
France

Ariel Many
Department of Obstetrics and Gynecology,
Maayne Hayeshua Medical Center, Tel
Aviv University, Tel Aviv, Israel

Aurélien Mattuizzi
Department of Obstetrics and Gynecology, Bordeaux University Hospital, Bordeaux, France

Cynthia Maxwell
Division of Maternal–Fetal Medicine, Department of Obstetrics and Gynecology, Mount Sinai Hospital, University of Toronto, Toronto, Ontario, Canada

Nir Melamed
Division of Maternal–Fetal Medicine, Department of Obstetrics and Gynecology, Sunnybrook Health Sciences Centre, University of Toronto, Toronto, Ontario, Canada

Dina Mohamed
Advanced Obstetric Fellow, Mount Sinai Hospital, University of Toronto, Toronto, Ontario, Canada

Mohamed Momtaz
Department of Obstetrics and Gynecology, University of Cairo, Cairo, Egypt

María del Mar Muñoz Muñiz
Pelvic Floor Unit, Department of Obstetrics and Gynecology, La Paz University Hospital, and Department of Obstetrics and Gynecology, Universidad Autonoma Madrid, Madrid, Spain

Hisham T. Nasief
Department of Obstetrics and Gynecology, University of Ottawa, Ottawa, Ontario, Canada

Kirsten M. Niles
Division of Maternal Fetal Medicine, Department of Obstetrics and Gynecology, University of British Columbia, Vancouver; and Department of Obstetrics and Gynecology, Fraser Health Authority, Surrey, British Columbia, Canada

Lawrence W. Oppenheimer
Department of Obstetrics and Gynecology, University of Ottawa, Ottawa, Ontario, Canada

Elisa Moreno Palacios
Department of Obstetrics and Gynecology, La Paz University Hospital, Madrid, Spain

Carlos López Ramón y Cajal
Obstetrics and Gynecology Service, Álvaro Cunqueiro Hospital, Vigo, Spain

Stefania Ronzoni
Sunnybrook Health Sciences Center and University of Toronto, Toronto, Ontario, Canada

Hadar Rosen
Fetal Medicine Unit, Department of Obstetrics and Gynecology, Sheba Medical Center, Tel Hashomer, Israel

Eliane Rozanes
Department of Obstetrics and Gynecology, Lis Maternity Hospital, Tel Aviv Sourasky Medical Center, Tel Aviv University, Tel Aviv, Israel

David Gómez Sánchez
Álvaro Cunqueiro Hospital, Vigo, Spain

Loïc Sentilhes
Department of Obstetrics and Gynecology, Bordeaux University Hospital, Bordeaux, France

María Luisa Morales Serrano
Burgos University Hospital, Burgos, Spain

Sara Serrano Velayos
Pelvic Floor Unit, Department of Obstetrics and Gynecology, La Paz University Hospital, Madrid, Spain

Orli Silverberg
Faculty of Medicine, University of Toronto, Toronto, Ontario, Canada

Mara Sobel
Department of Obstetrics and Gynecology, Temerty Faculty of Medicine, University of Toronto; and Department of Obstetrics and Gynecology, Mount Sinai Hospital, Sinai Health System, Toronto, Ontario, Canada

Rachel Spitzer
Department of Obstetrics and Gynecology, University of Toronto, Toronto, Ontario, Canada

Valentina Tosto
Giannina Gaslini Institute Department of Obstetrics and Gynecology, Genova (Italy) and University of Perugia, Department of Reproductive and Perinatal Medicine, Perugia (Italy)

Valentina Tsibizova
Institute of Perinatology and Pediatry of Almazov National Medical Research Centre, St Petersburg, Russia; and PREIS intl School, Firenze, Italy

María Serrano Velasco
Department of Obstetrics and Gynecology, La Paz University Hospital, Madrid, Spain

Dana Vitner
Rambam Health Care Campus, Haifa, Israel

Jenny Yang
Department of Obstetrics and Gynecology, University of Toronto, Toronto, Ontario, Canada

Yariv Yogev
Department of Obstetrics, Gynecology, and Fertility, Lis Hospital for Women, Tel Aviv Sourasky Medical Center, Sackler Faculty of Medicine, Tel Aviv University, Tel Aviv, Israel

Rita Zlatkin
Helen Schneider Hospital for Women, Rabin Medical Center, Petach Tikva, Israel

Preface

About 10 years ago I (Dan Farine) was chairing a session on normal pregnancy in an international meeting in Europe. To my surprise, an eminent professor in obstetrics and gynecology stood up in the discussion session and explained to the audience that prostaglandins in the semen were the cause of preterm birth. Furthermore, he stated that this was why he didn't care if his patients used condoms when they were not pregnant but that they had to use them when they were. In response, another professor explained that the cause was not the semen or the prostaglandins but the tonic contractions of the uterus during orgasm. He came up with a quite different statement saying that it was acceptable for his patients to have sex as long as they didn't enjoy it! When I researched both hypotheses, I was unable to find strong evidence to support them, nor the two recommendations provided by these two distinguished professors.

Upon returning to Toronto, I was approached by our residents who asked me to help them find a topic for grand rounds. They asked for a sexy topic related with pregnancy and that had not been presented before. The grand rounds on sex and pregnancy resulted in a review of the topic that comprised one-fifth of all medical articles quoted that year on the Internet.

Interestingly, to this day, not one medical textbook or resource has looked at the different aspects of sex in pregnancy. As a result, many obstetric caregivers have inadequate knowledge in this area, limiting their ability to provide accurate information to their patients.

A couple of years ago, Pablo Tobias and I had many discussions on how the Internet is changing obstetric care. While in the past patients relied on caregivers (or friends and family) to acquire information, nowadays they often have excessive and inaccurate information and our job is to direct them to the proper sources. For example, I had a patient who was mad at me for not being well informed about a paper from a developing country that was published in French and that was actually of poor quality. My image as an expert was shattered until I showed her that I did indeed search the topic and had read dozens of papers on this very remote anomaly. Another example came from a patient who insisted on a termination of pregnancy for an abnormality that was minimal (an extra digit) and which could easily be corrected surgically postpartum. Pablo and I initially thought to write a monograph or a review with the title "What did Dr. Google tell you?" but chose instead to write this book on sex and pregnancy. Coincidentally, Pablo and his wife Silvia became parents while "conceiving" this book. We decided to address the issue in this textbook in two different ways: First, there is a chapter on the Internet and how it should be used; and second, in the chapters addressing a specific clinical situation we initially wrote a standard chapter reviewing the medical information available and then added another section named "What did Dr. Google say?" that reviews the information available on the Internet and compares it to the standard information published in medical texts and articles. We believe this will address what our patients often read before they speak to us, and also reviews the internet information in the context of available medical information.

This book is addressed not only to obstetricians and other physicians who care for pregnant women, but also to other professions involved in the care of pregnant women: midwives, nurses, pregnancy educators, and others. Additionally, we think pregnant women would be interested in this book. Some of them will present the different complications outlined in this book and many of them will search the Internet for information.

In summary, this book, with its novel approach, addresses a niche that has never been properly explored in the medical literature and we believe it will be helpful for all the aforementioned potential readers.

Dan Farine

From Sex for Reproduction to Reproduction without Sex

Gian Carlo Di Renzo, Valentina Tosto, Valentina
Tsibizova, and Giuseppe Benagiano

1.1 Introduction

Throughout human history the connection between sexuality and reproduction has been
at the core of the life of the vast majority of men and women, although this has
manifested itself in various, sometimes conflicting ways, ranging from placing sexuality
at the center of a person's existence to its complete elimination in search of a higher level
of human achievement. In many ways, sexuality – historically driven by the imperative to
reproduce [1] – if properly used, can be at the core of human progress, whereas its abuses
can lead to totally dehumanizing and violent behaviors.

While sexual activity has been the norm, over the millennia there have always been
voices advocating abstinence for a variety of reasons. In the sixth century BC, Pythagoras
dictated that sex should be practiced in the winter but not the summer; in addition, he
believed that it was harmful to male, but not female, health [2]. During Christianity's
first 15 centuries of existence, abstinence was considered a means of achieving a higher
level of spirituality, and celibacy has a place in all the major religions [3,4].

Even centuries ago, well before the age of modern methods of family planning,
abstinence was also preached as a means of avoiding the risk of overpopulation [5]. At
the same time, well before the age of modern contraception, humans attempted to separate
sexual activity and reproduction by means other than abstinence, as evidenced by the
millenia-old descriptions of rudimentary contraceptive techniques in Egyptian papyri and
the writings of the Greek Soranus and the Romans Pliny the Elder and Dioscorides [6].

1.2 Sex without Reproduction

Separation of sex from reproduction remained a dream until the end of the nineteenth
century when Sigmund Freud wrote: "Theoretically, it would be one of the greatest
triumphs of humanity if the act responsible for procreation could be raised to the level of
voluntary and intentional behavior in order to separate it from the imperative to satisfy a
natural urge" [7]. Freud's dream became a reality around the middle of the twentieth
century when effective methods of family planning were developed. Research in this field
was driven by an event that will remain unique in the history of humanity, when, in only
one century, the human population increased from some 1.6 billion to more than
6 billion [8].

Besides bringing population growth under control, the availability of effective
methods of contraception made possible for the first time the separation of the two
acknowledged meanings of sexuality – procreation and recreation – producing the first
revolution in reproduction [5].

Credit for this advance should be given to the introduction, some six decades ago, of hormonal and intrauterine contraception. Granting women sexual freedom without the fear of an unwanted pregnancy, enabled them for the first time to take charge of their own reproductive potential. This in turn helped to shape a new place for women in society: Young women are now in a position to complete their education and develop careers in every field without abstaining from sexual activity, something that young men had always taken for granted.

Such a change deserves the title of "sexual revolution," one capable of challenging and transforming relationships between men and women. No progress, however, comes without a price: Delaying the first pregnancy by as much as 10 years, as is now the case in some Western countries, carries important consequences for reproduction. The decline in female fertility that starts in the thirties and increases rapidly after age 37 [9] will force more and more women to turn to Assisted Reproductive Technology (ART), with less and less satisfactory results. In addition, childbearing in the late thirties and early forties carries an increased risk of complications [10].

Clearly, the pleasure intrinsic in the sexual act has been the instrument through which reproduction took place, although in many cultures this pleasure has been regarded with disapproval. Today, the idea of sex for pleasure has gained such wide acceptance that some have concluded that sex is mostly for pleasure and not simply procreation. In this respect, Abramson and Pinkerton concluded that if it is undeniable that pleasure in sexual activity developed in order to promote procreation, it does not represent a simple by-product of the drive to procreate. Sexual pleasure facilitates interpersonal bonding, promotes interpersonal relationships, and can reduce social tensions [11].

In conclusion, starting during the twentieth century, the relationship between reproduction and sexuality has continuously evolved [12], each beginning to move independently and, in many ways, becoming separate. What seems surprising is that, after the first revolution separated sex from reproduction, within a few decades a new, even more dramatic revolution took place: reproduction without sex.

1.3 Reproduction without Sex

The new paradigm, made possible by the pioneering work of Edwards and Steptoe [13], eliminated the need for a sexual act to bring new life into the world, ending the ancient and seemingly untouchable meaning of sex as the indispensable ingredient of procreation, as every society in human history had believed.

Given this reality, it is not surprising that ART was initially regarded with great suspicion and even rejected outright [14]. However, within a few years, scientific progress, in association with marked sociocultural changes, led to an ever-increasing acceptance of ART in its various forms (see Chapter 9 for more details about ART). A global report published in 2018 (but referring to 2011) estimated that global utilization, including China, amounted to approximately 2.0 million cycles with 0.5 million babies born [15]. Of interest is the presence of an increasing trend: From 2010 to 2011, the number of reported oocyte aspirations and that of frozen embryo transfer cycles increased by 13.1% and 13.8%, respectively. The latest statistics from Europe are from 2016 and refer to 20 countries (with a total population of approximately 325 million inhabitants), in which ART clinics reported a total of 461 401 treatment cycles [16].

Data show a continuous increase in cycles performed, with a mean of 1410 cycles per million inhabitants (range 82–3088 per million inhabitants). This increased utilization led, at least in Europe, to overuse, as shown by an investigation from Ireland, published in 2010, where 14% of the women who had submitted to ART subsequently had a spontaneous pregnancy [17].

An important consequence of this trend to wider utilization of ART has been the application of these techniques to couples who are per se fertile, but who carry a genetically high risk of having offspring affected by serious pathological conditions. The methodology, known as preimplantation genetic diagnosis, was utilized for the first time some 30 years ago [18].

Recently, another technological advance has allowed the elimination of the consequences of maternally inherited mutations in mitochondrial DNA (mtDNA) that can cause fatal or debilitating mitochondrial disorders in offspring. The new technique, called mitochondrial replacement therapy, aims at preventing mtDNA transmission from oocytes to preimplantation embryos [19]. This technique produces what are commonly known as "three parent babies," because they are conceived using genetic material from two women (one providing the oocyte cytoplasm, the other the nucleus) and one man.

These scientific advances are progressively replacing the classic picture of sex for reproduction and bonding between partners, with reproduction totally separated from sexual activity. It should be obvious that these seemingly never-ending revolutions in human reproduction will continue, although the most important among them, human cloning, has been rejected by almost everyone [20] and unanimously condemned by the World Health Assembly [21].

1.4 New Family Paradigms

In parallel with these revolutions in reproduction, there have been several profound changes in the way of envisaging families. Concepts of traditional family and structure, traditional couples, and traditional unions are today challenged in the Western industrialized world, whereas they are still held valid in a majority of developing countries. In the West, same-sex unions and marriages are gradually becoming an accepted reality, whereas in Africa and Asia traditional unions are still strongly defended. One issue worthy of mention, as pointed out by Francesco Remotti, an Italian cultural anthropologist at the University of Turin, is that of the "irreducible multiplicity of solutions" proposed by humans in terms of families [22]. He mentions several examples of "traditional families" that do not conform to our classically accepted scheme.

Within the context of the United Nations (UN), support for family formation received an important endorsement during the 2011 UN General Assembly, when its Human Rights Council passed by majority vote a resolution stressing "the important role of family, community, society and educational institutions in upholding and transmitting these values, which contributes to promoting respect for human rights and increasing their acceptance at the grass roots, and calls upon all States to strengthen this role through appropriate positive measures." This text has been interpreted as an endorsement of traditional family structures, and it is likely that this is the reason why most of the votes against the resolution came from industrialized countries [23]. The problem with this resolution is that it implies a definition of "family" and therefore the existence of forms (one or more?) of "natural unions": The definition prevailing today around the world is that between one man and one woman, but possibly also between one man and several women, since among the countries voting in favor, some sanction polygamous unions.

1.5 Anthropological Aspects

The rapidly evolving relationship between sexuality and reproduction has created new needs and has inevitably met, and fought, cultural/religious objections. To understand the evolving scenario between reproduction and sexuality it is important to go beyond biology. Thus, anthropological facts, philosophical reflections, ethical norms, and religious dictates must be taken into consideration when looking at sexuality.

In humans, contrary to the vast majority of mammals, including primates, sexuality always had multiple meanings, first and foremost the need to reproduce and the creation of a bond within a couple. The fairly unique features of human sexuality and its important role in the life of most individuals has not only facilitated the evolution of *Homo sapiens*, but has also had a profound influence on human history, cultures, and societies everywhere.

The complex features involved in the evolution of the meaning of sexual intercourse in the human have been debated and summarized in the proceedings of an international conference published 25 years ago [24]. This contains an interesting historical overview of differences due to various cultural contexts, including the meaning of the sexual act in early Christianity and the subsequent Protestant reform, Buddhism, Judaism, and Islam.

Given that moral norms have always focused on sexuality and its regulation, the previously mentioned rapid evolution, after millennia of relative stability, drew the attention of ethicists, whether religious or secular, yielding conflicting outcomes. Catholic ethicists have been at the forefront of the battle against "dehumanizing" the reproductive process, whereas Judaism took a more open position. Early Christian teaching on sexuality focused on the practice of abstinence; this is because Christ himself defined celibacy as a better life choice for selected individuals striving for excellence. Drawing on this concept, early Christian Church fathers developed the concept, upheld by the Roman Catholic Church until the twentieth century, that intercourse is totally justifiable only in order to procreate [25]. This position was strongly opposed by Protestant reformers; in particular, Jean Calvin in his major book opposed celibacy with strong words [26]. Nowadays, some cautious overtures are being made within the Roman Catholic Church with the recognition that sexuality can also be an expression of love independent from procreation [27].

In the face of the new paradigms represented by these "revolutions," the positions of the major religions are fairly articulate. At present, the three monotheistic religions hold different positions toward ART, with no consensus on its potential advantages. Roman Catholicism, Orthodox churches, and some Protestant denominations (especially Evangelical churches) have staunchly defended the sexual act in its pristine naturality as the only ethical means to reproduce. In contradistinction to this position, some Islamic and Jewish scholars have affirmed the supremacy of childbearing over sex, to the point of opening a discussion even on reproductive cloning as a last attempt to give a child to a couple [12].

In anthropological terms, sexuality and reproduction have had a profound significance in determining the role of, and consideration for, women in a couple and in society. In many parts of the world, women are still vulnerable to gender-based violations of human and reproductive rights, limiting their role and potential [28]. In many social contexts, childlessness represents a real curse, and infertile women can be divorced simply on the grounds that they cannot provide an heir. Tragically, this curse is much more serious in the developing world, where access to ART is more limited [29]. In addition to the personal grief and the moral suffering it causes, the inability of an infertile woman to have children, especially in poor communities in the developing world, leads to shaming by her own family. This condition creates social stigma, economic hardship, social isolation, and violence, which may drive a woman to suicide or expose her to the risk of being killed [30,31]. A study conducted in Andhra Pradesh in India reported that approximately 70% of infertile women are being punished for their "disability" through physical violence [30]. To stress the existence of this problem and to search for technical innovations that can be used in the developing world, the European Society for Human Reproduction and Embryology (ESHRE) established the Task Force on Infertility and Developing Countries; the new attitude toward ART in developing countries is represented by a more constructive approach consisting of exploring new possibilities and innovative ways of ART that take into account the needs and the particular situations of low-resource settings [32].

A phenomenon that has accompanied the development of ART since the early days has been labeled "cross-border reproductive care" or "reproductive tourism"; it is the consequence of country-based legislation in ART, availability and quality of services, and economic issues [33].

1.6 Conclusions

Today the relative independence of sexuality from reproduction is well established, although the close relationship between the sexual act and having a child remains a cornerstone of every culture, especially among the more traditional societies. In other words, the intimate connection between the two aspects remains and the vast majority of pregnancies are, even today, achieved through sexual intercourse, a situation that is likely to remain for the foreseeable future.

Accordingly, what is important about "reproduction without sex" is not that it brings about complete separation between the two, but that it opens up new possibilities for achieving conception in infertile couples. According to Baldwin, ART, though a well-established option, does not – and for now will not – replace traditional sexual reproduction, given that most couples have no problem conceiving [34]. Others, like Suter, have predicted the potential end of sexual intercourse as a way of conceiving, arguing that emerging technologies may lead us down a path where sex as a means to conceive children will largely disappear, or at least decrease markedly [29]. Moreover, Greely has predicted that within the next 20–40 years, most people with access to good healthcare will no longer have sex to conceive their children [35].

Intriguingly, the most controversial encyclical letter of modern times, the *Humanae Vitae* by Pope Paul VI [36], has been called "prophetic" in light of its prediction of contraception as a tool for dismantling human sexuality, breaking of relationships, lowering of sexual standards, and increasing infidelity [37,38].

In this respect, it is a fact that the fear that women would become objects, mere instruments for the satisfaction of the desires of men, not only failed to materialize, but contraception brought about a "social revolution" that empowered women [39].

Finally, modern societies will have to deal with the emergence of new and different family structures brought about by the new technological advances that have made parenthood possible for people who in the past were excluded from achieving it [40].

References

1. G. Benagiano, S. Carrara, V. Filippi. Social and ethical determinants of human sexuality: 1. The need to reproduce. *Minerva Ginecol* 2010;**62**:349–59.

2. E. Abbott. *A History of Celibacy*. Boston: Da Capo Press, 2000: 43.

3. U. Ranke-Heinemann. *Eunuchs for the Kingdom of Heaven: The Catholic Church and Sexuality*. New York: Penguin Books, 1990.

4. C. Olson. *Celibacy and Religious Traditions*. Oxford: Oxford University Press, 2007.

5. G. Benagiano, M. Mori. The origins of human sexuality: procreation or recreation? *Reprod Biomed Online* 2009;**18**:50–9.

6. M. Potts, M. Campbell. History of contraception. In J. J. Sciarra, S. Dooley, R. Depp, et al., eds. *Gynecology and Obstetrics*. Philadelphia: Lippincott Williams & Wilkins, 2002: 1–23.

7. S. Freud. Die Sexualität in der Ätiologie der Neurose [Sexuality in the etiology of neurosis]. *Wiener Klinische Rundschau* 1898;**2**:21–2.

8. G. Benagiano, C. Bastianelli, M. Farris. Contraception today. *Ann NY Acad Sci* 2006;**1092**:1–32.

9. American College of Obstetricians and Gynecologists Committee on Gynecologic Practice and the Practice Committee of the American Society for Reproductive Medicine. Female age-related fertility decline. Committee Opinion No. 589. *Fertil Steril* 2014;**101**:633–4. (Replaces Committee Opinion No. 413, August 2008. Reaffirmed in 2020.)

10. A.-M. Nybo Andersen, J. Wohlfahrt, P. Christens, J. Olsen, M. Melbye. Maternal age and fetal loss: population based register linkage study. *BMJ* 2000;**320**:1708–12.

11. P. R. Abramson, S. D. Pinkerton. *With Pleasure: Thoughts on the Nature of Human Sexuality*. Oxford: Oxford University Press, 2002.

12. G. Benagiano, S. Carrara, V. Filippi. Sex and reproduction: an evolving relationship. *Hum Reprod Update* 2010;**16**:96–107.

13. P. C. Steptoe, R. G. Edwards. Birth after the reimplantation of a human embryo. *Lancet* 1978;**312**:366.

14. R. G. Edwards, P. Steptoe. *A Matter of Life: The Story of a Medical Breakthrough*. London: Morrow, 1980.

15. G. D. Adamson, J. de Mouzon, G. M. Chambers, et al. International Committee for Monitoring Assisted Reproductive Technology: world report on assisted reproductive technology, 2011. *Fertil Steril* 2018;**110**:1067–80.

16. C. H. De Geyter, C. Berg, C. Calhaz-Jorge, et al. ART in Europe, 2016: results generated from European registries by ESHRE. *Hum Reprod Open* 2020;**2020**: hoaa032.

17. B. Hennelly, R. F. Harrison, J. Kelly, S. Jacob, T. Barrett. Spontaneous conception after a successful attempt at in vitro fertilization/intracytoplasmic sperm injection. *Fertil Steril* 2000;**73**:774–8.

18. A. H. Handyside, E. H. Kontogianni, K. Hardy, R. Winston. Pregnancies from biopsied human preimplantation embryos sexed by Y-specific DNA amplification. *Nature* 1990;**344**:768–70.

19. J. Zhang, H. Liu, S. Luo, et al. Live birth derived from oocyte spindle transfer to prevent mitochondrial disease. *Reprod Biomed Online* 2017;**34**:361–8.

20. G. Benagiano, F. M. Primiero. Human reproductive cloning. *Int J Gynaecol Obstet* 2002;**79**:265–8.

21. World Health Organization. Cloning in human reproduction. Fiftieth World

Health Assembly. DOC WHA50.37. Geneva: World Health Organization, 1997.

22. F. Remotti. *Contro Natura: Una Lettera al Papa [Against Nature: A Letter to the Pope]*. Rome: Editori Laterza, 2008.

23. United Nations Human Rights Council. Promoting human rights and fundamental freedoms through a better understanding of traditional values of humankind: resolution adopted by the Human Rights Council, April 8, 2011. DOC A/HRC/RES/16/3. New York: United Nations, 2011. www.unhcr.org/ refworld/docid/4dc106fb2.html

24. G. Benagiano, G. C. Di Renzo, E. V. Cosmi. *The Evolution of the Meaning of Sexual Intercourse in the Human.* Cortona, Italy: International Institute for the Study of Man, 1996.

25. G. Benagiano, M. Mori. The evolution of thinking of the Catholic Church on the beginning of human life. *Reproductive BioMedicine Online* 2007;**14**(Suppl 1):162–8.

26. J. Calvin. *Institutio Christianae Religionis [Institutes of the Christian Religion].* Geneva: Oliua Robertus Stephanus. IV Edition, 1559; XII: 23–8.

27. Post-synodal Apostolic Exhortation. "Amoris Lætitia" of the Holy Father Francis. March 19, 2016. https://w2 .vatican.va

28. G. Benagiano, S. Carrara, V. Filippi. Reproductive rights as an integral part of women's rights. In J. G. Schenker, ed. *Ethical Dilemmas in Assisted Reproductive Technologies.* Berlin: De Gruyter, 2011: 29–42.

29. S. M. Suter. Book review of *The End of Sex and the Future of Human Reproduction. J Law Biosci* 2016;**3**:436–44.

30. A. S. Daar, Z. Merali. Infertility and social suffering: the case of ART in developing countries. In E. Vayena, P. Rowe, D.

Griffin, eds. *Current Practices and Controversies in Assisted Reproduction.* Geneva: World Health Organization, 2002: 15–21.

31. W. Ombelet. Global access to infertility care in developing countries: a case of human rights, equity and social justice. *Facts Views Vis Obgyn* 2011;**3**:257–66.

32. G. Pennings. Ethical issues of infertility treatment in developing countries. *ESHRE Monographs* 2008;**2008**(1):15–20.

33. M. Salama, V. Isachenko, E. Isachenko, et al. Cross border reproductive care (CBRC): a growing global phenomenon with multidimensional implications (a systematic and critical review). *J Assist Reprod Genet* 2018;**35**:1277–88.

34. T. Baldwin. Reproduction without sex: social and ethical implications. *EMBO Rep* 2012;**13**:1049–53.

35. H. T. Greely. *The End of Sex and the Future of Human Reproduction.* Boston: Harvard University Press, 2016.

36. Pope Paul VI. *Humanae Vitae [Of Human Life and the Regulation of Birth].* Vatican City: Tipografia Poliglotta Vaticana, 1968.

37. J. E. Smith. Paul VI, a prophet. In A. Reader, J. E. Smith, eds. *Why Humanae Vitae Was Right.* San Francisco: Ignatius Press, 1993: 519–31.

38. J. V. Turner, L. A. McLindon. Bioethical and moral perspectives in human reproductive medicine. *Linacre Q* 2018;**85**:385–98.

39. G. Benagiano, C. Bastianelli, M. Farris. Contraception: a social revolution. *Eur J Contracept Reprod Health Care* 2007;**12**:3–12.

40. G. Benagiano, S. Carrara, V. Filippi. Social and ethical determinants of sexuality: 4. Sexuality and families. *Eur J Contracept Reprod Health Care* 2012;**17**:329–39.

Chapter

Sex in Pregnancy
Beyond Reproduction

David Gómez Sánchez, Carlos López Ramón y Cajal,
and María Luisa Morales Serrano

2.1 Introduction

Sexuality is a central aspect of human existence, present throughout all phases of the life cycle. The World Health Organization defines sexual health as a state of physical, emotional, mental, and social well-being in relation to sexuality; it is not merely the absence of disease, dysfunction, or infirmity [1].

Pregnancy is one of the most important stages in the life of the woman and her partner. During this period, sexuality acquires an expression of its own. Multiple and profound changes occur in the couple, which can affect different areas of their relationship.

Sexuality is a reflection of our personality. It is unique and unrepeatable, providing a characteristic stamp of each couple. In order to enjoy adequate sexual health during pregnancy, there must be a process of acceptance and adaptation to these changes. Therefore, the couple will have to redirect their sexual enjoyment according to their possibilities and desires.

2.2 Changes in Sexual Function during Pregnancy

Pregnancy-associated changes will inevitably affect sexuality (see Chapter 3 for more details on changes during pregnancy). Each couple may react differently, influenced by multiple factors – physical, psychological, social, cultural, or religious. Although sexuality is different in each couple, a series of changes that are common during gestation can be established:

1. In the first trimester, there is often a decrease in sexual activity and desire. This is usually due to the appearance of bothersome physical symptoms, such as nausea, vomiting, tiredness, and abdominal pain. On the other hand, hormonal changes can cause greater emotional lability. Women frequently demand greater attention and demonstrations of love from their partner [2].

2. In the second trimester, some women report an improvement in their sexuality. Physical discomfort, especially nausea and vomiting, usually diminishes or disappears. In addition, initial fears, such as pregnancy loss, which occurs mostly in the first trimester, can vanish. During this stage, there is usually greater adaptation and a complete acceptance of the pregnancy by both partners [3].

3. In the third trimester, there is usually a decrease in sexual activity and desire [3,4]. The difficulty of adopting a comfortable posture, together with physical discomfort, fatigue, and worries related to childbirth and adapting to parenthood usually lead to a considerable decrease in sexual activity during this period.

2.3 Factors That Affect Sexuality during Pregnancy

Multiple aspects can influence the sexuality experienced by the pregnant woman and her partner.

Physical Changes: Because of increased blood flow, genital congestion occurs. Vaginal discharge also increases. There is a rise in sensitivity, which can produce greater sexual pleasure in some cases, but in others it can cause pain during sexual intercourse. There is also an increase in breast sensitivity, turning previously pleasant stimuli into painful. At the end of the pregnancy, the increase in the size of the belly produces a growing discomfort, making it difficult to adopt certain positions during intercourse. In addition, orgasmic contractions are usually more intense, which can be perceived as painful [2].

Body Dissatisfaction: During pregnancy, profound physical changes occur, such as breast and belly enlargement or variations in hair and skin color. In most cases, these modifications are perceived as positive – a symbol of the new motherhood – and may even increase the partner's sexual interest. However, some women experience these physical changes with deep dissatisfaction. This negative perception of their body image lowers their self-esteem, awakening the fear of losing their attractiveness to their partners, and which ends up diminishing sexual desire and satisfaction[5,6]. Possibly for this reason, overweight pregnant women have poorer sexual function [7].

Prepregnancy Sexuality: In most cases, the changes associated with gestation and the puerperium lead to a decrease in sexual activity and desire. Good sexuality prior to pregnancy acts as a protective factor against developing dysfunctions during this period [8].

Fear of Harming the Fetus: Although there is clear evidence that sexual activity is safe in a normal pregnancy [9], fear of a possible complication is one of the main reasons why couples avoid having intercourse during gestation [10]. These fears are much more noticeable in couples with a history of infertility (previous abortions, assisted reproductive techniques) or high-risk pregnancies, situations that increase perceived stress and the possibility of sexual dysfunction [11]. However, the quality of the couple's relationship is not necessarily affected; in these cases sexuality plays a secondary role, with the health of the future baby given priority. In such situations, the most important thing for women is to feel closeness and support from their partner [12].

Anxiety and Depression: Anxiety and depressive symptoms are frequent during pregnancy, and may appear or worsen in the postpartum period. Stress and depression are associated with sexual dysfunction and impaired relationship [13].

Cultural and Religious Background: Historically, the pregnant woman has been considered as asexual, focusing only on her reproductive function and ignoring her sexuality. In many cultures, beliefs regarding sex during pregnancy as dangerous, indecent, and even sinful still persist. These negative convictions can favor the appearance of sexual dysfunctions. Conversely, positive beliefs, such as the perception that sexual activity strengthens the couple's relationship, prevents infidelity, promotes fetal well-being, and makes labor easier, can help improve sexuality during pregnancy [14].

2.4 The Couple's Relationship

Pregnancy usually produces a series of changes in the sexual activity of the couple. In studies carried out on heterosexual couples, a marked decrease in the frequency of sexual intercourse has been observed [3,4].

As previously mentioned, the main cause of decreased sexual activity is the fear of harming the fetus, along with the physical changes experienced by the woman. These transformations can decrease her desire and make it difficult to adopt certain positions, turning intercourse uncomfortable and even painful.

In men, sexual desire remains constant, although attraction to their partners tends to decrease in the third trimester (see Chapter 10 for more details on the male partner's perspective). A process of adaptation to the new reality also takes place, and despite the decrease in intercourse frequency, sexual satisfaction is not usually impaired [3,15].

Most studies agree that the main factor related to sexual satisfaction is the quality of the couple's relationship. What men and women value most is the emotional closeness of their partner [15]. Caresses, hugs, kisses, complicity, and commitment to a common project are healthy expressions of sexuality that acquire much greater relevance than intercourse.

High-risk pregnancies, as well as those achieved by assisted reproductive techniques, are usually accompanied by great stress and concern (see Chapter 18 for more details on medical disorders in pregnancies). Here, emotional closeness acquires even more relevance: the woman needs to feel supported and understood by her partner [11,12].

Pregnancy is a period of special vulnerability, with changes, doubts, and uncertainties, which can cause increased stress. According to the theory of emotional capital, couples with shared positive experiences (including sexual ones) are more protected against stressful events. Therefore, maintaining satisfactory sexuality can help reduce stress and anxiety levels in both partners [16].

Finally, we must not forget the inequality and lack of rights suffered by women. In many societies, women's sexuality is still subordinated to men's wishes. For many women, sexual satisfaction may consist in not having problems with the partner. They agree to have sexual relations during pregnancy in order to maintain the stability of the marriage despite not obtaining pleasure from sexual intercourse.

Intimate partner violence is a worrying reality that still affects a large number of women, and is present in all countries and social classes. Psychological, physical, or even sexual violence are recognized as a cause of sexual dysfunction (see Chapter 26 for more details on sexual violence). Healthcare professionals must carry out a universal screening of intimate partner violence in order to detect and treat this serious problem [17].

2.5 Postpartum Sexuality

The postpartum is a period of profound changes in the life of the couple, in which there is usually a drastic decrease in desire and sexual activity (see Chapter 24 for more details on postpartum sexuality). Numerous factors can negatively affect sexuality at this stage, such as lack of sleep, fatigue, stress, the concerns that the new role as parents entails, depressive symptoms, lack of time for the partner, or the fear of painful relationships due to physical changes after childbirth [18].

Sometimes, the media conveys the idea that vaginal delivery can cause genital alterations, such as deformation of the vulva or excessive vaginal laxity, which can negatively affect sexuality [19]. A significant percentage of women think that a cesarean section can help prevent sexual dysfunction, especially in those societies that present a higher percentage of these interventions. However, these biases are not based on scientific evidence. Most studies state that the route of delivery or the practice of episiotomy does not have a significant influence on subsequent sexual function [18,20].

Breastfeeding has been associated with the appearance of sexual dysfunctions in the puerperium. Elevated prolactin levels produce a state of hypogonadism, with decreased levels of estrogens, progesterone, and testosterone. These hormonal changes can lead to decreased lubrication and vaginal atrophy, along with decreased sexual desire. However, studies show that if there is a negative effect on sexuality, it is very modest, with other factors such as the partner relationship much more important [13,21,22]. Furthermore, in experienced lactating mothers this effect is attenuated, showing the importance of adaptation and adjustment to this new situation. On the other hand, it has been postulated that the mother's physical contact with her baby during lactation could satisfy her needs for intimate contact, thus reducing the requirement for sexual relations with her partner [18].

Decreased desire and sexual activity in the postpartum period may simply be normal adaptive responses to this new situation, in which raising the baby is the primary goal. Therefore, they reflect normal transient changes that do not indicate sexual dysfunction and do not negatively affect the couple's relationship [13].

Sometimes, the media and also health professionals, in a well-intentioned way, encourage the couple to regain their prepregnancy sexuality as soon as possible. However, we may be falling into error. From the point of view of evolutionary psychology, the decrease in sexual interest and activity, far from being a dysfunction, reflects a satisfactory adaptation to the new role of parenthood, focusing attention and resources on a common goal. Thus, some studies show that couples with a better-quality relationship (greater degree of emotional closeness and mutual commitment) have less sexual activity in the postpartum period. These women feel that the postponement of sexual activity is a show of affection and commitment on the part of their partner, improving the quality of their relationship and their sexual satisfaction. In contrast, women with a worse relationship may be conditioned to resume their sexual activity earlier, as a way of seeking emotional connection and commitment from their partner [23].

2.6 Role of Healthcare Professionals

Historically, the subject of sexuality during pregnancy has been ignored by healthcare professionals. However, even though this situation has much improved in recent years, many pregnant women still dare not ask about aspects related to their sexuality, and some professionals are not comfortable or competent addressing this issue.

We must show interest in the pregnant woman's sexuality, with respect and empathy, by using a biopsychosocial perspective [18]. Maintaining adequate sexual health during pregnancy can help reduce stress, preserve self-esteem, and enhance the intimacy of the couple's relationship, thus improving overall well-being.

First, we must dismantle the prejudices and erroneous beliefs about sexuality, especially the fear of harming the fetus. In a normal gestation, sexual intercourse is healthy and is not associated with obstetric complications. On the other hand, during pregnancy we must normalize changes in sexuality, such as decreased desire or discomfort with certain postures, thus minimizing feelings of stress, guilt, or anxiety [10]. Active intervention by healthcare professionals, offering listening, information and advice, has been shown to improve sexuality and strengthen the couple's relationship during pregnancy [24].

Pelvic floor muscle exercise is beneficial for sexuality, especially in the postpartum period (see Chapter 25 for more details). Through hypertrophy of the muscle fibers, the levator ani muscle is strengthened, favoring the revascularization of damaged cells and tissues. In addition to the purely biological aspects, pelvic floor exercises offer a psycho-social benefit by promoting self-awareness, improving body self-image, favoring self-control, reducing stress, and enhancing the feeling of empowerment [25].

Pregnancy and the postpartum constitute a complex period, a time of hope but also of fears and uncertainties, in which the woman needs the support and closeness of her partner. Therefore, we must educate both partners in their emotional approach [12].

Whenever we deal with sexuality and the couple relationship, we must not forget to carry out a universal screening for gender violence, a serious problem that affects many women in all countries and social classes, offering the necessary support and resources to combat it [17].

2.7 Conclusions

Sexuality constitutes a cornerstone of a person's overall well-being, a source of pleasure, affection, and intimacy that is expressed differently in all phases of the life cycle.

Pregnancy represents an important stage for the woman and her partner. During this time, the couple experiences deep physical and mental changes that also affect sexuality. Some couples experience these modifications in a positive way, pregnancy being an opportunity to improve the emotional connection and complicity of the couple, thus strengthening their sexual health.

However, on many occasions, the physical, emotional, and social changes associated with pregnancy and the postpartum cause various difficulties that are also reflected in sexuality. During this time, sexual desire, pleasure, and activity often diminish. Sexual dysfunctions can also appear. Such problems can damage self-esteem, increase perceived stress, and negatively affect the couple's relationship.

Health professionals can be of great help in overcoming sexual difficulties that arise at this very important stage in a couple's life. They can provide information that normalizes the physical and emotional changes associated with this period, dismantling prejudices and erroneous beliefs about sexuality in pregnancy. Thus health professionals can dispel many fears and doubts, improving self-confidence and self-esteem, and reducing stress and anxiety.

In this stage full of changes and hopes, but also fears and uncertainties, the most important aspect for achieving a satisfactory sexuality is the quality of the couple's relationship. We must help both members to improve their emotional approach by promoting greater listening and understanding of each other's concerns and increasing the displays of affection. Therefore, with a greater commitment and involvement in a common project, sexuality and the couple's relationship will be strengthened.

In a normal pregnancy, sexual activity is safe and healthy. Active intervention by health professionals, based on respect and empathy, following a biopsychosocial approach can help improve sexuality. Adequate sexual health during pregnancy provides important benefits: it reduces stress levels, maintains adequate self-esteem, and enhances intimacy and complicity in the couple's relationship, thus improving overall well-being.

References

1. World Health Organization. *Sexual Health and Its Linkages to Reproductive Health: An Operational Approach.* Geneva: World Health Organization, 2017. www.who.int/publications/i/item/978924151288.

2. E. F. Pérez Campos. Cambios en la función sexual en el embarazo, puerperio y aborto. In C. Castelo-Branco, F. Molero, eds. *Manual de Sexología Clínica.* Madrid: Editorial Médica Panamericana, 2019: 242–3.

3. F. J. Fernández-Carrasco, L. Rodríguez-Díaz, U. González-Mey, et al. Changes in sexual desire in women and their partners during pregnancy. *J Clin Med* 2020;9:526.

4. A. Fuchs, I. Czech, J. Sikora, et al. Sexual functioning in pregnant women. *Int J Environ Res Public Health* 2019;16:4216.

5. P. M. Pascoal, P. J. Rosa, S. Coelho. Does pregnancy play a role? Association of body dissatisfaction, body appearance cognitive distraction, and sexual distress. *J Sex Med* 2019;16:551–8.

6. S. N. Radoš, H. S. Vraneš, M. Šunjić. Limited role of body satisfaction and body image self-consciousness in sexual frequency and satisfaction in pregnant women. *J Sex Res* 2014;51:532–41.

7. M. C. Ribeiro, M. U. Nakamura, M. R. Torloni, et al. Maternal overweight and sexual function in pregnancy. *Acta Obstet Gynecol Scand* 2016;95:45–51.

8. H. Yıldız. The relation between prepregnancy sexuality and sexual function during pregnancy and the postpartum period: a prospective study. *J Sex Marital Ther* 2015;41:49–59.

9. L. Kong, T. Li, L. Li. The impact of sexual intercourse during pregnancy on obstetric and neonatal outcomes: a cohort study in China. *J Obstet Gynaecol* 2019;39:455–60.

10. J. K. Beveridge, S. A. Vannier, N. O. Rosen. Fear-based reasons for not engaging in sexual activity during pregnancy: associations with sexual and relationship well-being. *J Psychosom Obstet Gynaecol* 2018;39:138–45.

11. C. Y. Huang, C. F. Liou, Y. C. Lu, et al. Differences in the sexual function and sexual healthcare needs of pregnant women who underwent in vitro fertilization and women who conceived naturally at each trimester: a prospective cohort study. *Sex Med* 2020;8:709–17.

12. K. Mirzakhani, T. Khadivzadeh, F. Faridhosseini, A. Ebadi. Pregnant women's experiences of the conditions affecting marital well-being in high-risk pregnancy: a qualitative study. *Int J Community Based Nurs Midwifery* 2020;8:345–57.

13. S. Wallwiener, M. Müller, A. Doster, et al. Sexual activity and sexual dysfunction of women in the perinatal period: a longitudinal study. *Arch Gynecol Obstet* 2017;295:873–83.

14. M. C. Ribeiro, M. de Tubino Scanavino, M. L. S. do Amaral, A. L. de Moraes Horta, M. R. Torloni. Beliefs about sexual activity during pregnancy: a systematic review of the literature. *J Sex Marital Ther* 2017;43:822–32.

15. S. Nakić Radoš, H. Soljačić Vraneš, M. Šunjić. Sexuality during pregnancy: what is important for sexual satisfaction in expectant fathers? *J Sex Marital Ther* 2015;41:282–93.

16. I. M. Tavares, H. E. Schlagintweit, P. J. Nobre, N. O. Rosen. Sexual well-being and perceived stress in couples transitioning to parenthood: a dyadic analysis. *Int J Clin Health Psychol* 2019;19:198–208.

17. E. Bahrami Vazir, S. Mohammad-Alizadeh-Charandabi, M. Kamalifard, et al. The correlation between sexual dysfunction and intimate partner violence in young women during pregnancy. *BMC Int Health Hum Rights* 2020;20:24.

18. L. E. Hipp, L. Kane Low, S. M. van Anders. Exploring women's postpartum sexuality: social, psychological, relational, and birth-related contextual factors. *J Sex Med* 2012;9:2330–41.

19. J. Cappell, C. F. Pukall. Perceptions of the effects of childbirth on sexuality among nulliparous individuals. *Birth* 2018;**45**:55–63.

20. D. Fan, S. Li, W. Wang, et al. Sexual dysfunction and mode of delivery in Chinese primiparous women: a systematic review and meta-analysis. *BMC Pregnancy Childbirth* 2017;**17**:408.

21. O. Gutzeit, G. Levy, L. Lowenstein. Postpartum female sexual function: risk factors for postpartum sexual dysfunction. *Sex Med* 2020;**8**:8–13.

22. L. M. Matthies, M. Wallwiener, C. Sohn, et al. The influence of partnership quality and breastfeeding on postpartum female sexual function. *Arch Gynecol Obstet* 2019;**299**:69–77.

23. T. K. Lorenz, E. L. Ramsdell, R. L. Brock. A close and supportive interparental bond during pregnancy predicts greater decline in sexual activity from pregnancy to postpartum: applying an evolutionary perspective. *Front Psychol* 2020;**10**:2974.

24. J. Malakouti, R. Golizadeh, M. Mirghafourvand, A. Farshbaf-Khalili. The effect of counseling based on ex-PLISSIT model on sexual function and marital satisfaction of postpartum women: a randomized controlled clinical trial. *J Educ Health Promot* 2020;**9**:284.

25. S. S. Sobhgol, H. Priddis, C. A. Smith, H. G. Dahlen. The effect of pelvic floor muscle exercise on female sexual function during pregnancy and postpartum: a systematic review. *Sex Med Rev* 2019;**7**:13–28.

Physiology of Pregnancy As Related to Sex

Silvia Barras Bermejo and Pablo Tobías González

3.1 Introduction

During pregnancy, the physiological changes a woman's body endures progressively affect her sexual function by means of different mechanisms. Through the three trimesters of pregnancy, there is a remarkable adaptation of the whole body to accommodate the growing uterus and fetus, as well for upcoming labor and delivery. Most of these physiological changes gradually regress over the postpartum, returning to prepregnancy levels after a period ranging from a few weeks to 6 months. The changes that occur in pregnancy have an important impact on a woman's sexual functioning (desire, arousal, orgasm, and sexual satisfaction).

The implications of the physiological changes that occur during pregnancy include effects on intimacy and sexual function, but these are seldom discussed by health professionals and care providers. It is not the usual practice during antenatal visits to record a sexual history due to lack of habit, knowledge gaps, and shame (in both mothers and health providers), among other reasons. As an example, in a small survey of 141 women in Canada, less than half of patients raised questions during visits and only one-third received information about sexual activity during pregnancy [1]. Indeed, patients may consult books, magazines, or friends before a physician, and many of those who did not discuss it during prenatal visits felt the subject should have been brought up [2].

Very briefly, the adjustments and changes in different systems throughout the pregnancy are explained in the following sections, mainly focusing on those that affect sexual function and their mechanisms.

3.2 Anatomical Changes

There is extensive anatomical adaptation to pregnancy in the woman's body beginning soon after conception in response to fetal and placental stimuli and demands. Basically, every organ undergoes changes that progressively become more noticeable as the pregnancy evolves.

3.2.1 Abdominal Wall and Skin

From the second trimester, up to 90% of women develop hyperpigmentation of some areas of the skin, noticeably on the midline of the abdomen (the linea alba). This acquires a darker tone (brown to black) to form the linea nigra. This phenomenon of skin color change can also present on the face and neck, forming chloasma. These pigmentation changes tend to disappear early in the postpartum period [3].

Also in the abdomen, striae gravidarum can arise in around half of pregnant women, more frequently in young females with significant weight gain during the pregnancy. These striae consist of depressed red streaks and can sometimes be present on the thighs and over the breasts.

Occasion, the rectus muscles may separate markedly from the midline because of increased tension caused by the gravid uterus, creating a diastasis recti. Eventrations or hernias are infrequent. The diastasis can sometimes persist after delivery, but is usually asymptomatic.

Angiomas shaped like a spider (called telangiectases) can develop on the skin of the face, neck, chest, and arms.

There is increased blood flow in the skin, which helps to dissipate the heat provoked by augmented metabolism.

3.2.2 Breasts

Breast tenderness beginning in the early weeks of pregnancy is frequent [1]. The breasts gradually increase in size and, as previously mentioned, striation can appear if there is major growth. Colostrum, the yellowish first milk produced during pregnancy, can be obtained after the first months. Nipples and areolae also become larger and more pigmented.

3.2.3 Perineum and External Genitalia

There is an increase in perianal vascularity, with associated congestion that softens the connective tissue. The labia majora commonly develop varicosities, more frequently in multiparous women, due to venous compression by the growing uterus; in most cases these are asymptomatic.

Hemorrhoids are also common because of the increased abdominal pressure. They can sometimes bleed or prolapse, but rarely develop thromboses and become painful. Abramowitz et al. [4] found that up to 9% of pregnant women had thrombosed hemorrhoids.

3.2.4 Vagina

The increased vascularity augments vaginal secretions, with higher lubrication in the second trimester. There is softening of the connective tissue, with an increase in mucosal thickness. Relaxin causes the vaginal lumen to increase, decreasing vaginal sensation during intercourse in some women. The pH of the vagina is normally moderately acidic (4.0–4.5) and is maintained at this level by the production of lactic acid by *Lactobacillus acidophilus* microorganisms in the vaginal fluid. Any factor that raises vaginal pH above 4.5 can produce itchiness and discomfort during pregnancy, along with vulvovaginitis in some women.

3.2.5 Uterus

The uterus, containing the fetus and placenta, becomes hugely enlarged during pregnancy, increasing from barely 70 g to more than 1 kg at term, with an average total volume of 5 L and uteroplacental blood flow of 500–600 mL/min by the end of the pregnancy [3]. The uterine walls initially become thicker, thinning toward the end of pregnancy (less than 1–2 cm thick). As pregnancy advances, the uterus exceeds the pelvis by week 12, displacing the abdominal organs and extending to the liver by the end of pregnancy.

The woman may perceive uterine contractions by the second trimester, these so-called Braxton Hicks contractions being irregular, sporadic, and nonrhythmic.

3.2.6 Cervix

Normally, the cervix undergoes eversion and the endocervical epithelium "moves" from the endocervix to the exocervix. The columnar epithelium appears reddish, and is more fragile and may bleed with minor trauma such as intercourse or digital examination. Cervical secretions are increased, giving a thicker discharge compared to before pregnancy.

3.3 Functional Changes

The profound transformations in the function of the different organs and systems can reach the pathological range, using the same criteria as for nonpregnant individuals; for example, cardiac remodeling occurs via similar mechanisms as those in patients with ventricular failure. Nevertheless, these changes can sometimes mask conditions that may be potentially harmful for the mother and fetus or even predict the start of diseases such as diabetes or hypertension, because of the whole-body stress the pregnancy induces.

3.3.1 Metabolism

Continuous augmentation of fetal and placental demands leads to an increase in basal metabolic rate by up to 10–20% by the third trimester [3].

There is increased water retention mediated by a fall in plasma osmolality of 10 mosmol/kg. Up to 6.5 L of extra water can be accumulated (3.5 L for the amniotic fluid, placenta, and fetus; 3 L for the added blood volume and uterus).

Glucose metabolism is characterized by hyperinsulinemia, with increased insulin resistance related to progesterone, estrogen, and placental lactogen, and higher concentrations of free fatty acids.

Increased lipolytic activity and lower lipoprotein lipase activity in adipose tissue cause maternal hyperlipidemia, with higher levels of cholesterol, triglycerides, and low-density lipoproteins, occasionally above the prepregnancy normal range.

3.3.2 Cardiovascular System

Blood volume rises over the course of pregnancy, increasing by 40% compared to before the pregnancy. This accommodates the uterine demands and compensates for the expected blood loss during delivery. Plasma augmentation is greater than cellular expansion, and as a result hemoglobin concentration decreases slightly to an average of 12.5 g/dL. Nevertheless, a certain degree of iron-deficiency anemia is common, requiring supplementation in some cases.

Heart function is modified early in pregnancy, with cardiac output increasing from the first month due to reduced vascular resistance and higher pulse rate [5]. Pulse increases by 10–15 beats/min, cardiac output increases by 1.2–2 L/min by the end of pregnancy, and blood pressure decreases, causing fatigue in some women, until mid pregnancy (24–26 weeks) and then rises progressively thereafter.

3.3.3 Respiratory System

During pregnancy, minute ventilation increases to 14 L/min and mean tidal volume to 0.8 L/min. The diaphragm rises while the thorax expands transversely. The increase in tidal volume lowers PCO_2, resulting in respiratory alkalosis. These changes are probably mediated by the hormones progesterone and estrogen. Some women may counterintuitively experience dyspnea due to the lowered PCO_2.

3.3.4 Musculoskeletal System

Through unclear mechanisms, likely hormonal stimuli, there is relaxation of the pelvic joints over the course of pregnancy. Relaxation of the symphysis pubis can become painful, essentially with walking and from pressure of the fetal head but can also affect intercourse, mostly in the third trimester. Sacroiliac mobility allows an increase in the diameter of the pelvic outlet in labor and delivery by up to 1–2 cm.

There is a forward shift in the center of gravity as the uterus grows, increasing lumbar lordosis, which may cause back pain and herniated disks as early as mid-pregnancy.

3.3.5 Gastrointestinal System

Hormonal changes during pregnancy, mainly an increase in human chorionic gonadotropin, are correlated with the frequent nausea and vomiting experienced during the first trimester. The growing gravid uterus continuously displaces the abdominal organs. As a result of stomach displacement, in addition to lower sphincter tone and increased intra-abdominal pressure, pyrosis or heartburn is common in pregnancy.

Bowel transit is slower during pregnancy because of the relaxed muscle tone secondary to progesterone. Therefore, constipation and bloating are common problems in pregnancy that add to the discomfort a woman suffers toward the end of pregnancy.

Congestion of the gums and softening produces bleeding with minor trauma such as toothbrushing.

3.3.6 Sleep Pattern

Worsening of sleep pattern has been described during pregnancy, with women experiencing difficulty going to sleep, fewer hours of deep sleep, and less sleep efficiency, but with a slight improvement in sleep characteristics [6]. These contribute to the tiredness and fatigue in pregnancy.

Although obstructive sleep apnea (OSA) seems to be more prevalent in the puerperium than during pregnancy, sleep disorders in pregnancy such as OSA increase the risk of adverse pregnancy outcomes (gestational diabetes mellitus, gestational hypertension, or cesarean section) [7].

3.4 Self Body Image

The appearance of a woman changes during pregnancy, in some cases affecting her self-esteem. With a recommended weight gain of 11–16 kg with a normal body mass index (BMI), weight gain can range between 3 and 45 kg. However, a worse body image seems to be more prevalent in the postpartum period rather than during pregnancy, is not related to BMI, and frequently returns to prepregnancy levels during the first months of the postpartum period [8].

3.5 Sexual Functioning and Activity

Studies assessing sexual functioning and activity in pregnancy are scarce, with low numbers of participants and inhomogeneous methodology, producing conflicting data and variation between populations. Many recent studies use the Female Sexual Function Index (FSFI), a validated 19-question questionnaire, to assess desire, arousal, lubrication, orgasm, satisfaction, and pain [9]. The total score ranges from 2 to 36, with less than 26.55 indicating sexual dysfunction. On the other hand, a reduction in sexual activity during the last weeks of pregnancy is quite common among the different studies [10,11]. In a metacontent analysis by von Sydow [12], 76–79% of women enjoyed intercourse before pregnancy, with a decrease in the first trimester to 59%, an increase in the second trimester to 75–84%, and a marked decrease to 40–41% in the third trimester (see Chapter 5 for more details on sexual function in pregnancy). The decrease in the first trimester seems to be due to psychological factors such as fear of harming the pregnancy and to physical factors such as fatigue, nausea, and vomiting. The described increase in the second trimester has been suggested to be due to pelvic congestion, less physical discomfort, increased vaginal lubrication, acceptance of the pregnancy, and less fear of affecting the pregnancy. The common decrease in the third trimester is due to discomfort, engagement of the fetal head, urinary incontinence, pubic symphysis diastasis, back pain due to marked lordosis, subluxation of the sacroiliac joints, and hemorrhoids [13–15].

Maternal testosterone and sex hormone-binding globulin increase during pregnancy, with a higher free androgen index during the first half of pregnancy, and this has been proposed as a cause of the occasional increase in sexual desire, although studies have not found a correlation between androgen levels and sexual function through the pregnancy [16].

Masters and Johnson, in their pioneering work of the 1960s, studied the performance of 101 women and reported an increase in sexual desire and function in the first and second trimesters, with a marked decrease in the third [17]. Nulliparous women described a decrease in sexual tension and responsiveness, with parous women noting rather small changes. During the second trimester, 80% of the women reported an increase in interest and responsiveness, exceeding prepregnancy levels in some individuals. Other studies have not found these differences between nulliparous and parous women [11,18]. There also seems to be no difference between maternal age, social class, planned pregnancy, religion, emotional lability, and breastfeeding regarding the decrease in sexual activity [1,18].

Problems not present before pregnancy that contribute to the decrease in sexual activity are many, such as changes in lubrication (37%), vaginal pain or soreness (11.6–22%), abdominal cramping (8.4–22%), and bleeding (10.6–13%) [1,2]. Low sexual frequency during pregnancy has been related to an equally low frequency before pregnancy [13].

During pregnancy there is also a shift to other positions rather than man-on-top as pregnancy evolves, such as side-by-side, on all fours, rear-entry, or woman-on-top, with some studies noting an increase in other practices such as anal sex, oral sex, and mutual masturbation [1,10,15,19].

3.5.1 Orgasm Response and Arousal

As previously noted, there is some variability between studies, some of them showing an increase in orgasm in mid pregnancy while others report a linear decrease in sexual interest, rate and quality of orgasm, and both coital and noncoital sex throughout the pregnancy [20] (see Chapter 4 for more details on orgasm). One of the suggested reasons for the stable orgasmic frequency and intensity is the increased pelvic congestion from the second trimester onwards [21]. The increased sensitivity to oxytocin, mostly in late pregnancy, is related to increased strength of uterine contractions during orgasm, which can sometimes be painful and contributes to the decrease in sexual interest and activity [19].

Sexual desire varies between women, increasing (5–37%), decreasing (29–60%), or remaining reasonably stable during the pregnancy (35–58%) [1,2,19]. The greatest variation in intercourse frequency occurs during the first trimester, ranging from inactivity to normal prepregnancy activity [22]. Interestingly, women who are ignorant of being pregnant display a higher frequency of sexual intercourse, probably due to the lack of fear of harming the pregnancy [23].

Masters and Johnson noticed slower genital vasocongestion and vaginal lubrication and distension during the first postpartum weeks, with a return to prepregnancy levels around 12 weeks postpartum [17]. During the postpartum, tension, fatigue, mastalgia, or soreness of episiotomy or perineal tears makes orgasmic attainment even more difficult than during pregnancy [10]. In fact, only 20% of women experience orgasm in the first intercourse after pregnancy, but 75% regain orgasm before 6 months postpartum [19]. There is a decrease in clitoral sensation (up to 94.2%), libido (92.6%), and orgasm (81%) that may persist during the first 6 months postpartum [15].

3.5.2 Fetal Repercussions

As early as Hippocrates, coitus was believed to be harmful for the fetus from the beginning of pregnancy [24], whereas today it is known that the main reason for spontaneous abortions at less than 12 weeks is chromosomal defects and very rarely because of trauma, injury, or physical activity. Nevertheless, 49% of women are concerned about harming the pregnancy if they have intercourse [1].

Some studies have presented the possibility that coitus during the last month of pregnancy could be associated with an increase in amniotic-fluid infection and perinatal mortality [20]. Prostaglandins present in the seminal fluid can stimulate uterine contractions, but do not clearly promote labor. Grudzinskas et al. [25] evaluated 70 couples and noted that sexually active women in the last 4 weeks of pregnancy had a higher incidence of meconium staining and Apgar score 6 at 1 minute, soft markers of fetal distress. Other studies have not found this association [26].

Initially, orgasm was also suspected to be associated with abortion, premature labor, and fetal distress. Uterine tension increases in the pre-orgasmic period with uterine contractions presenting during orgasm, which may be linked with fetal heart rate decelerations [27]. These decelerations have not been clearly associated with unexplained cases of fetal deaths in utero. The uterine activity may even be painful during orgasm and the activity tends to cease within 15 minutes after the orgasm. Given that frequent and intense uterine contractions are tolerated during labor, it is unlikely these decelerations imply fetal distress.

Most recent studies label sex as safe in pregnancy, with very few conditions or situations that may recommend avoiding it. •

References

1. E. Bartellas, J. M. Crane, M. Daley, K. A. Bennett, D. Hutchens. Sexuality and sexual activity in pregnancy. *BJOG* 2000;**107**:964–8.

2. W. Y. Fok, L. Y. Chan, P. M. Yuen. Sexual behavior and activity in Chinese pregnant women. *Acta Obstet Gynecol Scand* 2005;**84**:934–8.

3. M. M Corton, K. Leveno, S. Bloom, J. Hauth, D. Rouse, C. Spong. *Williams Obstetrics*, 23rd ed. New York: McGraw Hill Professional, 2009.

4. L. Abramowitz, I. Sobhani, J. L. Benifla, et al. Anal fissure and thrombosed external hemorrhoids before and after delivery. *Dis Colon Rectum* 2002;**45**:650–5.

5. J. M. Roberts, G. F. Cunningham, M. D. Lindheimer, eds. *Chesley's Hypertensive Disorders in Pregnancy*, 3rd ed. Academic Press, 2009.

6. K. A. Lee, M. E. Zaffke, G. McEnany. Parity and sleep patterns during and after pregnancy. *Obstet Gynecol* 2000;**95**:14–18.

7. M. Bazalakova. Sleep disorders in pregnancy. *Semin Neurol* 2017;**37**:661–8.

8. R. N. Pauls, J. A. Occhino, V. L. Dryfhout. Effects of pregnancy on female sexual function and body image: a prospective study. *J Sex Med* 2008;**5**:1915–22.

9. D. M. Carteiro, L. M. de Sousa, S. M. Caldeira. Clinical indicators of sexual dysfunction in pregnant women: integrative literature review. *Rev Bras Enferm* 2016;**69**:153–61.

10. K. Reamy, S. E. White. Sexuality in pregnancy and the puerperium: a review. *Obstet Gynecol Surv* 1985;**40**:1–13.

11. E. L. Ryding. Sexuality during and after pregnancy. *Acta Obstet Gynecol Scand* 1984;**63**:679–82.

12. K. von Sydow. Sexuality during pregnancy and after childbirth: a metacontent analysis of 59 studies. *J Psychosom Res* 1999;**47**:27–49.

13. R. Srisvastava, R. Thakar, A. Sultan. Female sexual dysfunction in obstetrics and gynecology. *Obstet Gynecol Surv* 2008;**63**:527–37.

14. J. Murtagh. Female sexual function, dysfunction, and pregnancy: implications for practice. *J Midwifery Womens Health* 2010;**55**:438–46.

15. C. E. Johnson. Sexual health during pregnancy and the postpartum. *J Sex Med* 2011;**8**:1267–84.

16. B. Erol, O. Sanli, D. Korkmaz, et al. A cross-sectional study of female sexual function and dysfunction during pregnancy. *J Sex Med* 2007;**4**:1381–7.

17. W. Masters, V. Johnson. *Human Sexual Response*. Boston: Little, Brown, 1966: 141–68.

18. S. A. Elliot, J. P. Watson. Sex during pregnancy and the first postnatal year. *J Psychosom Res* 1985;**29**:541–8.

19. H. Brtnicka, P. Weiss, J. Zverina. Human sexuality during pregnancy and the postpartum period. *Bratisl Lek Listy* 2009;**110**:427–31.

20. A. L. Herbst. Coitus and the fetus. *N Engl J Med* 1979;**301**:1235–6.

21. A. Kenny. Sexuality of pregnant and breastfeeding women. *Arch Sex Behav* 1973;**2**:215–29.

22. A. Fuchs, I. Czech, J. Sikora, et al. Sexual functioning in pregnant women. *Int J Environ Res Public Health* 2019;**16**:4216.

23. A. Corbacioglu, V. L. Bakir, O. Akbayir, B. P. C. Goksedef, A. Akca. The role of pregnancy awareness on female sexual function in early gestation. *J Sex Med* 2012;**9**:1897–903.

24. R. R. Limner. *Sex and the Unborn Child: Damage to the Fetus Resulting from Sexual Intercourse during Pregnancy.* New York: Julian Press, 1969.

25. J. G. Grudzinskas, C. Watson, T. Chard. • Does sexual intercourse cause fetal distress? *Lancet* 1979;**314**:692–3.

26. D. A. Solberg, J. Butler, N. N. Wagner. Sexual behavior in pregnancy. *N Engl J Med* 1973;**288**:1098–103.

27. R. C. Goodlin, W. Schmidt, D. C. Creevy. Uterine tension and fetal heart rate during maternal orgasm. *Obstet Gynecol* 1972;**39**:125–7.

General Issues

Does Orgasm Affect Fetal Well-Being?

Ayelet Dangot, Eliane Rozanes, and Ariel Many

4.1 Introduction

An orgasm is a variable transient sensation of intense and extreme pleasure, accompanied by an altered state of consciousness [1]. About 20% of women will experience orgasm for the first time during their pregnancies [2].

4.2 Physiology of Orgasm

In the past, sexual response in women was described as a four-stage sequence of physiological events: excitement/arousal, plateau, orgasm, and resolution. It is now known that sexual response in women is much more complex than this, and includes aspects of psychological, emotional, and social factors in addition to physiological events. During sexual arousal, there is vasocongestion of the genitalia due to increased blood flow. Vaginal lubrication is a result of a number of simultaneous processes, including plasma transudation through the vaginal epithelium and secretions from the uterus and vestibular and Bartholin glands. Relaxation of smooth muscles lengthens and dilates the vagina. Eversion and engorgement of the labia minora and protrusion of the clitoris is due to increased blood flow to the clitoral cavernosal and labial arteries. During orgasm, synchronous rhythmic muscle contractions occur in the vagina, uterus, and anus [3,4].

4.2.1 Hormonal Release and Sexual Arousal

Hormonal release and peptide function during sexual arousal has been well studied, yet few clear conclusions can be drawn about their function and effect. The most evidence exists for oxytocin, β-endorphin, and prolactin in both animal and human studies, and these hormones represent the main types of peptides relevant to sexual arousal.

4.2.1.1 β-Endorphin

Synthesis of β-endorphin takes place in the anterior pituitary, and in two cell groups in the brain: the arcuate nucleus of the hypothalamus and the nucleus of the solitary tract in the brainstem.

Animal studies have shown that β-endorphins have inhibiting effects on sexual arousal, mainly through their action on the preoptic area and the amygdala, the precise inhibiting effect depending on the site of infusion. The inhibitory effect is dose dependent, with low doses of opiate having facilitatory and high doses inhibitory effects [5].

Endogenous opiates have both facilitatory and inhibitory effects, but the exact mechanism and relation to dose remain elusive. As with oxytocin, there is a complex picture of potentially excitatory and inhibitory effects of endogenous opiates, interacting with gonadal steroids [6].

4.2.1.2 Prolactin

Prolactin is secreted by the anterior pituitary gland in a diurnal pattern, with maximum secretion at night. Low sexual desire is a common symptom of hyperprolactinemia.

During orgasm there is elevated secretion of prolactin and levels remain elevated for about 60 minutes after orgasm. These results have led researchers to speculate that the postorgasmic rise in prolactin levels acts via negative feedback to inhibit sexual drive; this contributes to the refractory period, a postorgasmic period characterized as relaxed and calm, attributed to the release of endorphins and the neurohormones oxytocin and prolactin as well [7].

4.2.1.3 Oxytocin

Oxytocin, popularly named the "love hormone" [8], is produced in the neurosecretory cells of the hypothalamus that project axons into the posterior pituitary from where the hormone is released into the peripheral circulation. It is generally accepted that oxytocin is involved in lactation as part of the milk ejection reflex. It is associated with uterine contractions during labor and animal studies show that it facilitates affiliative behavior, induces maternal behavior, and may be essential for initiating social interaction [9]. The evidence for oxytocin's role in sexual arousal is less consistent.

The results from animal studies suggest a peripheral and central role for oxytocin, peripherally of smooth muscle contraction and centrally as a neuromodulator in a variety of systems. Human studies found an increase in plasma oxytocin levels around the time of orgasm, levels remaining elevated for at least 5 minutes after orgasm. The authors suggested that oxytocin increases smooth muscle contractility in the reproductive tract, thus facilitating sperm and egg transport [10]. Conversely, other studies found only a short increase in oxytocin levels 1 minute after orgasm, returning close to baseline 5 minutes after orgasm [11].

It is unclear what effect oxytocin has on sexual arousal, or whether the increase in oxytocin around orgasm has any specific function or is simply a by-product of other changes. It is reasonable to assume that the rise in oxytocin will affect the experience of orgasm by influencing uterine, vaginal, and anal contractions.

Does this release of oxytocin have any effect on pregnancy? The subject is not often studied and data are lacking.

4.3 The Effect of Orgasm on Pregnancy Complications

4.3.1 Fetal Well-Being

In a study by Goodlin et al. [12] the effect of orgasm on fetal heart rate and uterine contractions was recorded in a 39 weeks' noncomplicated gravida patient with multiple orgasms. During these orgasmic periods, increasing uterine contractility was measured and fetal heart rate decelerations were observed (Figure 4.1). After the orgasmic episodes finished, fetal heart rate returned to normal, and the woman later delivered a healthy baby. These results were not seen in any other gravida studied so it is not clear if any conclusions can be drawn.

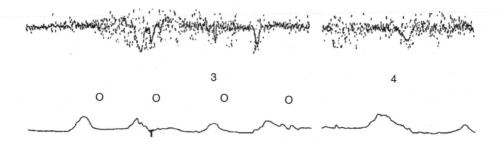

Figure 4.1 Recordings from a Smith-Kline fetal monitor with fetal heart rate recorded in the upper tracing and uterine tension in the lower. "O" refers to maternal orgasm. Basal fetal heart rate is approximately 155 beats/min and dips to 96 beats/min.

Sexual satisfaction changes during pregnancy due to physiological and psychological factors. Women can experience orgasms during pregnancy. The exact impact of orgasms on pregnancy, placental perfusion, uterine contractions, and fetal well-being have not been well studied. It seems that orgasm during pregnancy does not have detrimental effects on pregnancy, the woman, or the fetus. Further research is imperative in this field.

Data on intercourse during pregnancy is more prevalent, and may be used to draw conclusions about the safety of orgasm in pregnancy, especially when there is no evidence of harm. However, the specific effect of orgasm in high-risk pregnancies is not well established.

4.3.2 Preterm Labor and Orgasm

It is known that oxytocin plays a vital part in labor, both at term and preterm. Animal studies suggest it has a role in the initiation of labor: Plasma oxytocin concentrations and oxytocin receptor density were the same in rats with preterm labor and rats with term labor [13].

One study that addressed the issue of intercourse in high-risk pregnancies showed that the frequency of intercourse during early pregnancy does not significantly increase the risk of preterm birth in women with previous preterm delivery [14] (see Chapter 16 for more details on preterm birth).

According to Read et al. [15], frequent intercourse (defined a priori as once per week or more) during the second trimester significantly reduced the risk of subsequent preterm delivery in healthy women.

4.3.3 Placenta Previa and Pregnancy

While it is common practice to avoid digital examination of the uterine cervix due to fear of hemorrhage, and as a result there is a general recommendation to avoid sexual intercourse for fear that penile contact will elicit the same response, there is a paucity of prospective data to support or refute this recommendation, and there have been no attempts to examine the effect of orgasm without penetration on the incidence of hemorrhage with placenta previa and its safety (see Chapter 14 for more details on placenta previa).

References

1. C. M. Meston, R. J. Levin, M. L. Sipski, E. M. Hull, J. R. Heiman. Women's orgasm. *Annu Rev Sex Res* 2004;**15**:173–257. https://pubmed.ncbi.nlm.nih.gov/16913280/ (accessed March 22, 2021).

2. V. Polomeno. Sex and pregnancy: a perinatal educator's guide. *J Perinat Educ* 2006;**9**:15–27.

3. T. L. Woodard, M. P. Diamond. Physiologic measures of sexual function in women: a review. *Fertil Steril* 2009;**92**:19–34.

4. J. G. Bohlen, J. P. Held, M. O. Sanderson, A. Ahlgren. The female orgasm: pelvic contractions. *Arch Sex Behav* 1982;**11**:367–86.

5. J. Herbert. Peptides in the limbic system: neurochemical codes for co-ordinated adaptive responses to behavioural and physiological demand. *Prog Neurobiol* 1993;**41**:723–91.

6. J. Bancroft. The endocrinology of sexual arousal. *J Endocrinol* 2005;**186**:411–27.

7. M. S. Exton, T. H. C. Krüger, M. Koch, et al. Coitus-induced orgasm stimulates prolactin secretion in healthy subjects. *Psychoneuroendocrinology* 2001;**26**:287–94.

8. N. Magon, S. Kalra. The orgasmic history of oxytocin: love, lust, and labor. *Indian J Endocrinol Metab* 2011;**15**(Suppl 3): S156–61.

9. T. R. Insel. Oxytocin: a neuropeptide for affiliation. Evidence from behavioral, receptor autoradiographic, and comparative studies. *Psychoneuroendocrinology* 1992;**17**:3–35.

10. M. S. Carmichael, R. Humbert, J. Dixen, et al. Plasma oxytocin increases in the human sexual response. *J Clin Endocrinol Metab* 1987;**64**:27–31.

11. W. Blaicher, D. Gruber, C. Bieglmayer, et al. The role of oxytocin in relation to female sexual arousal. *Gynecol Obstet Invest* 1999;**47**:125–6.

12. R. C. Goodlin, W. Schmidt, D. C. Creevy. Uterine tension and fetal heart rate during maternal orgasm. *Obstet Gynecol* 1972;**39**:125–7.

13. M. Kobayashi, M. Akahane, K. Minami, et al. Role of oxytocin in the initiation of term and preterm labor in rats: changes in oxytocin receptor density and plasma oxytocin concentration and the effect of an oxytocin antagonist, L-366,509. *Am J Obstet Gynecol* 1999;**180**:621–7.

14. N. P. Yost, J. Owen, V. Berghella, et al. Effect of coitus on recurrent preterm birth. *Obstet Gynecol* 2006;**107**:793–7.

15. J. S. Read, M. A. Klebanoff. Sexual intercourse during pregnancy and preterm delivery: effects of vaginal microorganisms. *Am J Obstet Gynecol* 1993;**168**:514–19.

Demographics of Sexual Behavior in Pregnancy

Hanna R. Goldberg and Karthika Devarajan

5.1 Introduction

Sexual behavior in pregnancy is affected by biological, psychological, social, and environmental factors that vary throughout its course [1]. In general, the literature shows that sexual frequency and sexual function decline over the course of pregnancy [1–13], and this can have a significant impact on the relationship between partners and quality of life [2,11]. Questions around sex in pregnancy are common among patients, but traditionally this topic is rarely discussed during prenatal appointments [14]. As a result, myths, fears, and the Internet often shape patients' knowledge of sex in pregnancy. Changes in sexual behavior may make women feel less attractive or lead to extramarital relationships [15]. Therefore, it is important for antenatal care providers to be knowledgeable and proactive in sharing evidence-based information about sexual behavior in pregnancy and create an environment where patients feel comfortable discussing their questions.

In this chapter, we discuss the demographics of sex in pregnancy, including the frequency of sexual intercourse, types of sexual behaviors, sexual function, and the factors affecting sexual activity in pregnancy.

5.2 Defining Female Sexual Function and Dysfunction

Sexual dysfunction can be defined according to the criteria for female sexual interest/arousal disorder in the fifth edition of the *Diagnostic and Statistical Manual of Mental Disorders* (DSM-5) [16]. This definition encompasses significantly reduced sexual interest or arousal that causes clinically significant distress in an individual for at least 6 months [16]. The Female Sexual Function Index (FSFI) is a brief self-report measure of female sexual function that was developed to be used as a research tool for addressing the multidimensional nature of female sexual function [17]. The FSFI comprises five domains of sexual function, including (1) desire and subjective arousal, (2) lubrication, (3) orgasm, (4) satisfaction, and (5) pain/discomfort [17]. It is composed of 19 items and is psychometrically sound and easy to administer. Other scales include the Sexual Interaction Inventory, the Arizona Sexual Experiences Scale, and the Sexual Satisfaction Questionnaire [18].

5.3 Frequency of Sexual Intercourse and Sexual Function in Pregnancy

Difficulties with sexual functioning (73%), decreased sexual satisfaction compared to before pregnancy (55%), and sexual distress including negative emotions related to sexuality (42%) are common among pregnant women [19]. Many studies have used the FSFI to investigate the frequency of sexual intercourse during pregnancy and in the postpartum period [1–13]. Overall, the literature demonstrates a decline in frequency of sexual intercourse and sexual function over the course of pregnancy [1–13]. Most studies show a decrease in the first trimester, no change or an increase in the second trimester, and then a sharp decrease in the third trimester and early postpartum period [3].

Güleroglu et al. [5] administered the FSFI to 306 pregnant patients and found that 88.9% had sexual desire disorders, 86.9% had sexual arousal disorder, 42.8% had lubrication disorders, 69.6% had orgasm disorders, and 48% had sexual satisfaction disorders. Ninivaggio et al. [3] administered the FSFI to 623 nulliparous women in the first trimester, second trimester, and third trimester of pregnancy and found declining rates of sexual activity over time (94%, 90%, and 77%, respectively). Significantly lower FSFI scores were found in the third trimester as compared to the first and second. Esmer et al. [4] administered the FSFI to 363 women and found a decreased frequency of intercourse in 58.3%, 66.1%, and 76.5% of women in each trimester, respectively. Furthermore, the overall FSFI score was found to be significantly lower in the third trimester as compared to the first and second.

With regard to the types of sexual behaviors patients are engaging in, Von Sydow found that 41–53% of women prefer nongenital caressing, 25–32% clitoral stimulation, 23–30% breast stimulation, 15–30% vaginal stimulation, 6–16% cunnilingus, 4–11% fellatio, and 0–3% anal stimulation [11,20]. Use of the male-on-top sexual position declines during pregnancy, with female-on-top, side-by-side, and rear-entry positions being more favored as the pregnancy progresses [11].

Resuming sexual intercourse postpartum can be challenging (see Chapter 24 for more details of postpartum sexual function). Only 9–17% of couples engage in intercourse prior to the sixth week postpartum, whereas 88–95% have resumed sexual activity by 3 months postpartum [11]. During the first postpartum coitus, only 20% of women achieve orgasm, but 75% report orgasm by 3–6 months postpartum, which is similar to the prepregnancy relative orgasm rate [11,21].

5.4 Factors Affecting Sexual Activity in Pregnancy

In order to address the decline in sexual function over the course of pregnancy, it is important to understand and recognize the factors contributing to sexual dysfunction in pregnancy. Some of these factors include physiological changes, nausea, discomfort, fatigue, lack of interest, fear of miscarriage, fear of harming the fetus, fear of membrane rupture, fear of infection, physical awkwardness, and negative self-perception [1,14,22]. Potential benefits of sexual activity include managing back and pelvic pain, boosting intimacy, burning calories, and aiding in sleep [14].

5.5 Potential Complications of Sex in Pregnancy

Understanding the possible complications of sexual intercourse during pregnancy is necessary in order to address patients' fears. Many of the fears around sex in pregnancy are related to a lack of understanding of female anatomy, with many people believing that the penis can penetrate the uterus and thereby break the waters or hurt the baby [15]. For some couples sex in pregnancy is regarded as a moral sin as there is a third person present [15]. These fears tend to be cultural or religious and are less amenable to change (see Chapter 6 for more details on sexual activity in different cultures).

Jones et al. [23] discussed the potential complications of sex in pregnancy, including preterm labor, pelvic inflammatory disease (PID), antepartum hemorrhage in placenta previa, and venous air embolism.

- *Preterm labor*: Women with low-risk pregnancies, including those who have no signs or symptoms of lower genital tract infection, are *not* at increased risk of preterm labor [23]. Therefore, low-risk patients can be reassured that sex during pregnancy is safe [23]. While there is no clear benefit to restricting sexual activity in patients at increased risk for preterm labor, it is generally recommended to restrain from sexual activity in these cases given that it is a simple intervention with minimal harm [23]. There is even some evidence which suggests that women who have regular intercourse may be at decreased risk of preterm labor [14] (see Chapter 16 for more details on preterm birth).

- *PID*: It is possible for pregnant women to develop upper genital tract infections, particularly in the first trimester [23]. If patients are at high risk for acquiring sexually transmitted infections (STIs), they should be encouraged to use barrier methods when engaging in sexual intercourse (see Chapter 21 for more details on STIs).

- *Antepartum hemorrhage*: There is a paucity of evidence demonstrating a risk of hemorrhage following vaginal intercourse in patients with placenta previa; however, given the potential for significant bleeding, it is likely safest to abstain [23] (see Chapter 14 for more details on placenta previa).

- *Venous air embolism*: Venous air embolism is a rare, though potential complication of orogenital and penile–vaginal sex in pregnant patients [23] (see Chapter 19 for more details on air embolism).

Commonly accepted contraindications to sexual activity in pregnancy include placenta previa, placental abruption, uterine irritability, preterm premature rupture of membranes, incompetent cervix, current STIs, and antepartum hemorrhage [14].

5.6 Understanding the Barriers to Discussing Sexual Function with Patients

Physicians should create a supportive environment whereby patients feel comfortable discussing their concerns regarding sexuality in pregnancy. Many women report being too embarrassed to raise the topic of intercourse in pregnancy, so care providers could ask whether there are any questions about sex in order to address and correct any misconceptions [15]. Proactively addressing concerns may alleviate unnecessary abstinence and any attendant stress that this places on a relationship.

5.7 What Did Dr. Google Say?

5.7.1 Is It Safe to Have Sex in Pregnancy?

It's perfectly safe to have sex during pregnancy unless your doctor or midwife has told you not to. Having sex will not hurt your baby. Your partner's penis can't penetrate beyond your vagina, and the baby cannot tell what's going on. However, it's normal for your sex drive to change during pregnancy.

www.nhs.uk/pregnancy/keeping-well/sex/

5.7.2 What Kind of Sex Do People Have in Pregnancy?

As long as you're comfortable, most sexual positions are OK during pregnancy. Oral sex is also safe during pregnancy. As your pregnancy progresses, experiment to find what works best. Let your creativity take over, as long as you keep mutual pleasure and comfort in mind.

www.mayoclinic.org/healthy-lifestyle/pregnancy-week-by-week/in-depth/sex-during-pregnancy/art-20045318

5.7.3 Can You Have Oral Sex in Pregnancy?

"Oral sex can be part of a healthy sex life during pregnancy," Jamieson told Healthline. "As the body changes during pregnancy, some types of sex may become more uncomfortable and oral sex may be a great way for couples to express themselves sexually."

www.healthline.com/health-news/should-women-engage-in-oral-sex-during-pregnancy

5.7.4 Who Shouldn't Have Sex in Pregnancy?

You should not engage in any form of sexual activity if you are in preterm labor. Certain people are at a higher risk for preterm labor, such as people who are carrying more than one baby, people who have had problems with their cervix, or people who smoke while they are pregnant.

www.verywellfamily.com/pelvic-rest-reasons-you-can-t-have-sex-in-pregnancy-4111084

5.7.5 Can Sex Toys Be Used in Pregnancy?

Is it safe to use a vibrator while pregnant? Simply put, yes – it's probably safe to use your vibrator. For most low-risk pregnancies, sex, masturbation, and yes, internal or external use of your vibrator is safe.

www.healthline.com/health/pregnancy/can-you-use-a-vibrator-while-pregnant

References

1. J. Pauleta, N. Pereira, L. Graça. Sexuality during pregnancy. *J Sex Med* 2010;**7**:136–42.

2. S. Wallwiener, M. Müller, A. Doster, et al. Sexual activity and sexual dysfunction of women in the perinatal period: a longitudinal study. *Arch Gynecol Obstet* 2017;**295**:873–83.

3. C. Ninivaggio, R. Rogers, L. Leeman, et al. Sexual function changes during pregnancy. *Int Urogynecol J* 2017;**28**:923–9.

4. A. Corbacioglu Esmer, A. Akca, O. Akbayir, B. P. Goksedef, V. L. Bakir. Female sexual function and associated factors during pregnancy. *J Obstet Gynaecol Res* 2013;**39**:1165–72.

5. F. Tosun Güleroglu, N. Gördeles Beser. Evaluation of sexual functions of the pregnant women. *J Sex Med* 2014;**11**:146–53.

6. I. Gałązka, A. Drosdzol-Cop, B. Naworska, M. Czajkowska, V. Skrzypulec-Plinta. Changes in the sexual function during pregnancy. *J Sex Med* 2015;**12**:445–54.

7. K. Von Sydow, M. Ullmeyer, N. Happ. Sexual activity during pregnancy and after childbirth: results from the Sexual Preferences Questionnaire. *J Psychosom Obstet Gynaecol* 2001;**22**:29–40.

8. S. Chang, K. Chen, H. Lin, H. Yu. Comparison of overall sexual function, sexual intercourse/activity, sexual satisfaction, and sexual desire during the three trimesters of pregnancy and

assessment of their determinants. *J Sex Med* 2011;8:2859–67.

9. W. Fok, L. Chan, P. Yuen. Sexual behavior and activity in Chinese pregnant women. *Acta Obstet Gynecol Scand* 2005;**84**:934–8.

10. B. Erol, O. Sanli, D. Korkmaz, et al. A cross-sectional study of female sexual function and dysfunction during pregnancy. *J Sex Med* 2007;**4**:1381–7.

11. K. Von Sydow. Sexuality during pregnancy and after childbirth: a metacontent analysis of 59 studies. *J Psychosom Res* 1999;**47**:27–49.

12. G. Aslan, D. Aslan, A. Kizilyar, C. Ispahi, A. Esen. A prospective analysis of sexual functions during pregnancy. *Int J Impot Res* 2005;**17**:154–7.

13. J. Byrd, J. Hyde, J. DeLamater, E. Plant. Sexuality during pregnancy and the year postpartum. *J Fam Pract* 1998;**47**:305–8.

14. D. Cavalucci, Y. K. Fulbright. *Your Orgasmic Pregnancy*. Alameda, CA: HunterHouse, 2008.

15. M. C. Ribeiro, M. de Tubino Scanavino, M. L. S. do Amaral, A. L. de Moraes Horta, M. R. Torloni. Beliefs about sexual activity during pregnancy: a systematic review of the literature. *J Sex Marital Ther* 2017;**43**:822–32.

16. American Psychiatric Association. *Diagnostic and Statistical Manual of Mental Disorders*, 5th ed. Arlington, VA: American Psychiatric Publishing, 2013.

17. R. Rosen, C. Brown, J. Heiman, et al. The Female Sexual Function Index (FSFI): a multidimensional self-report instrument for the assessment of female sexual function. *J Sex Marital Ther* 2000;**26**:191–208.

18. A. Fuchs, I. Czech, J. Silkora, et al. Sexual functioning in pregnant women. *Int J Environ Res Public Health* 2019;**16**:4216.

19. A. K. Beveridge, S. A. Vannier, N. O. Rosen. Fear-based reasons for not engaging in sexual activity during pregnancy: associations with sexual relationship well-being. *J Psychosom Obstet Gynecol* 2018;**39**:138–45.

20. A. Tolor, P. V. DiGrazia. Sexual attitudes and behavior patterns during and following pregnancy. *Arch Sex Behav* 1976;**5**:539–51.

21. E. L. Ryding. Sexuality during and after pegnancy. *Acta Obstet Gynecol Scand* 1984;**63**:679–82.

22. E. O. Orji, I. O. Ogunlola, O. B. Fasubaa. Sexuality among pregnant women in South West Nigeria. *Obstet Gynecol* 2002;**22**:166–8.

23. C. Jones, C. Chan, D. Farine. Sex in pregnancy. *Can Med Assoc J* 2011;**183**:815–18.

Sexual Practices during Pregnancy in Different Cultures

Rachel Spitzer and Jenny Yang

6.1 Introduction

There is wide intercultural variation in sexual activity during pregnancy due to many factors that are complexly interrelated [1]. Universal factors affecting sexual activity in pregnancy such as fear of miscarriage or dyspareunia are influenced by culture-related factors such as degree of awareness of sexual health in pregnancy and extent of voluntary engagement in sexual activity [1]. Specific beliefs and "rules" in certain cultures and religions regarding the acceptability or unacceptability of sexual practices in pregnancy also affect rates of activity. This chapter describes the current evidence on rates of, and factors influencing, sexual activity in pregnancy in different cultures. This may help to reassure couples that a decrease in sexual activity in pregnancy may be a "normal" pregnancy-related trend and not necessarily indicative of relationship issues, but conversely may also identify areas of need that can be targeted to improve sexual health in pregnancy.

6.2 Frequency of Sexual Activity in Pregnancy

There is a diverse range of cultures researched with regard to rates of sexual activity in pregnancy, with studies conducted in countries across all the continents except Antarctica [1]. Despite limitations, this literature still effectively provides an overview of intercultural variation in frequency of sexual activity in pregnancy and also demonstrates the decrease in sexual activity in the third trimester observed universally in all populations studied [2].

Sexual activity in pregnancy is reported using a variety of parameters that hinders comparison of international data. These parameters include frequency of sexual activity in a select time period such as a week or month, percentage of women according to categorized frequency of sexual activity in a given period, percentage of women according to categorized change in frequency of sexual activity in each trimester or in pregnancy overall, percentage of women reporting any sexual activity in each trimester, and points from the relevant sections of questionnaires such as the Female Sexual Function Index (FSFI). Nevertheless, a similar trend in sexual activity in pregnancy is demonstrable in all studies regardless of cultural background or parameter used, with a decrease in sexual activity in the first trimester, stable level of activity in the second trimester, and a marked further decrease in activity in the third trimester, followed by an increase in sexual activity after delivery albeit to levels lower than those prior to pregnancy [2]. This trend is graphically portrayed by Gałązka et al. [3] who studied sexual practices in pregnancy in a Polish population (Figure 6.1).

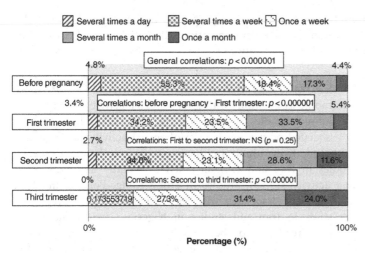

Figure 6.1 The frequency of sexual intercourse before pregnancy and in the subsequent trimesters [3].

Studies of average frequency of sexual activity in pregnancy overall show similar rates, ranging from 1.1 to 1.6 times per week in studies conducted in Nigeria, Pakistan, Burkina Faso, the USA, and Turkey [4–8]. Senkumwong et al. [9] found the most common frequency of sexual activity in pregnancy in a Thai cohort to be zero to once per week, with an increase in study participants reporting this frequency in each advancing trimester. Notable outliers in reported frequency of sexual activity in pregnancy include Ahmed et al. [10] who found higher average frequencies of 1.8 and 6.9 times per week in the third and second trimesters, respectively, in an Egyptian cohort, and Liu et al. [11] who conversely found much lower average frequencies of 0.4 and 1.7 times per month in the third and first trimesters, respectively, in a Taiwanese sample.

A decrease in sexual activity in pregnancy is reported by 55–93% of women in studies conducted in Nigeria and Hong Kong [12,13] and studies in Turkey and Canada report figures in between these [14,15]. Interestingly, 1–15% of women in these studies reported an increase in sexual activity in pregnancy [12–15]. Reported reduction in sexual activity appears to be more likely with advancing gestation, with studies in Canada and Turkey both finding that 76% of women in the third trimester reported decreased sexual activity compared with 48–58% who reported this finding in the first trimester [15,16].

The rate of abstinence in pregnancy is a more reliable and comparable parameter and may be more indicative of culture-related changes in sexual practices in pregnancy than frequency of sexual activity. There is wide variation in reported rates of abstinence in pregnancy, ranging from 0% in Nigeria to 46% in India, with rates of 9–14% reported in Canada, Poland, South Africa, and Burkina Faso [7,12,15,17–19]. Studies in Iran and Hong Kong have found rates of abstinence in pregnancy of 20 and 38% [13,20]. Studies assessing rates of abstinence in different trimesters demonstrate both a wide range in rates between different populations and a universally higher rate of abstinence in the third trimester. Rates of abstinence in the third trimester range from 17% in a Turkish study to 65% in a Taiwanese study, with an evenly ascending distribution of rates between these figures in studies conducted in Slovenia, the USA, Pakistan, South Africa, Sweden, Iran, and Hong Kong [8,11,13,18,20–24]. Overall, the current body of evidence suggests that levels of sexual activity in pregnancy are lower in Asian popula-tions compared with Caucasian and African populations. Potential cultural reasons for these trends are explored in subsequent sections.

6.3 Factors Associated with Level of Sexual Activity in Pregnancy

Attempts to identify demographic associations with level of sexual activity in pregnancy have revealed conflicting findings. Studies in Iran, Nigeria, and Turkey found multi-parity to be significantly associated with a lower level of sexual activity in pregnancy [4,5,20], whereas a study in Hong Kong found multiparous women to be more sexually active [13] and other studies in Iran and Canada failed to identify any association between parity and sexual activity [15,25]. Studies in Hong Kong, Poland, and Iran found increased maternal age to be associated with less sexual activity in pregnancy [19,20]; however, another study in Iran and studies in Nigeria, Canada, India, and Turkey failed to find any relationship between maternal age and activity [4,5,13,15,17,25]. Alizadeh et al. [25] found higher educational level to be associated with less reduction in sexual activity in pregnancy in an Iranian population, in contrast with Eryilmaz et al. [5] who reported higher educational level to be associated with reduced sexual activity in a Turkish cohort. Canadian, Indian, and Turkish studies failed to find any association between educational level and sexual activity [15–17], and two further Turkish studies also found conflicting associations between employment status and sexual activity in pregnancy, with Corbacioglu Esmer et al. [16] finding a greater reduction in activity with employment status but Eryilmaz et al. [5] failing to find any such association. Of note, Bartellas et al. [15] investigated the relationship between religion and sexual activity in pregnancy in a Canadian heterogeneously religious cohort, and did not find any association.

6.4 The Female Sexual Function Index and Female Sexual Dysfunction in Pregnancy

Sexual activity in pregnancy is also commonly assessed using the FSFI questionnaire, a 19-item self-administered questionnaire originally developed by Rosen and colleagues in 2000 and measures different aspects of sexual function in women, namely desire, arousal, lubrication, orgasm, satisfaction. and pain, and has been widely validated in studies representing a broad range of ethnicities [26,27]. Its widespread use in research on sexual activity in pregnancy has inadvertently identified previously unrecognized high rates of female sexual dysfunction (FSD) in pregnancy, and has provided insight into physical and nonphysical causes for change in sexual activity and FSD in pregnancy [1].

Domain-specific and total FSFI scores in each trimester parallel the reduction in frequency of sexual activity observed in the third trimester in all cultures studied, including Egypt, Turkey, USA, Taiwan, Poland, Iran, Burkina Faso, Brazil, Sweden, and Thailand [3,6,7,10,24,28–32]. Use of the FSFI reveals that this reduction in sexual activity is likely due to both physical factors such as dyspareunia and nonphysical factors such as reduced sexual desire, both of which were most common in the third trimester in all populations investigated [2]. As the FSFI identifies FSD at a total score of less than 26.55, use of the FSFI in pregnancy has revealed remarkably high rates of FSD during this reproductive life stage [27]. Rates of FSD in pregnancy are widely variable but are high, upwards of 34.2% [10,31], with one Iranian study finding FSD prevalences of 64.22 and 87.8% in the first and third trimesters, respectively, using a lower cutoff score of 21 [30], and studies in Taiwan and the USA reporting average total FSFI scores in the diagnostic range for FSD in all trimesters [23,29]. Ninivaggio et al. [23] suggest there may be a need to determine a pregnancy-specific cutoff for FSD in the pregnant population, although the low scores in all FSFI domains demonstrates there is a global decrease in sexual function during pregnancy.

As with frequency of sexual activity in pregnancy, researchers have attempted to identify causes of, and demographic factors associated with, lower FSFI scores in pregnancy with quite varied results and lack of overall consensus. Erol et al. [33] sought to identify whether a change in serum androgen levels with pregnancy is a biological explanation for reduced sexual desire but they failed to find such a correlation in a Turkish cohort. Ahmed et al. [10] proposed that female genital mutilation, which has an estimated prevalence of 74.5–95.8% in the Egyptian population, may be a major contributor to high rates of FSD in their study conducted in Egypt. Interestingly, Gałązka et al. [3] found low acceptance of pregnancy-related changes in appearance in a Polish cohort to be significantly associated with reduced FSFI and abstinence in pregnancy.

While unsurprisingly Yıldız [34] found prepregnancy FSD to be associated with FSD in pregnancy, FSD was also found to persist postpartum in 84.6% of those with FSD before pregnancy (Figure 6.2). Ahmed et al. [10] found older maternal age to be associated with lower FSFI scores in an Egyptian cohort, whereas studies in Canada, Iran, and Austria did not identify this association [30,35,36]. Ahmed et al. [10] also found longer duration of marriage to be associated with lower FSFI scores although this was not found in studies conducted in Canada and Turkey [16,35]. Lower FSFI was identified in those with higher parity in this Egyptian study, with lower parity in a Polish

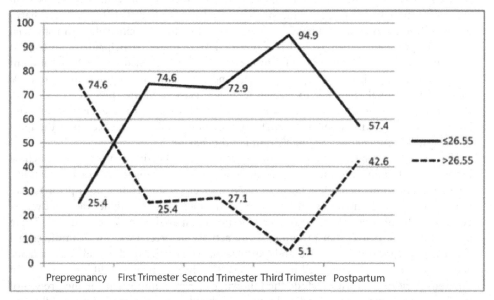

Figure 6.2 Percentages of sexual dysfunction in five assessments according to FSFI cutoff values. Values ≤26.55 indicate sexual dysfunction; values >26.55 indicate normal sexual function [34].

study, and unrelated to parity in a Turkish study [3,10,16]. Educational level was found to be significantly associated with lower FSFI in a Taiwanese study [29], whereas no association was identified in studies conducted in Egypt, Canada, Turkey, and Austria [10,16,35,36]. Interestingly, Chang et al. [29] found lower FSFI scores in pregnancy to be associated with higher prepregnancy body image scores, suggesting a differential reaction of individuals to pregnancy-related physical changes in those with poor versus favorable body image. In any case, small datasets limit accurate cultural representation and identification of true associations between demographic factors and FSFI scores in the different cultural contexts.

6.5 Reasons for Altered Sexual Activity in Pregnancy Reported in Different Cultures

Physical reasons provided for decreased sexual activity in pregnancy across cultures that are separate from those assessed in the FSFI include fatigue, feeling awkward, inability to find a suitable position, nausea, vaginal bleeding, swelling of external genitalia, and abdominal cramps or labor pains [5,18,22,24]. Despite the available evidence offering reassurance that sexual activity is safe in low-risk pregnancies [1], fear of harm to the fetus or pregnancy by causing miscarriage, preterm labor, or premature rupture of membranes is still reported by 5–65% of women across various cultures [5,7,9,14,15,20,35,37] and by 82.9% of women in a study performed in Hong Kong [13]. Beveridge et al. [35] found 58.6% of women reported fear as a reason for abstaining in the prior month and fear-based reasons to be associated with sexual distress, although not with sexual function, sexual satisfaction, or relationship satisfaction.

Certain cultures express specific fears of harm from sexual activity in pregnancy. A study in Burkina Faso identified fears of pain to the fetus, causing a black spot on the baby's skin at birth, and fetal abnormalities [7]. Of the 45% of women in a Pakistani study who thought sex was harmful for the fetus, five specified that they believed harm was only limited to female fetuses [8]. There are also culture-specific rules against sexual activity in pregnancy, such as the belief reported by 24.6% of participants in an Iranian study that sexual intercourse is sinful in pregnancy due to a third person being present [38]. In a South African study, 5% of respondents followed religious rules and 4% followed traditional rules not to engage in sexual activity during pregnancy [18]. Liu et al. [11] state that Chinese prohibitions on sexual activity in pregnancy stem from beliefs rooted in Chinese medicine that sex may be a malign influence upon the fetus directly or by influencing a woman's mind and behavior.

Other culture-related factors influencing rate of sexual activity in pregnancy include lower rates of coital interest in expectant mothers with stronger religious affiliations, Chinese populations being less likely to orgasm or enjoy intercourse both prior to and during pregnancy compared with Europeans and Americans, and higher rates of dyspareunia in Hispanic and African-American women compared with Caucasians [2]. There are also cultural beliefs that promote sexual activity in pregnancy, for example sexual activity in pregnancy is positive and purposeful, widens the birth canal, makes labor easier, and improves fetal well-being [4,8,17,37]. Beliefs held by different tribes in different African countries include the following: sperm is important for the growth of the fetus, sperm turns into blood and nourishes the bloodstream of the future child, and that sex is necessary to help the child grow [7].

Several studies report reasons for maintaining sexual activity in pregnancy that are related to the nature of the spousal relationship, which is heavily influenced by cultural context such as acceptance and practice of polygamy, adultery, and sexual autonomy in the relationship. Naim and Bhutto [8] describe Pakistani society as male-dominated, and found that 40.7% of women engaged in sex to fulfill marital obligations. Leite et al. [31] state that the women of the Alagoas ethnic group in Brazil "do not hold a strong position during sexual negotiations" and "probably have difficulty saying no to partners" and postulate that these factors may contribute toward higher levels of both sexual activity in pregnancy and FSD.

In their study conducted in Pakistan, Naim and Bhutto [8] further note that less women feared their husband's infidelity where relationships were highly monogamous, with only 13.3% stating they felt sex served to keep their husband around, compared with a Nigerian study [4] where only 15.9% reported not fearing this. Up to 25.3% of women in a study conducted in Burkina Faso stated they had sex to avoid spousal infidelity, with 21.3% having sex to obtain pleasure for their spouse only and not themselves, and 4.8% having sex to satisfy marital obligations [7]. Pressure from partners to have sex in pregnancy was reported by 9 and 19% of women in studies performed in Hong Kong and Canada, respectively [13,15].

Some studies report avoidance of sexual activity in pregnancy being driven by the spouse due to reasons such as fear of harming the fetus, reduced attraction, and being inhibited by the growing womb [14]. One Austrian study reported that 62% of spouses showed signs of worry [36]. Cultural customs such the woman staying at her mother's residence during pregnancy separate from her husband, described in an Indian study, also contributes toward decreased sexual activity in pregnancy [17].

6.6 Practices of Different Sexual Positions and Activities in Pregnancy in Different Cultures

Studies in a range of cultural settings, including Nigeria, Canada, the USA, Hong Kong, Poland, Turkey, South Africa, Sweden, Thailand, and Germany, have found variable results regarding altered sexual positions and practice of nongenital sexual activities in pregnancy that might change due to pregnancy-related physical changes impeding genital–genital intercourse or fears of risks with such intercourse [3,6,9,12,13,15,18,19,21,24,32]. Many studies have reported a change in sexual position so that a male (or nonpregnant) partner was progressively less likely to be on top in each trimester, suggesting position changes to indeed be driven by growth of the womb [9,19,21,32].

Gałązka et al. [3] did not find a difference in genito-anal or genito-oral contacts or masturbation frequency in pregnancy; however, they propose that this may be due to the religious beliefs of Polish women, among whom 51% are Catholic [19], or the feeling that such practices are embarrassing or inappropriate to report, which highlights the difficulty in accurately assessing such practices. Other studies assessing masturbation by women or their partners during pregnancy did not find any significant differences either, but similarly may have been subject to underreporting [6,13,19]. Livingstone et al. [17], who conducted their study in a Christian medical college, specifically comment that they could not enquire about other forms of sexual activity, homosexual activity, or activity with persons other than husbands due to having to respect local cultural sentiments.

6.7 Postpartum Resumption of Sexual Activity

Similar to reported changes in sexual position during pregnancy, resumption of sexual activity following delivery also appears to be largely driven by physical factors (see Chapter 24 for more details on the postpartum period). Average time to resumption ranged from 7.1 to 11.4 weeks in studies conducted in the USA, Austria, and Turkey [34,36], although one Nigerian study reported a later average time to resumption of 16.5 weeks with reasons for this including factors related to breastfeeding and family planning, or lack thereof [4,6]. It must be noted that longer time to resumption is associated with vaginal delivery (compared with cesarean section) and with breastfeeding, likely due to consequent hypoestrogenic dyspareunia [6], and rates of these vary highly between different countries [39,40].

6.8 Attitudes toward Antenatal Sexual Health Assessment and Education

Lack of antenatal sexual health assessment and education is a significant factor contributing to reduced sexual activity in pregnancy, as is the issue that sex is a taboo subject in many cultures and this impedes the dispelling of misconceptions regarding the harm of sexual activity in pregnancy and women from seeking treatment of sex-related issues. Sex is reported as taboo in up to 31.3% of women in one study in Burkina Faso [7], and an Indian study on sexual practices in pregnancy had a 47.6% rate of refusal to participate and 20% nonresponse rate for questions regarding sexual activity, demonstrating the difficulty of investigating this subject in conservative cultures [17]. In this study, 23.1% of respondents stated they would continue to bear problems with sexual activity without discussing it with anyone else [17], and 78.1% of women with sexual problems in a Nigerian study did not discuss these with their care providers [12].

Discussion of sexual issues in pregnancy with health practitioners was reported by 3% of women in a South African study [18] and by 29% of women in a Canadian study [15]. In the Canadian study, though the rate of discussion was relatively higher than in other studies, only 34% of women reported they felt comfortable to raise the topic themselves [15]. Interestingly, one Thai study reported that 22% of women received information about sexual activity in pregnancy [32], whereas another Thai study reported that 62% of women received information about sexuality in pregnancy from health physicians [9]. Despite low rates generally, high rates of women report the desire for this discussion. All the 75.8% of women in a Turkish study who reported being too shy to discuss sexual activity in pregnancy indicated that they wanted to discuss this with health professionals, while 74 and 76% of women who had not discussed sexual issues in pregnancy with their doctor in studies in Hong Kong and Canada, respectively, felt they should be discussed [13,15].

Another issue that may be a consequence, and which compounds the impact, of the lack of sexual education provided by health practitioners is that most women obtain advice regarding sexual activity in pregnancy from sources such as partners, friends, family, the media, and even religious leaders [8,17]. In Pakistan, 70% of families live in joint family systems that have been proposed to perpetuate the provision of ill-informed advice from family members [8]. One study in Taiwan reported that 3.3% of women stopped having sex in pregnancy due to the advice of their mother-in-law and 3.3%

stopped due to advice by their mothers [11]. Even when advice is given by health practitioners, avoidance of sexual activity due to medical advice was reported by 29% of women in a Polish study, which may reflect low levels of education regarding sexual health in pregnancy even among health practitioners [19].

6.9 Efficacy of Sexual Education in Pregnancy

A few studies have investigated the impact of antenatal sex education on sexual function in pregnancy. Several studies in Iran investigating antenatal sex education interventions revealed such education to be beneficial as measured by FSFI scores in comparison with control groups who did not receive education [41–44]. In contrast, a study conducted in Thailand failed to find a significant improvement in FSFI score with antenatal sex education [45].

Bahadoran et al. [42] also found that male sexual function improved as measured by the Brief Form of Sexual Inventory questionnaire, which is deemed to be the male equivalent of the FSFI; this was particularly the case with face-to-face education, which the authors thought was due to the ability to ask individualized questions and express erroneous beliefs more easily, with less fear of humiliation. Heidari et al. [43] also noted that although sex education in Iran is taboo, only 5% of couples discontinued education due to unwillingness, suggesting a role for sex education in even conservative societies.

6.10 Limitations of Evidence on Sexual Practices in Pregnancy

As mentioned previously, accurately capturing data on a subject that is taboo or uncomfortable to discuss in many cultures is inherently challenging. Although self-administration of questionnaires is used as a strategy to increase privacy and hence accurate responses, the limitation this imposes on such research is that views captured are limited to those who are both literate and speak the same language as that used in the questionnaires. Furthermore, the vast majority of studies have recruited women in antenatal clinics and hence do not capture the views of women who have late or no antenatal care, which is more likely in the geographically isolated and lower socio-economic groups [46].

Selection bias is also likely due to voluntary participation in studies, with those uncomfortable with discussing sexual activity in pregnancy being able to decline study participation even though this is one of the aspects being investigated. In one study conducted in a Christian medical college in India, 47.8% of those approached declined to participate [17]. Another issue with recruiting women in antenatal clinics is that studies which assessed prepregnancy sexual activity obtained these data retrospectively, subjecting such data to recall bias [21,24,36]. Similarly, the accuracy of trends in sexual activity with advancing gestation may be questionable due to the cross-sectional nature of these studies, which extrapolate trends from different rates in different women in the different trimesters [3,5,7–9,12,13,15,17,18,20,22,25,29,33,35]. Despite the many weaknesses of these studies, largely due to the challenges inherent in researching such an issue, such efforts to research sexual practices in pregnancy may in itself facilitate normalization of such discussions, leading to better quality data, increased discussion of sexual health in pregnancy antenatally, and improved recognition and treatment of FSD in pregnancy.

6.11 Conclusion

There is a broad cultural representation in the literature of sexual practices in pregnancy that demonstrates a universal reduction in sexual activity and increase in FSD particularly in the third trimester. Reasons for decreased sexual activity due to culture-related prohibitions and pregnancy-related physical changes are difficult to address; however, the significant proportion of couples reporting decreased activity due to ill-informed fears of risks to pregnancy can be helped by increasing antenatal sex education and assessment of sexual issues, routinely incorporating this into provision of antenatal care. There is evidence to demonstrate that such measures are both desired by pregnant women and couples across various cultures and may be effective in improving sexual function. Improving sexual health in pregnancy may reap benefits for the well-being of both pregnant patients and their partners, and helps create a nurturing environment for the development of children and families.

References

1. T. Zakšek. Sexual activity during pregnancy in childbirth and after childbirth. In A. P. Mivšek, ed. *Sexology in Midwifery*. London: IntechOpen, 2015: 111–33.

2. K. von Sydow. Sexuality during pregnancy and after childbirth: a metacontent analysis of 59 studies. *J Psychosom Res* 1999;**47**:27–49.

3. I. Gałązka, A. Drosdzol-Cop, B. Naworska, M. Czajkowska, V. Skrzypulec-Plinta. Changes in the sexual function during pregnancy. *J Sex Med* 2015;**12**:445–54.

4. J. Adinma. Sexual activity during and after pregnancy. *Adv Contracept* 1996;**12**:53–61.

5. G. Eryilmaz, E. Ege, H. Zincir. Factors affecting sexual life during pregnancy in eastern Turkey. *Gynecol Obstet Invest* 2004;**57**:103–8.

6. J. S. Hyde, J. D. DeLamater, E. A. Plant, J. M. Byrd. Sexuality during pregnancy and the year postpartum. *J Sex Res* 1996;**33**:143–51.

7. S. Kiemtorè, I. Ouèdraogo, A. Ouattara, et al. Sex during pregnancy: opinions, attitudes and practices among pregnant women. *J Women's Health Care* 2016;**5**:1–5.

8. M. Naim, E. Bhutto. Sexuality during pregnancy in Pakistan women. *J Pak Med Assoc* 2000;**50**:38–44.

9. N. Senkumwong, S. Chaovisitsaree, S. Rugpao, W. Chandrawongse, S. Yanunto. The changes of sexuality in Thai women during pregnancy. *J Med Assoc Thai* 2006;**89**(Suppl 4):S124–9.

10. M. R. Ahmed, E. H. Madny, W. A. Sayed Ahmed. Prevalence of female sexual dysfunction during pregnancy among Egyptian women. *J Obstet Gynaecol Res* 2014;**40**:1023–9.

11. H. Liu, P. Hsu, K. Chen. Sexual activity during pregnancy in Taiwan: a qualitative study. *Sex Med* 2013;**1**:54–61.

12. A. Anzaku, O. Ngozi, B. Dabu, E. Edet. Frequency, perceptions and complications of sexual activity during pregnancy among a group of Nigerian women. *Int Arch Integrated Med* 2015;**2**:54–63.

13. W. Fok, L. Chan, P. Yuen. Sexual behavior and activity in Chinese pregnant women. *Acta Obstet Gynecol Scand* 2005;**84**:934–8.

14. R. Babazadeh, K. Mirzaii, Z. Masomi. Changes in sexual desire and activity during pregnancy among women in Shahroud, Iran. *Int J Gynecol Obstet* 2013;**120**:82–4.

15. E. Bartellas, J. Crane, M. Daley, K. A. Bennett, D. Hutchens. Sexuality and sexual activity in pregnancy. *Br J Obstet Gynaecol* 2000;**107**:964–8.

16. A. Corbacioglu Esmer, A. Akca, O. Akbayir, B. Goksedef, V. Bakir. Female

sexual function and associated factors during pregnancy. *J Obstet Gynaecol Res* 2013;**39**:1165–72.

17. J. D. Livingstone, L. Ralte, J. T. Magar, et al. Sexual behaviour in pregnancy among antenatal women attending a secondary hospital in southern India. *Int J Community Med Public Health* 2018;**5**:3501–5.

18. J. Moodley, S. Khedun. Sexual activity during pregnancy: a questionnaire-based study. *South Afr J Epidemiol Infect* 2011;**26**:33–5.

19. M. Staruch, A. Kucharczyk, K. Zawadzka, M. Wielgos, I. Szymusik. Sexual activity during pregnancy. *Neuro Endocrinol Lett* 2016;**37**:101–6.

20. F. Torkestani, S. Hadavand, Z. Khodashenase, et al. Frequency and perception of sexual activity during pregnancy in Iranian couples. *Int J Fertil Steril* 2012;**6**:107–10.

21. S. Gökyildiz, N. Beji. The effects of pregnancy on sexual life. *J Sex Marital Ther* 2005;**31**:201–15.

22. T. Košec, A. Jug Došler, M. Kusterle, A. P. Mivšek. Sex life during pregnancy. *Slovenian Nurs Rev* 2019;**53**:280–7.

23. C. Ninivaggio, R. Rogers, L. Leeman, et al. Sexual function changes during pregnancy. *Int Urogynecol J* 2017;**28**:923–9.

24. E. Ryding. Sexuality during and after pregnancy. *Acta Obstet Gynecol Scand* 1984;**63**:679–82.

25. S. Alizadeh, H. Riazi, H. Alavi Majd, G. Ozgoli. Factors affecting the variation in sexual activity and response before and during pregnancy among pregnant women in Rasht City, Northern Iran. *Galen Med J* 2019;**8**:e1531.

26. R. Rosen, C. Brown, J. Heiman, et al. The Female Sexual Function Index (FSFI): a multidimensional self-report instrument for the assessment of female sexual function. *J Sex Marital Ther* 2000;**26**:191–208.

27. M. Wiegel, C. Meston, R. Rosen. The female sexual function index (FSFI):

cross-validation and development of clinical cutoff scores. *J Sex Marital Ther* 2005;**31**:1–20.

28. G. Aslan, D. Aslan, A. Kizilyar, C. Ispahi, A. Esen. A prospective analysis of sexual functions during pregnancy. *Int J Impot Res* 2005;**17**:154–7.

29. S. Chang, K. Chen, H. Lin, H. Yu. Comparison of overall sexual function, sexual intercourse/activity, sexual satisfaction, and sexual desire during the three trimesters of pregnancy and assessment of their determinants. *J Sex Med* 2011;**8**:2859–67.

30. Z. Khalesi, M. Bokaie, S. Attari. Effect of pregnancy on sexual function of couples. *Afr Health Sci* 2018;**18**:227–34.

31. A. Leite, A. Campos, A. Dias, et al. Prevalence of sexual dysfunction during pregnancy. *Rev Assoc Med Bras (1992)* 2009;**55**:563–8.

32. W. Uwapusitanon, T. Choobun. Sexuality and sexual activity in pregnancy. *J Med Assoc Thai* 2004;**87**(Suppl 3):S45–9.

33. B. Erol, O. Sanli, D. Korkmaz, et al. A cross-sectional study of female sexual function and dysfunction during pregnancy. *J Sex Med* 2007;**4**:1381–7.

34. H. Yıldız. The relation between prepregnancy sexuality and sexual function during pregnancy and the postpartum period: a prospective study. *J Sex Marital Ther* 2015;**41**:49–59.

35. J. Beveridge, S. Vannier, N. Rosen. Fear-based reasons for not engaging in sexual activity during pregnancy: associations with sexual and relationship well-being. *J Psychosom Obstet Gynaecol* 2018;**39**:138–45.

36. G. Trutnovsky, J. Haas, U. Lang, E. Petru. Women's perception of sexuality during pregnancy and after birth. *Aust NZ J Obstet Gynaecol* 2006;**46**:282–7.

37. M. C. Ribeiro, M. de Tubino Scanavino, M. L. S. do Amaral, A. L. de Moraes Horta, M. R. Torloni. Beliefs about sexual activity during pregnancy: a systematic review of the literature. *J Sex Marital Ther* 2017;**43**:822–32.

38. S. Jamali, L. Mosalanejad. Sexual dysfunction in Iranian pregnant women. *Iran J Reprod Med* 2013;**11**:479–86.

39. F. Althabe, C. Sosa, J. Belizán, et al. Cesarean section rates and maternal and neonatal mortality in low-, medium-, and high-income countries: an ecological study. *Birth* 2006;**33**:270–7.

40. A. Eidelman. The impact of culture on breastfeeding rates. *Breastfeeding Med* 2016;**11**: 215.

41. M. Afshar, S. Mohammad-Alizadeh-Charandabi, E. Merghti-Khoei, P. Yavarikia. The effect of sex education on the sexual function of women in the first half of pregnancy: a randomized controlled trial. *J Caring Sci* 2012;**1**:173–81.

42. P. Bahadoran, M. MohammadiMahdiabadzade, H. Nasiri, A. GholamiDehaghi. The effect of face-to-face or group education during pregnancy on sexual function of couples in Isfahan. *Iran J Nurs Midwifery Res* 2015;**20**:582–7.

43. M. Heidari, F. Aminshokravi, F. Zayeri, S. Azin. Effect of sexual education on sexual function of Iranian couples during pregnancy: a quasi experimental study. *J Reprod Infertil* 2018;**19**:39–48.

44. E. Mahnaz, B. Nasim, O. Sonia. Effect of a structured educational package on women's sexual function during pregnancy. *Int J Gynaecol Obstet* 2020;**148**:225–30.

45. S. Wannakosit, V. Phupong. Sexual behavior in pregnancy: comparing between sexual education group and nonsexual education group. *J Sex Med* 2010;**7**:3434–8.

46. I. N. Okedo-Alex, I. C. Akamike, O. B. Ezeanosike, C. J. Uneke. Determinants of antenatal care utilisation in sub-Saharan Africa: a systematic review. *BMJ Open* 2019;**9**:e031890.

Chapter 7

What Do Obstetric Guidelines Say?

Vered B. Lamhot, Ola Gutzeit, and Dana Vitner

7.1 Introduction

Women's sexual health is an important component of women's well-being at any age. Pregnancy, in particular, brings about biological, psychological, and social changes that may alter sexual well-being [1]. However, the subject of sexual intercourse during pregnancy is not well defined in obstetric guidelines. Table 7.1 summarizes the information from the leading obstetric societies worldwide.

As depicted in Table 7.1, sex during normal pregnancy is permitted. The reasons for avoiding sex in pregnancy differ in different guidelines, as do the situations in which nonvaginal sex is permitted. Most of these resources concur that in cases of placental problems such as placenta previa [5,6,8] or heavy bleeding [3,7], sex should be avoided. There also seems to be an agreement that sex should be avoided in cases of ruptured membranes [5,7,8] or pregnancies in which there is a high likelihood of premature labor [3,5–8]. Some of the resources suggest that sexual intercourse should be avoided in cases of nonsingleton pregnancies [3,4,7] or even of hypertension [4]. It is a consensus that orgasms are safe [2,3,7,8] and all sexual positions are permitted as long as the woman is comfortable, though it is preferable to lay on the side [2–4,6–8]. Condoms should be used by women who are nonmonogamous and with new partners [3,6–8]. There are contradictory instructions as to sex with a partner with a sexually transmitted infection (STI), namely avoidance versus condom use [6]. The exact effect of pregnancy on sexual desire differs between guidelines but the tone in all guidelines is the same: all women are different and all changes in sexual desire are normal and should be accepted.

7.2 What Did Dr. Google Say?

Though official medical guidelines regarding sex during pregnancy are lacking, thankfully Dr. Google has a lot to say on the subject. Healthline [9–13], Parents [14,15], WebMD [16], the BUMP [17], What to expect [18], as well as many other sites targeted at pregnant women, have at least 10 different articles on the subject covering many topics, including penetration, spotting, masturbation, sexual positions, sex drive and even bondage/discipline, dominance/submission, and sadism/masochism (BDSM).

7.2.1 Sex Safety

All these sites recommend the continuation of sexual intercourse throughout pregnancy unless restricted by the physician. Possible reasons that may cause the physician to ban sex include multiple birth pregnancy, incompetent cervix, signs of preterm labor, or placenta previa. These sites also acknowledge that sexual drive may change throughout

Table 7.1. Obstetric society guidelines

	ACOG [2]	NHS [3]	SOGC [4]	Australian Government Department of Health [5]	Mayo Clinic [6]	Tommy's [7]	HealthLink British Columbia [8]
Can you have sex during pregnancy?	Most sexual activity is safe for women having healthy pregnancies. This includes sexual intercourse or penetration with fingers or sex toys	Unless told otherwise by physician Sex should be avoided if: • Heavy bleeding • Waters have broken • Cervical problems • Multiple pregnancy • History of premature labor	Yes, if pregnancy is normal Avoid sex if at risk for preterm labor (multiple pregnancy, high blood pressure)	In low-risk pregnancies there is a low risk of adverse outcomes from sexual activity and it is unlikely to be associated with preterm birth Though there is no evidence to suggest a clear benefit from restricting sexual activity in women who are at risk of preterm labor (e.g. previous spontaneous preterm birth) or antepartum hemorrhage because of placenta previa, it may be advisable for them to abstain from sexual activity	Yes Avoid if at risk for preterm labor or have placental problems Avoid if partner has a sexually transmitted infection (STI)	Yes, unless told otherwise by physician Sex should be avoided if: • Any heavy bleeding during pregnancy • Waters have broken • Cervical problems • Multiple pregnancy • History of premature labor • Partner has an STI	Yes Sex should be avoided if: • Placenta previa • Waters have broken • Contractions before 37 weeks • Vaginal bleeding
Is it safe to have an orgasm?	Orgasm can cause cramps. If cramps are severe and persistent, or if there is heavy bleeding, obstetrics/gynecology should be contacted	Orgasm may cause Braxton Hicks contractions				Yes, may cause Braxton Hicks contractions Orgasm intensity may change during pregnancy	Yes. Orgasm close to due date may start uterine contractions
Best sexual positions	Different positions should be attempted in order to find the most comfortable	As long as comfortable It may be better to lie on the sides either facing each other or with the partner behind	As long as comfortable		As long as comfortable	As long as comfortable It may be better to lie on side, either facing each other or with partner behind Water-based lubricants may help with dryness	Most comfortable lying on side

Anal and oral sex	Oral sex is allowed. Partner should not blow air into vagina, as it can cause an air embolism that can be potentially fatal to mother and fetus Anal sex is allowed as long as it is not followed by vaginal sex	Oral sex is safe Avoid vaginal, anal and oral sex if partner has an STI	Safe to have oral sex in pregnancy If partner has sores in mouth or lips, protection should be used Partner should not blow air into vagina as it can cause an air embolism that can be potentially fatal to mother and fetus If sex is prohibited for any of the reasons listed, all sexual activity should be avoided, including anal sex, masturbation, and use of sex toys Vaginal sex should not follow anal sex unless partner washes his genitals and changes condoms	Condoms should be used with a new partner or a partner who may have an STI
Are condoms necessary?	If in nonmonogamous relationship.	Use condom if nonmonogamous or have new partner during pregnancy	Use condom if you or your partner have an STI, if nonmonogamous, or have new partner during pregnancy	
Sex drive	Sex drive may change. It may decrease during first and third trimesters	Desire may decrease or increase	It is normal for sex drive to change during pregnancy Some couples enjoy sex during pregnancy; others avoid it	Desire for sex commonly decreases as the pregnancy progresses	Everyone is different As a very general guide, most women find that their sexual desire goes down in the first trimester, goes up again in the second trimester, and then goes down again in the third trimester

ACOG, American College of Obstetricians and Gynecologists; NHS, National Health Service; SOGC, Society of Obstetricians and Gynaecologists of Canada.

pregnancy [9,10,14,16,17]. Condoms should be used if the STI status of partners is unknown [9,13]. Sexual contact with partners who have lesions or pain in their lower back, buttocks, thighs, or knees that might be caused by herpes should be avoided until a few days after their symptoms have resolved [12]. If sex becomes uncomfortable, other methods should be found to achieve intimacy [9].

7.2.2 Desire

Most women suffer from a lack of desire during the first trimester due to nausea and exhaustion. The second trimester is typically the trimester in which women show an increased libido and an increase in sexual pleasure. This is secondary to the alleviation of first-trimester symptoms. The third trimester may bring with it a decrease in sexual intercourse due to the growing discomfort brought on by the enlarging uterus, the edema, and the joint pain that often accompanies late pregnancy [9,10,14,16,17]. Of course, each woman and each pregnancy are different and therefore a woman's sexual interest may not follow this rule of thumb.

7.2.3 Orgasm

On the whole, masturbation is permitted but if the physician has forbidden intercourse, orgasms may be forbidden as well [10,11,14,16]. The physician should address this topic too. If not specifically forbidden, orgasms during pregnancy may even benefit the pregnancy due to calming hormones and increased cardiovascular blood flow. The vagina may feel less tight and the vulva and clitoris may be engorged because of the increase in blood flow [9]. This can feel pleasurable, irritating, or something in between. Orgasmic dreams may occur during pregnancy and are normal.

7.2.4 Positions and Anal and Oral Sex

Sexual positions should be chosen to keep pressure off the abdomen. Lying on the back should be avoided after the first trimester due to decreased blood flow [9,14,16–19]. A list of the best sexual positions is detailed on all these websites. During penetration the penis will not reach the baby or harm it but some positions can allow the parturient to control the depth of penetration, which can keep her more comfortable [14]. Oral sex is generally permitted throughout pregnancy. It should be avoided in the event of a partner with oral herpes or a history of oral herpes [12,14]. Air should not be blown into the vagina to avoid air embolism, which while rare may prove fatal [9,14]. In the event of anal sex, washing the penis or sex toy prior to moving it from the anus to the vagina is advisable. In order to avoid anal tears and secondary infections, use of water-based lubricants and slow movements during anal penetration are recommended [15]. Importantly, if vaginal intercourse is prohibited, so is anal intercourse.

If BDSM is part of the sexual ritual, spanking of the belly or abdomen should be avoided. If bondage is preformed, it is important to take into account the swollen extremities and the discomfort tight bondage may cause. It is important for the woman to be able to express her discomfort and needs. Erotic asphyxiation is forbidden during pregnancy. Role-playing that includes excessive fear should be avoided as it causes the release of stress hormones [18].

7.2.5 Contractions and Spotting

Sex does not cause miscarriage. Mild contractions can occur after sex and are safe [10,11,14]. Spotting after sex may be normal due to irritability of the cervix during pregnancy [9,10,14,16,17]. If the bleeding is inconsistent or accompanied by abdominal pain, it is abnormal and may be a sign of placenta previa or ectopic pregnancy [10].

Having sex will not cause labor to begin before the body is ready for delivery. In the event that the body is ready for delivery, intercourse may augment the process through the actions of prostaglandins in the semen, which can help ripen the cervix and induce contractions, and of oxytocin, the hormone released during orgasm and which causes uterine contractions [13,14]. Having said that, actual research on the subject is contradictory. Some evidence points to earlier onset of delivery at term in sexually active women [19,20], whereas other studies do not show a positive correlation between sexual activity and earlier labor [21,22].

7.3 Conclusion

Medical guidelines addressing sexual intercourse during pregnancy are lacking. However, patients can surf the Web and find an abundance of information on the topic. In short, sex during normal pregnancy is permitted. The most common reasons for abstaining from sex in pregnancy are placental problems, ruptured membranes, and pregnancies in which there is a high likelihood of premature labor. Orgasms are safe as long as intercourse is not forbidden, as are different sexual positions.

Because of the importance of the matter and the need for patient and medical practitioner education on the subject, it is our sincere hope that guidelines on the subject will be provided to medical personnel and to their patients accordingly.

References

1. O. Gutzeit, G. Levy, L. Lowenstein. Postpartum female sexual function: risk factors for postpartum sexual dysfunction. *Sex Med* 2020;8:8–13.

2. American College of Obstetricians and Gynecologists. Is it safe to have sex during pregnancy? 2021. www.acog.org/womens-health/experts-and-stories/ask-acog/is-it-safe-to-have-sex-during-pregnancy (accessed April 7, 2021).

3. National Health Service. Sex in pregnancy. 2021. www.nhs.uk/pregnancy/keeping-well/sex/ (accessed April 7, 2021).

4. Society of Obstetricians and Gynaecologists of Canada. Sex and pregnancy. www.pregnancyinfo.ca/your-pregnancy/healthy-pregnancy/sex-and-pregnancy/ (accessed April 7, 2021).

5. Australian Government Department of Health. Pregnancy care guidelines: sexual activity. 2018. www.health.gov.au/resources/pregnancy-care-guidelines/part-c-lifestyle-considerations/sexual-activity (accessed April 7, 2021).

6. Mayo Clinic. Sex during pregnancy: What's OK, what's not. 2020. www.mayoclinic.org/healthy-lifestyle/pregnancy-week-by-week/in-depth/sex-during-pregnancy/art-20045318 (accessed April 7, 2021).

7. Tommy's Pregnancy Hub. Sex in pregnancy. 2019. www.tommys.org/pregnancy-information/im-pregnant/sex-pregnancy (accessed April 7, 2021).

8. HealthLink British Columbia. Sex during pregnancy. 2021. www.healthlinkbc.ca/pregnancy-parenting/pregnancy/your-health-during-pregnancy/sex-during-pregnancy (accessed April 7, 2021).

9. L. Shinn. Will it hurt the baby? Plus 9 more questions about safe pregnancy sex. Healthline, 2018. www.healthline.com/health/pregnancy/pregnant-sex (accessed April 11, 2021).

10. S. Bradley. Can sex in the first trimester cause miscarriage? Early pregnancy sex questions. Healthline, 2020. www.healthline.com/health/pregnancy/sex-first-12-weeks-of-pregnancy (accessed April 11, 2021).

11. J. Timmons. Masturbating while pregnant: is it safe? Healthline, 2016. www.healthline.com/health/pregnancy/masturbation (accessed April 11, 2021).

12. H. Grey. Should women engage in oral sex during pregnancy? Healthline, 2019. www.healthline.com/health-news/should-women-engage-in-oral-sex-during-pregnancy (accessed April 11, 2021).

13. A. Marcin. Get it on and get it…out? Can having sex induce labor? Healthline, 2020. www.healthline.com/health/pregnancy/sex-to-induce-labor (accessed April 11, 2021).

14. N. Dworkin-McDaniel. Sex during pregnancy: what every pregnant person should know. Parents, 2021. www.parents.com/pregnancy/my-life/sex-relationship/pregnancy-sex-guide/ (accessed April 11, 2021).

15. N. Harris. Is anal sex safe during pregnancy? Parents, 2019. www.parents.com/pregnancy/my-life/sex-relationship/is-anal-sex-safe-during-pregnancy/ (accessed April 11, 2021).

16. R. B. Taylor. Sex during pregnancy. WebMD, 2021. www.webmd.com/sex-relationships/guide/sex-during-pregnancy (accessed April 11, 2021).

17. K. Miller. Sex during pregnancy: what you need to know. The BUMP, 2021. www.thebump.com/a/sex-during-pregnancy (accessed April 11, 2021).

18. H. Murkoff. Bondage and S&M during pregnancy. What to expect, updated 2022. www.whattoexpect.com/pregnancy/sex-and-relationships/bondage-bdsm-during-pregnancy/ (accessed April 13, 2021).

19. P. C. Tan, A. Andi, N. Azmi, M. N. Noraihan. Effect of coitus at term on length of gestation, induction of labor, and mode of delivery. *Obstet Gynecol* 2006;**108**:134–40.

20. M. Kafaei Atrian, Z. Sadat, M. Rasolzadeh Bidgoly, F. Abbaszadeh, M. Asghari Jafarabadi. The association of sexual intercourse during pregnancy with labour onset. *Iran Red Crescent Med J* 2014;**17**: e16465.

21. J. Schaffir. Sexual intercourse at term and onset of labor. *Obstet Gynecol* 2006;**107**:1310–14.

22. P. C. Tan, C. M. Yow, S. Z. Omar. Effect of coital activity on onset of labor in women scheduled for labor induction: a randomized controlled trial. *Obstet Gynecol* 2007;**110**:820–6.

Using the Internet to Educate on Sex and Pregnancy
Grading Internet Information

Noa Gilad, Yariv Yogev, and Michael Lavie

The origins of the Internet date back to the development of a method of grouping data and transmitting it over a digital network by the United States Department of Defense in the 1960s to enable time-sharing of computers. The funding of the National Science Foundation Network as a new backbone in the 1980s, as well as private funding for other commercial extensions, led to worldwide participation in the development of new networking technologies, and the merger of many networks. The linking of commercial networks and enterprises by the early 1990s marked the beginning of the transition to the modern Internet, and generated a sustained exponential growth as generations of institutional, personal, and mobile computers were connected to the network.

As other information started to spread widely through the Internet, so did health information. In the beginning we thought we could manage it. In an article published in 1998, Eysenbach and Diepgen [1] tried to establish a labeling system operated by doctors that would rank the quality of information by the name of PICS or Platform for Internet Content Selection. In 2002 Eysenbach et al. [2] tried to establish a methodological method on how quality on the web is being evaluated in practice. They acknowledged their failure mostly because of the vast amount of information that flooded the Web with no medical supervision. In 2003, Powell et al. [3] stated that the Internet has a profound impact on health and healthcare: it has the potential to improve the effective and efficient delivery of healthcare, empower and educate consumers, support decision-making, enable interaction between consumers and professionals, support the training and revalidation of professionals, and reduce inequalities in health. However, there is also a need for vigilance regarding new and emerging threats to health posed by the Internet.

The threat to security is always in place, with the user losing control of the device that transfers information or theft of data from a data aggregation system, or even impersonation of the device's IP address [4–7]. The threat to privacy is another issue [4]. Papoutsi et al. [8] found that 79% of patients had concerns about the security of the data within their electronic health record. All the devices that connect through a Wi-Fi network allow access from wherever the manufacture or the hacker are, as these devices are often poorly secured [9]. Also, maintenance and update of the health information may allow poor health information to be used improperly. Patients might trust misleading information or might make important health decisions based on sensationalized or emotionally charged stories that are not relevant to their health context [10], or financial conflicts of interest and reporting bias may lead corporations to manipulate health evidence and mislead consumers [11].

Despite all these hazards, we know that both healthcare professionals and ordinary people use medical information gathered from the Internet. Pregnancy, although a natural event in a woman's life, is a leading cause for information search as pregnancy care generally involves medical monitoring and prenatal testing, which can lead to anxiety. Consequently, many pregnant women utilize the Internet as a source of information, as a means of helping them deal with doubts and to navigate pregnancy-related decisions [12,13].

Furthermore, women using assisted reproductive technologies start using the Web even before they conceive. In a study from the Netherlands by Tuil et al. [14] that followed 51 couples, 25 420 page views were generated and 11 403 utterances were posted. The authors found that significant individual changes occurred in the intensity of use during the different stages of the treatment. During the stages in which there was no contact between the patient and the clinic, patients made use of the website's communication functions. This reflects the patients' need for continued communication and support during the last stages of treatment, a service that in vitro fertility (IVF) clinics traditionally cannot or do not provide.

Listening to Mothers II, a nationwide survey of women who gave birth in 2005, revealed that 16% of first-time mothers and 13% of experienced mothers rated the Internet as their most important information source [15]. Among respondents who used the Internet during pregnancy, frequent use was the norm. The average woman reported 20 visits online in order to receive information about pregnancy or labor. However, nearly one in five (19%) reported at least 100 such Internet visits during pregnancy [15]. In another study by Larsson [16], a vast majority (91%) of pregnant women had access to the Internet and, to a great extent (84%), used it to retrieve information, most often in the early stages of their pregnancy. Fetal development and stages of childbirth were the two most frequently mentioned topics of interest. Most participants considered the information to be reliable, and the two most important criteria for judging the trustworthiness of web-based information were if the facts were consistent with information from other sources and if references were provided.

Internet users appear to consider the health information they find online to be reliable, as according to a Harris Poll, 86% of medical information seekers said the information they found was "very" or "somewhat" reliable [17].

Medical professionals such as doctors and researchers also use the Internet on a daily basis. A systematic review from 2008 found that up to 90% of medical professionals in North America had access to the Internet, and this was steadily increasing [18].

Most of the internet activity of medical professionals focuses on email and searching in journals and databases. In 1997, Feingold et al. [19] described the essential internet tools that obstetricians and gynecologists used in those years. These tools have changed over the years, but Table 8.1 describes the relevant and up-to-date convenient sites that doctors use on a daily basis in order to expand their knowledge and to provide the best medical solution for their patients. The daily use of internet services is no longer a privilege but a necessity.

When patients want to search the Internet for an answer about a symptom or a disease, the amount of information they encounter is vast. In order for it to be efficient and reliable, patients should work according to the following steps.

8.1 Consider the Source

Look for an "About Us" page in order to understand who wrote the information. In addition look for the extension of the web page:

- .gov (government websites)
- .edu (educational websites)
- .org (non-profit organization).

Table 8.1. Internet sites used by doctors

Journals

Ultrasound in Obstetrics and Gynecology	https://obgyn.onlinelibrary.wiley.com/journal/14690705
BJOG: An International Journal of Obstetrics and Gynaecology	https://obgyn.onlinelibrary.wiley.com/journal/14710528
American Journal of Obstetrics and Gynecology	www.ajog.org/
Fertility and Sterility	www.fertstert.org/
International Journal of Gynecology and Obstetrics	https://obgyn.onlinelibrary.wiley.com/journal/18793479

Medical calculators

Fetal growth	https://intergrowth21.tghn.org/standards-tools/
Perinatology: ultrasound calculators	www.perinatology.com/calculators2.htm
QxMD	Application

Medical websites and societies

ACOG, American College of Obstetricians and Gynecologists	www.acog.org/
SOGC, Society of Obstetricians and Gynaecologists of Canada	https://sogc.org/
PubMed	https://pubmed.ncbi.nlm.nih.gov/
CDC, Centers for Disease Control and Prevention	www.cdc.gov/
Orphanet, the portal for rare diseases and orphan drugs	www.orpha.net/consor/cgi-bin/index.php
UpToDate	www.uptodate.com/home
NIH, National Institutes of Health	www.nih.gov/

Women's hospital public information

Mount Sinai, Toronto	www.mountsinai.on.ca/patients/patient-education-resources
Children's Hospital of Philadelphia	www.chop.edu/conditions-diseases
UHN, University Health Network Toronto	www.uhn.ca/PatientsFamilies/Health_Information/Pages/default.aspx
Mayo Clinic	www.mayoclinic.org/patient-care-and-health-information
St. Michael's Hospital	www.stmichaelshospital.com/programs/obstetrics/

8.2 Focus on Quality

- Check the date the information was updated; it should be at least from the last 10 years.
- Look for any evidence of peer-review published data as opposed to testimonials.
- Look at the site's editorial policy.
- Look for reviews or comments to see if any doctors have responded to the information.

8.3 Website Funding

- What is the purpose of the site? Who is providing the funding?
- Keep an eye out for advertisements that look like health information. Advertisements should be labeled. Be cautious when clicking on advertisements, understanding that often companies are there for their own profit and are not necessarily a valid source of information.

8.4 Protecting Your Privacy

- Privacy policy: read the website's privacy policy. It is usually at the bottom of the page or on a separate page titled "Privacy Policy" or "Our Policies."
- Cookies: If a website says it uses "cookies," your information may not be private. While cookies may enhance your web experience, they can also compromise your online privacy.
- If you are asked to share personal information, be sure to find out how the information will be used. Secure websites that collect personal information responsibly have an "s" after "http" in the start of their website address (https://) and often require that you create a username and password.
- Be careful about sharing your ID number.
- Use a strong password.
- Do not enter sensitive information over public Wi-Fi that is not secure.

8.5 There Are No Magical Solutions

- Be careful of websites or companies that claim any one remedy will cure a lot of different illnesses. Question dramatic writing or cures that seem too good to be true.
- Make sure you can find other websites with the same information. Even if the website links to a trustworthy source, it doesn't mean that the site has the other organization's endorsement or support.

References

1. G. Eysenbach, T. L. Diepgen. Towards quality management of medical information on the internet: evaluation, labelling, and filtering of information. *BMJ* 1998;**317**:1496–502.

2. G. Eysenbach, J. Powell, O. Kuss, E. R. Sa. Empirical studies assessing the quality of health information for consumers on the World Wide Web: a systematic review. *JAMA* 2002;**287**:2691–700.

3. J. A. Powell, M. Darvell, J. A. M. Gray. The doctor, the patient and the world-wide web: how the internet is changing healthcare. *J R Soc Med* 2003;**96**:74–6.

4. C. Showell. Risk and the internet of things: Damocles, Pythia, or Pandora? *Stud Health Technol Inform* 2016;**221**: 31–5.

5. D. Kozlov, J. Veijalainen, Y. Ali. Security and privacy threats in IoT architectures. Workshop on Security Tools and Techniques for Internet of Things (SeTTIT), Oslo, September 24–26, 2012. http://dx.doi.org/10.4108/icst.bodynets .2012.250550 (accessed December 25, 2020).

6. S. Vidalis, O. Angelopoulou. Assessing identity theft in the Internet of Things. *IT Convergence Practice* 2014;**2**:15–21.

7. S. Reback, T. Costello. Deconstructing the Internet of Things. The system promises substantial benefits, but privacy and security concerns may prompt new rules. 2014. www.multivu.com/players/English/ 7371431-bloomberg-visa-the-digital-trust-securingcommerce/flexSwf/ impAsset/document/166030bd-bc8d-40ed-97c2-5f60a0270bbd.pdf (accessed December 25, 2020).

8. C. Papoutsi, J. E. Reed, C. Marston, et al. Patient and public views about the security and privacy of Electronic Health Records (EHRs) in the UK: results from a mixed methods study. *BMC Med Inform Decis Mak* 2015;**15**:86.

9. Z. Whittaker. New security flaws found in popular IoT baby monitors. 2015. www .zdnet.com/article/security-vulnerability-flaw-internet-things-baby-monitors/ (accessed December 25, 2020).

10. T. Tonsaker, G. Bartlett, C. Trpkov. Information sur la santé dans internet: mine d'or ou champ de mines? *Can Fam Physician* 2014;**60**:419–20.

11. M. Bes-Rastrollo, M. B. Schulze, M. Ruiz-Canela, M. A. Martinez-Gonzalez. Financial conflicts of interest and reporting bias regarding the association between sugar-sweetened beverages and weight gain: a systematic review of systematic reviews. *PLoS Med* 2013;**10**: e1001578.

12. A. M. Romano. A changing landscape: implications of pregnant women's Internet use for childbirth educators. *J Perinat Educ* 2007;**16**:18–24.

13. B. M. Lagan, M. Sinclair, W. G. Kernohan. What is the impact of the Internet on decision-making in pregnancy? A global study. *Birth* 2011;**38**:336–45.

14. W. S. Tuil, M. van Selm, C. M. Verhaak, P. F. de Vries Robbé, J. A. M. Kremer. Dynamics of Internet usage during the stages of in vitro fertilization. *Fertil Steril* 2009;**91**:953–6.

15. E. R. Declercq, C. Sakala, M. P. Corry, S. Applebaum. Listening to Mothers II: Report of the Second National U.S. Survey of Women's Childbearing Experiences. *J Perinat Educ* 2007;**16**:9–14.

16. M. Larsson. A descriptive study of the use of the Internet by women seeking pregnancy-related information. *Midwifery* 2009;**25**:14–20.

17. H. Taylor. Harris Poll #76, July 31, 2007. Harris Poll shows number of "cyberchondriacs" – adults who have ever gone online for health information – increases to an estimated 160 million nationwide.

18. K. Masters. For what purpose and reasons do doctors use the Internet: a systematic review. *Int J Med Inform* 2008;**77**:4–16.

19. M. Feingold, R. Kewalramani, G. E. Kaufmann. Internet and obstetrics and gynecology. *Acta Obstet Gynecol Scand* 1997;**76**:718–24.

Chapter

9

Sex and Assisted Reproductive Technologies

Trish Dinh and Crystal Chan

9.1 Sex and Pregnancy Outcomes

Assisted reproductive technologies (ART), including in vitro fertilization (IVF), can help patients with infertility, recurrent miscarriage, and hereditary conditions to conceive healthy children. IVF involves ovarian stimulation followed by oocyte retrieval, fertilization of oocytes in the laboratory, and transfer of resultant embryos to the uterine cavity. Given the high costs and expectations of the treatment, there can be significant patient concern that activities such as intercourse and orgasm may impede or disrupt embryo implantation, leading to treatment failure or miscarriage. Patients undergoing IVF also commonly ask their physician if intercourse is safe during treatment.

Patients are often advised to abstain from sexual intercourse when undergoing ART despite unclear evidence. The abstinence approach has been based on the theoretical possibility that intercourse may be detrimental via two mechanisms: induction of uterine contractions and possible increased risk of infection. On the other hand, more recent studies have suggested that penile–vaginal intercourse may actually promote implantation due to factors in seminal plasma.

In this chapter, we explore these topics and offer evidence-based recommendations regarding sex during ART treatment. We also discuss the impact of undergoing ART can have on couples' sexuality and sexual function.

9.1.1 Studies on Sex and Pregnancy Outcomes

In spontaneously conceived non-ART pregnancies, Steiner et al. [1] performed a prospective study examining the impact of sexual intercourse around the time of implantation, defined as 5–9 days after ovulation via the calendar method. The study included 564 women who conceived naturally without risk factors for infertility. They discovered that couples with two or more days of intercourse during the peri-implantation window had poorer fecundability rates compared with those who were abstinent (fecundability ratio 0.65, 95% confidence interval [CI] 0.42–0.91). However, limitations of this study included use of the calendar method to define the implantation window.

A study performed by Stanford et al. [2] produced the opposite results and reported that peri-implantation intercourse does not lower pregnancy rates. Studying 661 women and 2606 cycles from five different European countries, they found no significant association between three or more acts of intercourse and fecundability (fecundability ratio 1.00, 95% CI 0.76–1.13). Both studies used prospectively collected data based on patient diaries of sexual activity and excluded subfertile or infertile couples. However, in the Steiner et al. study, all women were actively trying to conceive whereas in the

Stanford et al. study, many couples were avoiding pregnancy [1,2]. Therefore, in the latter study, 61% of cycles in the study period were excluded as there was no chance of pregnancy. It is unclear why these two observational studies using otherwise similar methodologies had discrepant findings.

Specifically looking at ART and cycles involving embryo transfer, a randomized controlled study performed by Aflatoonian et al. [3] showed no significant differences in pregnancy rates with or without intercourse in those undergoing embryo transfer. The study included 390 women with at least 5 years of infertility, where women were randomized to either having intercourse at least once at 12 hours after embryo transfer versus remaining abstinent. The authors found the implantation rate was 6.5% in the intercourse group compared with 5.5% for the control group. Furthermore, clinical pregnancy rates were not significantly higher in the intercourse group compared to the control (14.2% vs. 11.7%). The authors concluded that intercourse during the peri-transfer period is unlikely to increase pregnancy outcomes but also does not appear to be detrimental either.

In contrast, a study by Crawford and Steiner [4] demonstrated that intercourse may have a negative impact on pregnancy outcomes. The study included 125 women who underwent embryo transfer and recorded the frequency of intercourse from embryo day 6 to 12. The authors found that women who had intercourse at least once during this period had 1.59 times the odds of miscarriage (95% CI 0.26–9.78) compared to those who did not engage in intercourse. Furthermore, any intercourse during this period resulted in a lower likelihood of live birth (odds ratio [OR] 0.67, 95% CI 0.15–2.91). Specifically, when comparing timing of intercourse, those who had intercourse on embryo day 10 had a significantly increased risk of miscarriage ($p = 0.031$) and decreased likelihood of live birth ($p = 0.0018$).

Given these variable findings, larger sample sizes are needed to further elucidate these results and a single, blinded, randomized controlled trial is in the recruitment process to assess whether unprotected vaginal intercourse 24 hours after frozen embryo transfer truly does affect pregnancy rates within 10–14 days post transfer [5].

9.1.2 Uterine Contractility

In the physiological menstrual cycle, increased uterine contractions have been observed mid-cycle, putatively to assist with sperm transport to the oocyte [6]. In the postovulatory secretory phase, a progressive decline in contractile activity to achieve uterine quiescence has been observed, perhaps to set the stage for successful embryo–endometrial contact and implantation. In ART, embryo transfer occurs to coincide with the mid-secretory phase, and uterine contractility around this time has been the subject of investigation.

Studies on the impact of unprovoked uterine contractility on ART outcomes have had varied conclusions. A study by Fanchin et al. [7] included 209 infertile women undergoing 220 cycles of IVF and assessed the frequency of uterine contractions visualized on ultrasound 5 minutes prior to embryo transfer. They reported poorer rates of pregnancy and implantation in those with higher uterine contractile frequencies compared to those with lower frequencies. The authors theorized that frequent myometrial contractile activity may physically disrupt the interaction between the embryo and endometrium and hinder implantation. Conversely, an earlier study by Woolcott and

Stanger [8] reported improved IVF outcomes when increased uterine contractile activity was observed by ultrasound post embryo transfer. Endometrial wave-like movement was visualized in 36% of transfers, where 28% of these showed active movement of the embryo-associated air bubble in the cervix-to-fundal direction. However, endometrial contractions were not observed in 64% of embryo transfers. Overall, the authors found that pregnancy occurred in those with observed endometrial activity in 45.5% of embryo transfers compared to 15.6% of those without ($p < 0.001$). They proposed that the presence of endometrial activity may reflect a favorable state of endometrial receptivity and therefore may be of prognostic significance.

However, it is difficult to extrapolate the results of these studies to determine whether intercourse-induced uterine contractility affects implantation post embryo transfer. Intercourse has been shown to increase uterine contractions, particularly during female orgasm [9], but the nature of these contractions and their impact on embryo transfer have not been specifically studied. It is also unclear whether the timing of intercourse and/or orgasm relative to the day of embryo transfer makes a difference.

9.1.3 Risk of Infection

The second mechanism by which intercourse could disrupt implantation is through the introduction of pathological microorganisms and infection. The vagina and cervix are colonized by normal flora; however, pathogens from the lower genital tract may be inadvertently introduced into the uterine cavity at the time of embryo transfer. The cervical mucous barrier that usually protects against ascending bacteria may be disrupted due to passage of an embryo transfer catheter.

Although no study has specifically investigated intercourse-related infection and ART outcomes, a study by Fanchin et al. [7] examined whether the presence of cervical microorganisms at the time of embryo transfer affects IVF outcomes. The study included 279 women undergoing controlled ovarian hyperstimulation for IVF. Just prior to embryo transfer, a test catheter was inserted into the endocervix to the internal os under sterile conditions and sent for bacterial culture. None of the women had clinical evidence of vaginitis or cervicitis. Results showed that 51% of cultures were positive (143/279 patients), where the most common organisms cultured were *Escherichia coli* (64%) and *Streptococcus* spp. (8%). The study found that the clinical pregnancy rate (24% vs. 37%), ongoing pregnancy rate (17% vs. 28%), and implantation rates (9% vs. 16%) were significantly lower in the positive culture group than in the negative culture group.

Possible reasons proposed by the authors for these poorer outcomes included subclinical infection leading to induction of uterine contractions, subclinical endometritis and subsequent poor implantation, and lastly direct contamination of embryos from pathogens limiting their inherent capacity to implant. However, although intercourse has been linked with ascending uterine infection during late pregnancy, this study did not assess the direct relationship of intercourse around the time of embryo transfer and whether it is a risk factor for cervical colonization.

9.1.4 Effect of Seminal Plasma

Recent studies have suggested a possible beneficial feature of penile–vaginal intercourse during ART, namely that exposure to seminal plasma may improve pregnancy rates [10]. Seminal plasma acts as a transport and nutrient medium for spermatozoa, and its components may play a key role in promoting embryo development and implantation. As intercourse is the first exposure of the female immune system to seminal fluid, this triggers an inflammatory response leading to the development of immune tolerance to seminal antigens; this stimulating event is key in priming the female immune system to prepare for embryo implantation, as similar antigens that are present within the seminal fluid will also be present within the implanting embryo. Ultimately, studies have shown that these immune changes play a crucial role in promoting fertility [11].

First described by Bellinge et al. [12], high vaginal insemination of semen was found to improve implantation rates in IVF by greater than twofold (53% vs. 23% in the control group; $p < 0.05$). The implantation rate was not significantly different in patients who had known tubal occlusion or previous bilateral salpingectomy, suggesting that the site of sperm influence was on the endometrium as opposed to the tubes. The authors proposed that the presence of sperm may lead to a leukocytic invasion and improve endometrial receptivity in preparation for the arrival of the developing embryo.

Tremellen et al. [13] performed a multicenter, prospective, randomized controlled trial that included women undergoing frozen or fresh embryo transfers who were randomized to either abstinence or engagement in vaginal intercourse around the time of embryo transfer. The study included two centers, in Australia and Spain. The Australian center patients were randomized to either engagement in intercourse over a 4-day period including the 2 days before and after embryo transfer or abstinence from intercourse. The Spanish center patients were directed to have intercourse on at least two occasions, once in the 12 hours prior to oocyte collection and again in the 12 hours following embryo transfer. The authors found that the transfer of 1343 embryos during 478 cycles of IVF resulted in 107 pregnancies (22.4%), with 125 viable embryos remaining by 6–8 weeks' gestational age. They found no significant difference between groups with regard to pregnancy rate (23.6% and 21.2%, respectively). However, the proportion of embryos viable at 6–8 weeks was significantly higher in those who had been exposed to semen compared to those who had not (OR 1.48, 95% CI 1.01–2.19). The authors therefore concluded that exposure to semen around the time of embryo transfer may increase the success of embryo implantation and development.

A systematic review and meta-analysis performed by Saccone et al. [14] was performed to evaluate the beneficial effects of seminal plasma in IVF treatment at time of oocyte aspiration or embryo transfer. The study included eight randomized controlled trials (RCTs) for a total of 2128 patients in which women randomized to the semen-exposed group (either through seminal plasma/semen injection or sexual intercourse) had a significantly higher clinical pregnancy rate compared with controls (30.0% vs. 25.1%; relative risk [RR] 1.20, 95% CI 1.04–1.39). No significant differences were found in live birth rate, biochemical pregnancy, miscarriage, multiple pregnancies, and birthweight. The authors then carried out a subgroup analysis of four RCTs that included only those studies where undiluted seminal plasma was injected (either intracervical or intravaginal) and also found an improvement in clinical pregnancy rates compared with controls (46.3% vs. 37.2%; RR 1.23, 95% CI 1.05–1.45). They concluded that local application of seminal plasma in IVF cycles at the time of oocyte pickup may be considered a potential treatment for improving implantation.

9.1.5 Other Potential Risks of Sex during ART

With controlled ovarian hyperstimulation, the ovaries become enlarged and often more sensitive close to the time of oocyte retrieval. Therefore, it is expected that sexual activity would be uncomfortable or even painful for many patients. Other than discomfort, there may be an increased risk of adnexal or ovarian torsion related to sexual activity, as larger ovaries have a higher propensity to tort [15]. However, studies on whether intercourse during ART specifically increases the risk of torsion are lacking due to the rare nature of this complication. With due regard to the risks involved, patients with particularly enlarged ovaries or those with a history of ovarian torsion should be advised to abstain from intercourse during ART.

Ultimately, the question of whether sexual intercourse is advisable in those undergoing ART remains controversial. Patients should be aware that there is no evidence that strict abstinence improves outcomes. It is unclear if the possible risks of coitus-induced uterine contractions or subclinical infection outweigh the benefits recently described with exposure to seminal plasma and possible promotion of implantation. Therefore, the decision to engage in sexual intercourse should ultimately be based on patient choice after thorough counseling with a healthcare practitioner. Ultimately, when couples undergoing infertility treatment are interviewed about issues related to treatment satisfaction, informed choice and a sense of personal control are major factors influencing a positive outlook toward infertility treatments [16]. If a couple feels uncomfortable, either for physical or psychological reasons, abstinence should be supported. On the other hand, couples may feel benefit in engaging in intercourse as a way to promote an emotional connection and actively participate in their conception process.

9.2 Impact of ART on Couples' Sexuality

In most species, sex and reproduction are intertwined, with the former being performed solely for the purpose of the latter. Humans, on the other hand, have evolved to the point that sex and reproduction can be mutually exclusive of each other. Human sexuality is complex, and sex is performed without reproductive purpose in many scenarios including, but not limited to, sex using contraception, sex after menopause, sex for pleasure, and sex between same-sex couples. ART has also allowed the opposite to be true, which is for reproduction to happen without the need for sex. However, we are just beginning to learn how facilitating artificial reproduction without sex may affect the psychosocial health of a couple and their sexuality.

A large, prospective, cross-sectional survey was conducted on 1045 French patients with a history of infertility and medically assisted reproduction in order to evaluate the psychosocial impacts of infertility and ART [17]. Subjects in this study were recruited at various time points with respect to ART treatment; 19% were currently undergoing treatment, half had previously undergone ART and conceived successfully, and the remainder had either undergone failed treatment or were about to undergo treatment. Subjects reported several areas of sexuality and relationship health that were impacted, with 57% stating that undergoing ART had affected their sexual life either "moderately" or "a lot," while 21% reported not having sex for several weeks or months. Interestingly, there was no gender difference observed with this finding, with 21.1% of women and 21.8% of men reporting no sexual intercourse for a prolonged period. From this study, it is unclear if the decrease in sexual activity is related to the infertility status or the fertility treatment, but the two stressors are likely inextricably tied.

Focusing on female sexual function, an Italian study assessed 269 female patients aged 24–45 years attending an infertility clinic [18]. Sexual dysfunction, sexual distress, dyspareunia (painful intercourse), and frequency of intercourse during the 30 days prior to ovarian stimulation treatment were assessed using validated scores. Sexual dysfunction was described using the Female Sexual Function Index (FSFI), a 19-item questionnaire assessing six dimensions including desire, arousal, lubrication, orgasm, pain, and satisfaction. These scores were correlated with infertility-related distress measured using the Fertility Problem Inventory (FPI), a 46-item questionnaire that evaluates five specific domains: social concern, sexual concern, relationship concern, rejection of child-free lifestyle, and need for parenthood. This study found that 30% of infertile patients reported sexual dysfunction. Furthermore, women with sexual dysfunction exhibited significantly greater overall infertility-related distress. The domains of social, relationship, and sexual concerns were particularly associated with sexual dysfunction. Subjects were recruited for this study at the time of egg retrieval, and likely the ART treatment itself had some effect on the outcomes studied. However, this study did not include a control group of women who were not infertile or not undergoing treatment with ART. Contrary to the previous study, subjects reported high sexual frequency in the month leading up to their IVF cycle (5.6 ± 3.7 episodes of intercourse). One key difference is that all the women in this study were actively undergoing ART, whereas the majority of subjects in the previous study had previously undergone treatment. The frequency of intercourse in this study may be more reflective of prescribed treatment than innate sexuality or desire.

As sex has become no longer essential to reproduction, the psychosocial impact of replacing this basic human act with ART has to be studied more closely. Although frequency of sex may be maintained during treatment, sexual dysfunction rates are high (30%). Long-term impact on sexual function has been poorly studied, and available studies are limited by the lack of control groups. ART practitioners should be cognizant and ready to support patients and consider referral for sexual therapy.

9.3 What Did Dr. Google Say?

This section includes some common questions that have been searched on Google regarding sex and ART. We provide a summary of the information that is discussed on the Internet and provide evidence-based information to address these questions.

1. My partner and I used to have sex all the time but since starting fertility treatment, we have stopped. Is there something wrong with us?

   Response: Don't worry, you are not alone. When sex goes from "recreational" to "procreational," this is a common experience. Studies have shown that people undergoing ART have high rates of sexual dysfunction. It is important to recognize that ART may be a risk factor for poor sexual function, and communicate with your partner early on and consider seeking out resources such as sex therapy.

2. Is it safe to have sexual intercourse when undergoing intrauterine insemination?

   Response: After insemination has been performed, sexual intercourse on the same day can increase the chance for pregnancy. This may help increase the chances of *fertilization by adding to the sperm that was introduced during the insemination. This is supported by the literature but mostly in instances where insemination occurs with a lower motile sperm count. A study by Huang et al. [19] showed how engaging in timed intercourse 12–18 hours post insemination led to an increased pregnancy rate (27.7% vs. 10.5%; p = 0.023) in patients with lower motile sperm number (<40 × 10⁶), but no increased pregnancy rate (25.7% vs. 22.7%, p = 0.671) in patients with higher sperm number (≥40 × 10⁶). Given there is minimal harm in engaging in sexual intercourse post insemination, it is often encouraged if patients feel comfortable.*

3. How long should we abstain from intercourse/ejaculation to ensure a "good" sperm sample for ART treatments?

   Response: The most recent guidelines from the World Health Organization recommend that the minimum period of ejaculatory abstinence prior to semen collection should not be less than 2 days and no more than 7 days.

References

1. A. Z. Steiner, D. A. Pritchard, S. L. Young, A. H. Herring. Peri-implantation intercourse lowers fecundability. *Fertil Steril* 2014;**102**:178–82.

2. J. B. Stanford, J. L. Hansen, S. K. Willis, N. Hu, A. Thomas. Peri-implantation intercourse does not lower fecundability. *Hum Reprod* 2020;**35**:2107–12.

3. A. Aflatoonian, S. Ghandi, N. Tabibnezhad. The effect of intercourse around embryo transfer on pregnancy rate in assisted reproductive technology cycles. *Int J Fertil Steril* 2009;**2**:169–72.

4. N. M. Crawford, A. Z. Steiner. Intercourse after embryo transfer and pregnancy outcomes. *Fertil Steril* 2014;**101**:28–9.

5. ClinicalTrials.gov. The impact of vaginal intercourse on pregnancy rates after frozen embryo transfer (updated June 4, 2019). https://clinicaltrials.gov/ct2/show/study/NCT03974295.

6. E. A. Lyons, P. J. Taylor, X. H. Zheng, et al. Characterization of subendometrial myometrial contractions throughout the menstrual cycle in normal fertile women. *Fertil Steril* 1991;**55**:771–4.

7. R. Fanchin, C. Righini, F. Olivennes, et al. Uterine contractions at the time of embryo transfer alter pregnancy rates

after in-vitro fertilization. *Hum Reprod* 1998;**13**:1968–74.

8. R. Woolcott, J. Stanger. Potentially important variables identified by transvaginal ultrasound-guided embryo transfer. *Hum Reprod* 1997;**12**:963–6.

9. C. A. Fox, H. S. Wolff, J. A. Baker. Measurement of intra-vaginal and intra-uterine pressures during human coitus by radio-telemetry. *J Reprod Fertil* 1970;**22**:243–51.

10. G. Crawford, A. Ray, A. Gudi, A. Shah, R. Homburg. The role of seminal plasma for improved outcomes during in vitro fertilization treatment: review of the literature and meta-analysis. *Hum Reprod Update* 2015;**21**:275–84.

11. D. J. Sharkey, A. M. Macpherson, K. P. Tremellen, S. A. Robertson. Seminal plasma differentially regulates inflammatory cytokine gene expression in human cervical and vaginal epithelial cells. *Mol Hum Reprod* 2007;**13**:491–501.

12. B. S. Bellinge, C. M. Copeland, T. D. Thomas, et al. The influence of patient insemination on the implantation rate in an in vitro fertilization and embryo transfer program. *Fertil Steril* 1986;**46**:252–6.

13. K. P. Tremellen, D. Valbuena, J. Landeras, et al. The effect of intercourse on pregnancy rates during assisted human

reproduction. *Hum Reprod* 2000;**15**:2653–8.

14. G. Saccone, A. Di Spiezio Sardo, A. Ciardulli, et al. Effectiveness of seminal plasma in in vitro fertilisation treatment: a systematic review and meta-analysis. *BJOG* 2019;**126**:220–5.

15. H. Gorkemli, M. Camus, K. Clasen. Adnexal torsion after gonadotrophin ovulation induction for IVF or ICSI and its conservative treatment. *Arch Gynecol Obstet* 2002;**267**:4–6.

16. E. A. F. Dancet, W. L. D. M. Nelen, W. Sermeus, et al. The patients' perspective on fertility care: a systematic review. *Hum Reprod Update* 2010;**16**:467–87.

17. B. Courbiere, A. Lacan, M. Grynberg, et al. Psychosocial and professional burden of medically assisted reproduction (MAR): results from a French survey. *PLoS ONE* 2020;**15**: e0238945.

18. F. Facchin, E. Somigliana, A. Busnelli, et al. Infertility-related distress and female sexual function during assisted reproduction. *Hum Reprod* 2019;**34**:1065–73.

19. F. J. Huang, S. Y. Chang, J. C. Chang, et al. Timed intercourse after intrauterine insemination for treatment of infertility. *Eur J Obstet Gynecol Reprod Biol* 1998;**80**:257–61.

The Male Partner's Perspective

Marcos Luján Galán

10.1 Introduction

Sexual function is considered a key feature in the health and personality of women and men. An adequate sexual activity (especially penile–vaginal intercourse) is associated with better physiological and psychological health indices [1].

Pregnancy poses a life crisis for pregnant women and their male partners. Psychosocial and physical needs may produce insecurity, anxiety, and physical discomfort, and a variety of changes in the physical, hormonal, psychological, social, and cultural context may lead to a decrease in sexual function. The general evidence is that sexual function decreases in women during pregnancy (desire, orgasm, even pain impairment) and the first 6 months after delivery, but may persist for up to 4 years after giving birth [2,3]. Approximately half of women feel sexual distress during pregnancy, and the decrease in sexual function (avoidance of sex and feelings of nonsensuality) has been found to be greater in women than in their male partners [4], in whom pregnancy may also impact to a certain degree.

In this chapter I attempt to describe such changes in sexual function from the male's perspective.

10.2 Sexual Activity and Sexual Satisfaction during Pregnancy

Sexual dysfunction is greater during the second and third trimester of pregnancy [5] (see Chapter 5 for more details of sexual functioning in pregnancy). Studies that explored some aspects of sexuality (sexual desire, frequency, and satisfaction) in expectant fathers showed that a majority decreased their sexual activity during pregnancy, but less than one-third experienced loss of libido while their perception of sexual satisfaction remained quite high [6,7].

Some aspects of the relationship with their pregnant partner are the most important determinants of sexual satisfaction, especially closeness and communication. Even though satisfaction with body image and body image self-consciousness have also been related to sexual satisfaction (mainly in female partners), communication and nearness are much more important predictors of sexual satisfaction than body image variables [8].

Fear of hurting the fetus may be an important reason for avoiding intercourse during pregnancy in up to 80% of men [7,8]. Although in some studies this is not considered a significant determinant of sexual satisfaction, it can be a leading predictor of sexual frequency [8].

It has also been hypothesized that sexual position during intercourse can impact on sexual satisfaction during pregnancy. Although the most current sexual position used by couples during pregnancy is man-on-top face-to-face, it has been suggested that the woman-on-top face-to-face position could provide better sexual satisfaction for pregnant women, especially during the last months of pregnancy, where the male partner might find the missionary position somewhat uncomfortable [9].

Other conditions that occur with greater frequency during pregnancy include vaginismus, where vaginal spasms make penetration difficult during intercourse [10]. Believed to be largely underdiagnosed, its estimated prevalence is 1% but has been found to be higher during pregnancy [4]. Vaginismus, dyspareunia, and (again) decreased communication between partners are likely to contribute to the decreased sexual function observed during pregnancy.

Unfortunately, in the real world most couples focus on other aspects of pregnancy and few seek appropriate counseling with regard to sexual health. These issues should be considered by health services when counseling and supporting couples during pregnancy. Some evidence also shows that men who participate in childbirth courses exploring men's feelings about pregnancy, childbirth, and parenting tend to be more involved with their female partners through pregnancy [11].

Although these aspects of pregnancy may alter sexual satisfaction in the expectant couple, some pathological conditions can specifically affect the male partner and are considered next.

10.3 Erectile Dysfunction

10.3.1 Physiology of Erection

Briefly, the mechanism of erection involves the endothelial cells of the cavernous tissue and arterial smooth muscle cells [12]. Sexual stimulation (involving the central nervous system and somatic and autonomic pathways) releases neurotransmitters (mainly nitric oxide) in these cells causing their relaxation (via reduction of cytosolic calcium) and increasing blood flow into the corpus cavernosum, stretching its tunica and leading to venous occlusion and completion of the erection phase.

10.3.2 Causes of Erectile Dysfunction

The pathophysiology of erectile dysfunction (ED) is often multifactorial (a combination of more than one factor, organic and/or psychogenic). Psychogenic factors were previously thought to be the most prevalent cause of ED but organic causes should also be considered, especially where aging males are concerned. Psychogenic causes are most common in young patients (in whom other organic factors attributable to the aging process are less prevalent). The presence of a psychogenic etiology in the male partner of a pregnant woman is also important because pregnancy can undoubtedly be considered a major life event that may disrupt mental and behavioral function[13]. Organic causes, including neurogenic (multiple sclerosis, Parkinson's disease, stroke, etc.), endocrine (hypogonadism, hyperprolactinemia, etc.), vasculogenic (atherosclerosis, smoking, diabetes, etc.), and drug induced (antidepressants, thiazide diuretics, beta-blockers, etc.), should also be considered when assessing ED in male partners of pregnant women.

As mentioned earlier, major life events such as pregnancy can be a risk factor for psychogenic ED [13], and religious and sociocultural issues, such as taboos and restriction of communication between female and male partners (as seen in some countries), can account for differences in its presentation [14]. Other factors, such as low level of education, unwanted pregnancy, older age, or long marriage, might account for sexual dysfunction [15].

However, not only psychological changes occur in expectant fathers; hormonal changes have been detected in men during pregnancy and after delivery. Serum testosterone levels may decrease from the first trimester of their partner's pregnancy, and the lowest levels can be found days after delivery, and recovery to nonpregnancy levels can be delayed up to 10 months after delivery [16,17]. Testosterone levels recovery gradually after birth and are related to the quality of parental care [18]. A correlation has also been described between low testosterone levels and paternal attitude and engagement with children [19]. This association may be of an adaptive nature, where the father's physiology responds to, for example, the increased involvement in parental engagement with children and decreased male–male competition.

Another factor that might account for this link between low testosterone and parental involvement is sleep disturbance, as testosterone is produced foremost during sleep. While some observational studies have found a relationship between sleep deprivation and low testosterone levels [20], other studies have not confirmed such findings. Paternal postpartum depression (which can be linked to psychogenic loss of libido and ED) is also associated with low testosterone levels [21]. Higher levels of prolactin and estradiol have also been detected in male partners from before delivery [22]. Such hormonal changes may again be related to the father's attitude with regard to household and caring issues.

Maternal and paternal stress patterns during pregnancy can also influence cortisol levels in both partners [23]. Lower paternal cortisol levels may buffer maternal cortisol excess, but higher paternal levels can account for amplified maternal cortisol levels. Therefore, interpersonal psychological and physiological stress from both parents can mutually influence hormone changes during pregnancy. Changes in cortisol levels can also be observed in gay fathers (lower levels compared with gay nonfathers), suggesting that the psychosocial stress response can be mitigated in some way in fatherhood [24].

10.3.3 Therapies for Erectile Dysfunction

Oral phosphodiesterase (PDE)5 inhibitors (sildenafil, tadalafil, vardenafil, avanafil) are considered first-line therapy in patients with no specific contraindication to their use [25]. On-demand intracavernosal injections of alprostadil could be selected when there is failure of oral PDE5 inhibitors. Intraurethral or topical alprostadil should only be considered with concomitant condom use during pregnancy. A penile prosthesis might be considered as a last resort when there is failure of other first- and second-line therapies.

10.4 Premature Ejaculation

Premature ejaculation (PE) is defined as the inability to delay ejaculation that occurs within 1 minute of vaginal penetration (or even before penetration). This condition usually leads to negative personal disturbances (anxiety, frustration, avoidance of sexual intimacy, etc.) [26]. The etiology is multivariate and complex. The natural time to ejaculation may vary broadly between individuals, even between cultures. Causes of acquired ED may be categorized as organic (urological, neurological, endocrine, etc.) and psychogenic, with PE coexisting in one-third of patients with ED. The pathophysiology of both conditions are also linked: On the one hand, any attempt to control ejaculation can induce anxiety that might account for psychogenic ED; on the other, to increase excitation intentionally in order to improve erection response may lead to PE.

Male partners of women with vaginismus suffer from a high incidence of sexual dysfunction, and PE can be found in 50% of these men and ED in 28% [27].

Therapeutic options for PE involve cognitive–behavioral therapy, and/or pharmacological treatment [26]. Dapoxetine (a short half-life selective serotonin reuptake inhibitor) has been approved for this current use in some European countries.

10.5 Couvade Syndrome

Couvade syndrome (CS) is an entity that deserves to be described separately. Pregnancy may cause physical, psychological, and social impacts on the expectant father [28]. Originally named from the antique French *couvade* meaning "breeding," CS is described as a group of physical and psychological symptoms presented by some fathers with regard to their female partner's pregnancy. Frequency has been established at 20–80% in Western countries, with a possibly higher incidence in first-time fathers [22,28]. Psychosomatic symptoms (up to 39 described in the literature) have been reported, for example nausea, vomiting, abdominal pain, changes in appetite, increased concern with skin lesions, and lower limb pain. Changes in social and family activities have also been described, with 33% of these men presenting with deterioration of the couple's relationship during pregnancy and a general decrease in sexual activity (especially during the third trimester) and a parallel decrease in libido. Preventive measures, including medical interviews or group discussions among expectant fathers during prenatal classes, have been proposed in order to minimize consequences.

10.6 Paternal Perinatal Depression

Paternal perinatal depression is a recent diagnostic entity not acknowledged in the fifth edition of the *Diagnostic and Statistical Manual of Mental Disorders*, and is therefore not yet an official mental disorder [29]. The onset of this condition can be observed from the beginning of pregnancy, with a short period of improvement after childbirth, but can extend up to 1 year after delivery in both mother and father. The difference in men with respect to women is that other symptoms not typical of depression (fatigue, self-criticism, irritability, restlessness, or anger episodes) prevail over classic depression symptoms or low mood [29].

10.7 Sexual Function and Postpartum

From 6 months to 1 year after childbirth, many women present with decreased interest in sexual activity (46.3%), less vaginal lubrication (43%), and dyspareunia (37.5%), with loss of body image and breastfeeding among the most important causes [30] (see Chapter 24 for more details on the postpartum period). These sexual issues should be kept in mind when couples are planning future pregnancies and they should consider seeking adequate help.

Mode of delivery (e.g. cesarean, vaginal with episiotomy) could be hypothesized as a disadvantage for future satisfaction during intercourse (see Chapter 25 for more details on sex after pelvic floor injuries). There is no clear relationship between mode of delivery and impairment of sexual function [2]. It has been hypothesized that vaginal delivery could loosen the vaginal walls and therefore impair the couple's satisfaction during subsequent intercourse. Studies with measurement of intravaginal pressure during coitus showed a decrease in pressure in patients with previous vaginal delivery when compared to patients who had undergone cesarean section, but no significant differences were found with regard to sexual satisfaction [31].

In a study by Gungor et al. [32], although men with a nulliparous partner showed the least impairment in sexual function, there were no significant differences in male sexual function regardless of the previous type of delivery of the female partner. To my knowledge, the male partner's future sexual function is not taken into account when a decision about mode of delivery is made, and the choice is exclusively based on obstetric issues.

Therefore, we can conclude that type of delivery, breastfeeding, intimacy, and partner's contribution to housework do not significantly affect sexual function [6].

10.8 What Did Dr. Google Say?

When you type "sex pregnancy male partner" into a Google search bar, more than 100 million matches are obtained. Advice for parents-to-be are found on general interest websites focused on pregnancy issues, for example raisingchildren.net.au, motherforlife.com, whattoexpect.com, healthline.com, parents.com, and so forth. Additionally, cosmopolitan.com shows a variety of personal experiences from couples who found their sex life worsened, unchanged, or even improved during pregnancy [33]. Another interesting article on babycenter.com shows what male partners think (their true opinion) about their pregnancy and their views on sexual life during pregnancy [34]. Menshealth.com gives advice for male partners so that the pregnant couple's sex life can remain as unaltered as possible [35].

Other major information on the web (e.g. theguardian.com or cnn.com) addresses this topic and provides guidance for future parents with regard to sex life during pregnancy [36,37].

Some government websites post information addressed to future parents. As an example, the National Health Service of the United Kingdom website offers tips for male partners to improve their involvement during pregnancy and birth [38].

References

1. S. Brody. The relative health benefits of different sexual activities. *J Sex Med* 2010;7:1336–61.

2. A. O. Yeniel, E. Petri. Pregnancy, childbirth, and sexual function: perceptions and facts. *Int Urogynecol J* 2014;25:5–14.

3. M. Aydin, N. Cayonu, M. Kadihasanoglu, et al. Comparison of sexual functions in pregnant and non-pregnant women. *Urol J* 2015;12:2339–44.

4. D. S. Dwarica, G. G. Collins, C. M. Fitzgerald, et al. Pregnancy and Sexual Relationships Study Involving wOmen and meN (PASSION Study). *J Sex Med* 2019;16:975–80.

5. A. Fuchs, I. Czech, J. Sikora, et al. Sexual functioning in pregnant women. *Int J Environ Res Public Health* 2019;16:4216.

6. T. T. Saotome, K. Yonezawa, N. Suganuma. Sexual dysfunction and satisfaction in Japanese couples during pregnancy and postpartum. *Sex Med* 2018;6:348–55.

7. S. Nakić Radoš, H. Soljačić Vraneš, M. Šunjić. Sexuality during pregnancy: what is important for sexual satisfaction in expectant fathers? *J Sex Marital Ther* 2015;**41**:282–93.

8. S. N. Radoš, H. S. Vraneš, M. Šunjić. Limited role of body satisfaction and body image self-consciousness in sexual frequency and satisfaction in pregnant women. *J Sex Res* 2014;**51**:532–41.

9. J. T. Lee, C. L. Lin, G. H. Wan, C. C. Liang. Sexual positions and sexual satisfaction of pregnant women. *J Sex Marital Ther* 2010;**36**:408–20.

10. R. Achour, M. Koch, Y. Zgueb, U. Ouali, R. Ben Hmid. Vaginismus and pregnancy: epidemiological profile and management difficulties. *Psychol Res Behav Manag* 2019;**12**:137–43.

11. M. Friedewald, R. Fletcher, H. Fairbairn. All-male discussion forums for expectant fathers: evaluation of a model. *J Perinat Educ* 2005;**14**:8–18.

12. R. C. Dean, T. F. Lue. Physiology of penile erection and pathophysiology of erectile dysfunction. *Urol Clin North Am* 2005;**32**:379–95.

13. R. Shamloul, H. Ghanem. Erectile dysfunction. *Lancet* 2013;**381**:153–65.

14. M. D. Akyuz, E. C. Turfan, S. C. Oner, T. Sakar, D. M. Aktay. Sexual functions in pregnancy: different situations in near geography: a case study on Turkey, Iran and Greece. *J Matern Fetal Neonatal Med* 2020;**33**:222–9.

15. K. Abouzari-Gazafroodi, F. Najafi, E. Kazemnejad, P. Rahnama, A. Montazeri. Demographic and obstetric factors affecting women's sexual functioning during pregnancy. *Reprod Health* 2015;**12**:72.

16. R. S. Edelstein, B. M. Wardecker, W. J. Chopik, et al. Prenatal hormones in first-time expectant parents: longitudinal changes and within-couple correlations. *Am J Hum Biol* 2015;**27**:317–25.

17. R. Corpuz, D. Bugental. Life history and individual differences in male testosterone: mixed evidence for early environmental calibration of testosterone response to first-time fatherhood. *Horm Behav* 2020;**120**:104684.

18. R. Corpuz, S. D'Alessandro, G. K. S. Collom. The postnatal testosterone rebound in first-time fathers and the quality and quantity of paternal care. *Dev Psychobiol* 2020;**63**:1415–27.

19. L. T. Gettler. Becoming DADS: considering the role of cultural context and developmental plasticity for paternal socioendocrinology. *Curr Anthropol* 2016;**57**:38–51.

20. T. Akerstedt, J. Palmblad, B. de la Torre, R. Marana, M. Gillberg. Adrenocortical and gonadal steroids during sleep deprivation. *Sleep* 1980;**3**:23–30.

21. P. Kim, J. E. Swain. Sad dads. Paternal postpartum depression. *Psychiatry (Edgmont)* 2007;**4**:35–47.

22. K. E. Wynne-Edwards. Why do some men experience pregnancy symptoms such as vomiting and nausea when their wives are pregnant? *Scientific American* 2004. www.scientificamerican.com/article/why-do-some-men-experienc/ (accessed December 19, 2020).

23. S. H. Braren, A. Brandes-Aitken, A. Ribner, R. E. Perry, C. Blair. Maternal psychological stress moderates diurnal cortisol linkage in expectant fathers and mothers during late pregnancy. *Psychoneuroendocrinology* 2020;**111**:104474.

24. E. E. Burke, R. G. Bribiescas. A comparison of testosterone and cortisol levels between gay fathers and non-fathers: a preliminary investigation. *Physiol Behav* 2018;**193**:69–81.

25. I. Eardley, C. Donatucci, J. Corbin, et al. Pharmacotherapy for erectile dysfunction. *J Sex Med* 2010;**7**:524–40.

26. D. Rowland, C. G. McMahon, C. Abdo, et al. Disorders of orgasm and ejaculation in men. *J Sex Med* 2010;**7**:1668–86.

27. S. Dogan, M. Dogan. The frequency of sexual dysfunctions in male partners of women with vaginismus in a Turkish sample. *Int J Impot Res* 2008;**20**:218–21.

28. P. Laplante. The Couvade syndrome: the biological, psychological, and social impact of pregnancy on the expectant father. *Can Fam Physician* 1991;**37**:1633–60.

29. A. Bruno, L. Celebre, C. Mento, et al. When fathers begin to falter: a comprehensive review on paternal perinatal depression. *Int J Environ Res Public Health* 2020;**17**:1139.

30. D. O'Malley, A. Higgins, C. Begley, D. Daly, V. Smith. Prevalence of and risk factors associated with sexual health issues in primiparous women at 6 and 12 months postpartum: a longitudinal prospective cohort study (the MAMMI study). *BMC Pregnancy Childbirth* 2018;**18**:196.

31. L. Cai, B. Zhang, H. Lin, W. Xing, J. Chen. Does vaginal delivery affect postnatal coitus? *Int J Impot Res* 2014;**26**:24–7.

32. S. Gungor, I. Baser, T. Ceyhan, E. Karasahin, S. Kilic. Does mode of delivery affect sexual functioning of the man partner? *J Sex Med* 2008;**5**:155–63.

33. P. Gilmour. What sex during pregnancy feels like for men and women. 2017. www.cosmopolitan.com/uk/love-sex/sex/a13026981/sex-during-pregnancy-stories/ (accessed February 23, 2021).

34. S. McGinnis. Dads confess their true feelings about pregnant bodies. 2018. www.babycenter.com/pregnancy/hear-from-moms/dads-confess-their-true-feelings-about-pregnant-bodies_20001112 (accessed February 10, 2021).

35. C. Borzillo. How to have great sex when she's pregnant. The 6 things every man needs to know. 2016. www.menshealth.com/sex-women/g19534938/pregnancy-sex/?slide=4 (accessed February 23, 2021).

36. A. Barbieri. Pregnancy: problem solved. 2011. www.theguardian.com/lifeandstyle/2011/mar/05/annalisa-barbieri-pregnancy-sex-husband (accessed February 23, 2021).

37. I. Kerner. Is pregnancy putting your sex life on pause? 2011. https://thechart.blogs.cnn.com/2011/11/17/is-pregnancy-putting-your-sex-life-on-pause/comment-page-1/ (accessed February 10, 2021).

38. National Health Service. Tips for your birth partner. 2017. www.nhs.uk/pregnancy/labour-and-birth/what-happens/tips-for-your-birth-partner/ (accessed February 23, 2021).

Chapter

Sex in the First Trimester

Kirsten M. Niles

11.1 Introduction

Pregnancy represents a unique period during which significant physical, psychosocial, and hormonal changes occur. Healthy sexuality and sexual interactions during pregnancy are important factors that assist couples in navigating pregnancy and the changes it brings to their family [1]. The first trimester of pregnancy, typically defined from conception until the completion of the 12th week of gestation, is often when couples identify the pregnancy, which for some represents the first moments of their transition to parenthood. The identification of a pregnancy may invoke a multitude of emotional responses depending on cultural and psychosocial factors, the desirability of the pregnancy, and events leading up to conception. Additionally, in the first trimester, women experience rapid physiological and hormonal changes that can induce breast tenderness, prompt nausea and vomiting of pregnancy, impact mood, and result in significant fatigue. Given the breadth of changes that occur during the first trimester, it is therefore not surprising that it has the potential to impact all intimate aspects of a relationship including sexual interactions (see Chapter 3 for more details of physiological changes). Research into sexuality in pregnancy, particularly in the first trimester, may be limited by the timing at which individuals are approached, dependence on recall, and rates of nonresponse potentially due to the sensitivity of the subject [1].

Initial studies on sexual activity in pregnancy published in the 1970s and 1980s demonstrated a decline in sexual activity during the first trimester of pregnancy [2]. While these early studies laid the foundation for our understanding of the overall safety of sexual activity in pregnancy, these publications may now be dated as definitions of sexual function have continued to evolve, societal attitudes toward sexual activity during pregnancy have altered, and the medical advice provided to couples has changed [3]. More recent studies have focused not only on the frequency of sexual activity but also on the potential factors that impact it in pregnancy. This chapter addresses sexual activity, function, attitudes, and safety and discusses the role of medical professionals in advising pregnant individuals in the first trimester of pregnancy.

11.2 Prevalence of Sexual Activity in the First Trimester

The definition of sexual activity differs between studies. Some studies specifically evaluate vaginal intercourse while others consider all forms of sexual activity including noncoital activities such as fantasy, kissing, embracing, breast fondling, masturbation, oral sex, and anal intercourse. Approximately 86–100% of pregnant individuals report participating in some form of sexual activity in pregnancy [4]. The overall frequency of sexual activity declines in the first trimester compared with before pregnancy, with 46.8–93% of pregnant individuals specifically reporting a reduction in sexual activity in the first trimester [3,5–7]. Some pregnant individuals, however, may experience no change or even an increase in the frequency of sexual activity in the first trimester. When compared with before pregnancy, a Portuguese study utilizing a survey of 188 women at the time of delivery demonstrated that 17.5%, 28.7%, and 46.8% of women reported increased, decreased, and unchanged sexual activity in the first trimester, respectively [6]. When considering the frequency of individual noncoital sexual activities, a systematic review by Jawed-Wessel and Sevick [8] determined that there was no statistically significant change in the first trimester.

Vaginal intercourse is consistently the most common form of sexual activity in pregnancy and its frequency declines during pregnancy [8,9]. Overall, 55.6–96% of pregnant individuals report participating in vaginal intercourse in the first trimester compared to nearly 100% of couples prior to pregnancy [3,5,7]. Although Pauleta et al. determined that 44.7% of pregnant women reported that vaginal intercourse was most frequent in the first trimester compared with other trimesters in pregnancy, the frequency was reduced compared with prepregnancy levels in up to 90% of pregnant women [6,7]. Aslan et al. [9] demonstrated a monthly coital frequency of 8.6 ± 3 before pregnancy and 6.9 ± 2.5 in the first trimester. Oruc et al. [10] found similar results, with a reduction in monthly coital frequency from 12.4 ± 5.9 before pregnancy to 8.09 ± 4.30 in the first trimester. When reviewing twin gestations, Stammler-Safar et al. [2] determined that 82.0% of women reported participating in vaginal intercourse in the first trimester. Complete avoidance of vaginal intercourse in the first trimester was reported by 10–38.6% of pregnant individuals [1,5,7,10,11].

11.3 Sexual Function in the First Trimester

Sexual function refers to how the human body reacts during the phases of the sexual response cycle, including desire, arousal, pain/discomfort, and orgasm (see Chapter 5 for more details on sexual function). Dysfunction represents any interruption of normal sexual functioning at one or more points within this cycle. Sexual function is a particularly personal experience, making it challenging to evaluate. Studies of sexual function in pregnancy utilize a mixture of author-designed questionnaires and validated research tools such as the Female Sexual Function Index (FSFI) questionnaire, which allows for comparisons between diverse populations. The FSFI includes 19 questions regarding sexual activity in the 4 weeks prior to its administration that evaluate six domains including desire, arousal, lubrication, orgasm, satisfaction, and pain. Lower scores are associated with a higher degree of sexual dysfunction.

In the first trimester, 59% of pregnant women enjoy intercourse as compared to 76–79% before pregnancy [1]. This is consistent with the numerous studies that show a decline in sexual function as measured by the FSFI in pregnancy [5,9,12,13]. Individual domain and total FSFI scores all show a reduction in the first trimester when compared with before pregnancy [9]. Sexual dysfunction was identified in 36.3% of pregnant women in the first trimester [13]. In contrast, a recent study by Fuchs et al. [14] of 624 women in Poland did not identify clinically relevant sexual dysfunction in the first trimester. For studies that did not utilize the FSFI questionnaire, similar themes were identified. Changes in vaginal lubrication and pain were reported by 37% and 22% of pregnant women, respectively, and 60% of women reported a reduction in sexual desire and enjoyment during pregnancy [3,7].

However, the general trend toward sexual dysfunction in the first trimester of pregnancy may not be relevant to all couples or all aspects of sexual function. A systematic review demonstrated that sexual interest in the first trimester of pregnancy was relatively unchanged or only slightly decreased for both members of the couple [1]. Increased sexual desire, pleasure during lovemaking, and frequency of orgasm during lovemaking in pregnancy was reported by 14% of women [3]. In a study by Fok et al. [7] that reported some of the highest reductions in vaginal intercourse and sexual activity, 5% of women reported an increase in sexual desire and enjoyment during pregnancy. These studies highlight the importance of considering individual experiences by also evaluating the prevalence of positive and negative changes in sexual function as compared to only reporting overall trends in average scores.

11.4 Factors Influencing Sexual Activity and Function in the First Trimester

Evidence suggests that most pregnant women have a favorable view of sexual activity in pregnancy. In a review of 59 studies between 1950 and 1996, 82% of pregnant women believed that intercourse should be practiced during the whole pregnancy [1]. A more recent questionnaire-based study of 286 Turkish pregnant women supported this finding, with 77.5% indicating that they believed sexual intercourse is appropriate during noncomplicated pregnancy [15]. Finally, 70% of women with twin pregnancies believed that a change in sexual behavior would only be of importance when pregnancy was complicated [2] (see Chapter 17 for more details on twin pregnancies). However, the evidence presented earlier in this chapter of reduced frequency of sexual activity and increased sexual dysfunction during the first trimester of pregnancy contradicts these attitudes. Numerous cultural, psychosocial, emotional, physical, demographic, and medical factors relevant to both members of a partnership have the potential to influence sexual activity and function, particularly in pregnancy. Assessing the role of these variables independently is extremely challenging.

Physical aspects that have been reported to influence sexual function in the first trimester include fatigue, nausea and vomiting, and breast tenderness. Breast discomfort with breast fondling was reported by 56% of women in the first trimester [3]. Dyspareunia has been reported to be less common in the first trimester as compared with the remainder of pregnancy, although comparison with prepregnancy experiences was not completed [10]. As the gravid uterus is still contained within the pelvis, some of the physical challenges of the enlarging uterus that affect sexual activity in later stages of pregnancy are likely to have minimal impact. Surprisingly, 65.9% of men and women indicated that there were several sexual positions that they could no longer use due to the pregnancy even prior to 13 weeks' gestation [8]. The impetus behind this adjustment was not explored, but it may be related to subtle changes in cervical position and sensitivity as well as nonphysical factors.

The first trimester presents a unique opportunity to better differentiate the impact of physical and nonphysical variables on sexual activity in pregnancy by evaluating the behavior of those who have yet to become aware of their pregnancy. Once awareness occurs, emotional, cultural, and social influences may influence participation in sexual activity. Corbacioglu et al. [16] administered a general survey on demographic information and the FSFI questionnaire to 57 women who were aware of their pregnancy and 63 women who were not yet aware of their pregnancy. Interestingly, women who were unaware of their pregnancy had a significantly higher frequency of coitus as well as higher overall FSFI scores. Arousal, lubrication, orgasm, and satisfaction scores were also negatively affected by awareness of the pregnancy. No significant differences were identified in pain or desire [16].

In the study by Corbacioglu et al. [16], 45.6% of the women who were aware of their pregnancy indicated a concern about the adverse effects of sexual activity on the pregnancy, including 12.3% who avoided intercourse due to fear of miscarriage and hurting the fetus. Identified in multiple studies, this concern demonstrates the most prevalent factor influencing sexual activity in the first trimester. Fear of miscarriage, reported by 12.0–53.1% of pregnant individuals, was the most common reported etiology for decreased frequency of vaginal intercourse in the first trimester [5,11,16–18]. A fear of bleeding was reported by 57–74.8% of pregnant individuals, although only 12–13% of them experienced bleeding complications [3,7]. In different regional cohorts concerns regarding harm to the pregnancy varied significantly. Fok et al. identified that up to 82.9% of pregnant women in China reported worries of possible adverse effects of vaginal intercourse during pregnancy, while only 5–9% of women in a Canadian cohort and 6–12% of women in a Nigerian cohort expressed similar concerns [3,7,18]. Partners were also reported to have expressed similar concerns regarding the safety of sexual activity during pregnancy in 28–81% of cases, although it is unclear how frequently these opinions were discordant from those of the pregnant individual as studies of the partner are limited [3,5,8,18]. A prior history of miscarriage or pregnancy complications negatively affected sexual function in pregnancy [15] (see Chapter 26 for more details on stillbirth and miscarriage). Faisal-Cury et al. [19] demonstrated a 50% increase in sexual dysfunction among pregnant women with a prior history of miscarriage. Chang et al. [12] identified that a history of infertility and spontaneous abortion had a negative effect on sexual function and sexual desire, respectively.

Multiple additional factors have been evaluated in relation to sexual function in pregnancy with conflicting results, including maternal level of education [10,12–14,20], maternal employment status [5], maternal age [4,7,10,13], parity [7,16], unwanted pregnancy [20], and need to ensure fidelity of the partner [18]. These studies demonstrate the complexity in determining factors that influence decisions regarding sexual activity in pregnancy.

11.5 Safety of Sexual Activity in the First Trimester

As discussed earlier in this chapter, concern regarding the impact of sexual activity on the pregnancy is one of the most voiced reasons for the reduction of sexual activity in the first trimester. Sexual activity during pregnancy has generally been considered safe, with no clear evidence of association with preterm birth or pregnancy complications [1,2]. In a study performed in the UK comparing 603 women with a recent miscarriage to 6116 women with a pregnancy that progressed beyond 12 weeks' gestation, participation in intercourse during pregnancy was not associated with an increased risk of first trimester miscarriage unless bleeding occurred. Bleeding during intercourse was associated with an adjusted odds ratio of 1.96 (1.31–2.92) [21]. Self-reported coitus during early pregnancy was not associated with preterm birth in a cohort of 165 pregnancies with a preexisting increased risk of preterm birth [22]. These studies provide reassurance that, with the exception of pregnant individuals experiencing vaginal bleeding, sexual activity in the first trimester does not increase the risk of adverse pregnancy outcomes and can be safely supported.

11.6 Role of Healthcare Professionals

Healthcare professionals are often considered a reliable source of information in pregnancy; however, they address sexual activity in pregnancy infrequently or only in settings where restrictive advice may be required [1]. Of pregnant individuals surveyed, 9.4–48.7% of women obtained their information regarding sexual activity during pregnancy from their healthcare provider [3,7,15,17]. Up to 54% of these individuals raised the subject themselves but only 66% of those who initiated discussions felt comfortable doing so [3,7]. Conversely, up to 76% of those who did not discuss sexual activity in pregnancy with their care provider felt that it should be discussed [3,7].

Introduction of a sexual education package to women recruited between 8 and 14 weeks' gestation demonstrated improvements in all domains of the FSFI even though there was no significant difference in the frequency of sexual activity between the control and intervention groups [23]. A significant difference was noted in the sexual positions utilized during vaginal intercourse, with increased frequency of the woman-on-top and reduced frequency of the man-on-top positions, which may have impacted sexual function [23]. In contrast, a sexual education package provided to women recruited between 14 and 27 weeks' gestation did not demonstrate any significant change in sexual desire, arousal, satisfaction from coitus, orgasm from coitus, or frequency of coitus [17]. Further studies are required to determine the impact of sexual education on sexual function in pregnancy.

There is growing evidence that sexual satisfaction, including during pregnancy, is important to a healthy relationship. While not all couples will want to participate in sexual activity in pregnancy, for those that do, access to adequate information is critical. Of those individuals who did not obtain advice from their care provider, the majority relied on books and friends [7,17].

11.7 What Did Dr. Google Say?

Online resources have expanded significantly over the last decade, and in many instances have replaced books as a source of information. Search terms such as "sex in pregnancy" and "sex in the first trimester" identify several online resources, including those built by national obstetric societies and/or edited by medical professionals, which provide reliable information regarding expectations and safety of sexual activity in pregnancy. Couples using online search engines may also find and peruse nonmedical websites and articles, the majority of which support the safety of sex in the first trimester. Finally, the above search terms resulted in additional search suggestions, including safety of sex in pregnancy, reasons to consider sex during pregnancy, optimal positions, and answers to some of the questions couples may be afraid to ask such as "where does sperm go during pregnancy."

Many websites direct pregnant individuals to review their questions with their care provider to ensure assessment of clinical contraindications to sexual activity or identify other health concerns. Obstetric care providers are therefore uniquely positioned to address sexuality in pregnancy including safety concerns, contraindications, normalization of the varied experiences of sexuality in pregnancy, its importance to couples, and alternative sexual activities or positions that may promote intimacy and improve sexual function. As many pregnant individuals feel uncomfortable raising the subject of sexuality in pregnancy themselves, questions exploring their interest in further information, provision of reliable online or print resources that couples can explore independently, and inclusion in routine conversations regarding pregnancy will allow for a supportive environment to address concerns.

11.8 Conclusions

The first trimester of pregnancy represents a major transition for pregnant individuals and their partners. Sexual activity frequency decreases during the first trimester and is accompanied by increased sexual dysfunction, particularly once the pregnancy is identified. Factors influencing sexual activity in the first trimester include physical factors such as fatigue and nausea and vomiting and a fear of miscarriage or harm to the pregnancy. Sexual activity in the first trimester has not been demonstrated to result in miscarriage, adverse obstetric outcomes, or fetal harm. However, warning against vaginal intercourse is advisable if vaginal bleeding is occurring. Sexual satisfaction, including during pregnancy, is an important aspect of a healthy relationship. Nevertheless, pregnancy represents a unique period during which significant physical, psychosocial, and hormonal changes occur, which may add tension to intimate relationships. Obstetric care providers can offer support to couples seeking information regarding sexual activity in early pregnancy by including discussions of the safety of sexual activity, expectations during pregnancy, and alternative mechanisms of intimacy as part of routine pregnancy care.

References

1. K. von Sydow. Sexuality during pregnancy and after childbirth: a metacontent analysis of 59 studies. *J Psychosom Res* 1999;47:27–49.

2. M. Stammler-Safar, J. Ott, S. Weber, E. Krampl. Sexual behaviour of women with twin pregnancies. *Twin Res Hum Genet* 2010;13:383–8.

3. E. Bartellas, J. M. Crane, M. Daley, K. A. Bennett, D. Hutchens. Sexuality and sexual activity in pregnancy. *BJOG* 2000;107:964–8.

4. A. P. Leite, A. A. Campos, A. R. Dias, et al. Prevalence of sexual dysfunction during pregnancy. *Rev Assoc Med Bras (1992)* 2009;55:563–8.

5. A. Corbacioglu Esmer, A. Akca, O. Akbayir, B. P. Goksedef, V. L. Bakir. Female sexual function and associated factors during pregnancy. *J Obstet Gynaecol Res* 2013;39:1165–72.

6. J. R. Pauleta, N. M. Pereira, L. M. Graca. Sexuality during pregnancy. *J Sex Med* 2010;7:136–42.

7. W. Y. Fok, L. Y. Chan, P. M. Yuen. Sexual behavior and activity in Chinese pregnant women. *Acta Obstet Gynecol Scand* 2005;84:934–8.

8. S. Jawed-Wessel, E. Sevick. The impact of pregnancy and childbirth on sexual behaviors: a systematic review. *J Sex Res* 2017;54:411–23.

9. G. Aslan, D. Aslan, A. Kizilyar, C. Ispahi, A. Esen. A prospective analysis of sexual functions during pregnancy. *Int J Impot Res* 2005;17:154–7.

10. S. Oruc, A. Esen, S. Lacin, et al. Sexual behaviour during pregnancy. *Aust NZ J Obstet Gynaecol* 1999;39:48–50.

11. F. Torkestani, S. H. Hadavand, Z. Khodashenase, et al. Frequency and perception of sexual activity during pregnancy in Iranian couples. *Int J Fertil Steril* 2012;**6**:107–10.

12. S. R. Chang, K. H. Chen, H. H. Lin, H. J. Yu. Comparison of overall sexual function, sexual intercourse/activity, sexual satisfaction, and sexual desire during the three trimesters of pregnancy and assessment of their determinants. *J Sex Med* 2011;**8**:2859–67.

13. C. Ninivaggio, R. G. Rogers, L. Leeman, et al. Sexual function changes during pregnancy. *Int Urogynecol J* 2017;**28**:923–9.

14. A. Fuchs, I. Czech, J. Sikora, et al. Sexual functioning in pregnant women. *Int J Environ Res Public Health* 2019;**16**:4216.

15. M. Seven, A. Akyuz, S. Gungor. Predictors of sexual function during pregnancy. *J Obstet Gynaecol* 2015;**35**:691–5.

16. A. Corbacioglu, V. L. Bakir, O. Akbayir, B. P. Cilesiz Goksedef, A. Akca. The role of pregnancy awareness on female sexual function in early gestation. *J Sex Med* 2012;**9**:1897–903.

17. S. Wannakosit, V. Phupong. Sexual behavior in pregnancy: comparing between sexual education group and nonsexual education group. *J Sex Med* 2010;**7**:3434–8.

18. E. O. Orji, I. O. Ogunlola, O. B. Fasubaa. Sexuality among pregnant women in South West Nigeria. *J Obstet Gynaecol* 2002;**22**:166–8.

19. A. Faisal-Cury, H. Huang, Y. F. Chan, P. R. Menezes. The relationship between depressive/anxiety symptoms during pregnancy/postpartum and sexual life decline after delivery. *J Sex Med* 2013;**10**:1343–9.

20. K. Abouzari-Gazafroodi, F. Najafi, E. Kazemnejad, P. Rahnama, A. Montazeri. Demographic and obstetric factors affecting women's sexual functioning during pregnancy. *Reprod Health* 2015;**12**:72.

21. N. Maconochie, P. Doyle, S. Prior, R. Simmons. Risk factors for first trimester miscarriage: results from a UK-population-based case-control study. *BJOG* 2007;**114**:170–86.

22. N. P. Yost, J. Owen, V. Berghella, et al. Effect of coitus on recurrent preterm birth. *Obstet Gynecol* 2006;**107**:793–7.

23. M. Afshar, S. Mohammad-Alizadeh-Charandabi, E. S. Merghti-Khoei, P. Yavarikia. The effect of sex education on the sexual function of women in the first half of pregnancy: a randomized controlled trial. *J Caring Sci* 2012;**1**:173–81.

12

Sex in the Second and Third Trimesters

Rita Zlatkin and Hadar Rosen

12.1 Epidemiology and Pathophysiology

Sexual activity is an important part of a woman's well-being and general health and is unequivocally affected by the physiological and psychological processes that occur during pregnancy [1]. The frequency of sexual intercourse declines during pregnancy, more so in the third trimester, alongside a decrease in female libido and enjoyment from intercourse [2–7]. This decrease is often explained by dyspareunia or fear of harming the baby [2,7,8] and usually is not discussed during antenatal visits [7,9]. However, in some cases, intercourse is restricted by the attending physician due to obstetric reasons, such as premature contractions, a history of preterm birth, or placenta previa.

The rationale for the restriction of sexual intercourse during pregnancy is derived mainly from the following pathophysiological mechanisms.

1. *Prostaglandin secretion*: Direct contact with the cervix might cause endogenous prostaglandin secretion that could cause cervical ripening and uterine contractions, as has been demonstrated in vaginal examinations and cerclage placements [10–12]. Exogenous prostaglandins F2α and E2 that can be found in the semen might also contribute to this process, either by absorption into the maternal circulation via the vaginal mucosa or by directly affecting the cervix [13,14]. Interestingly, despite the biological logic behind this proposed pathophysiology, the Cochrane Library review of sexual intercourse and induction of labor mentioned only one study that sought to investigate this topic and found no effect on Bishop score after ejaculation [15].

2. *Oxytocin release*: Female orgasm, genital stimulation, and/or nipple stimulation can cause endogenous oxytocin release that may prompt uterine contractions.

   a. Nipple stimulation: Despite not being considered a formal method for induction of labor, nipple stimulation can produce comparable uterine contractions to exogenous oxytocin [16–18] (see Chapter 23 for more details on nipple stimulation). This method can cause contractions that resolve after 15–90 minutes and are of limited intensity [19].

   b. Genital stimulation: The Ferguson reflex is activated when pressure is placed on the cervix and vaginal walls, resulting in oxytocin release and myometrial contraction [20].

   c. Female orgasm: Previous research has established that female orgasm causes endogenous oxytocin release which may result in uterine contractions that are similar in pattern to contractions occurring during labor [21–26] (see Chapter 4 for more details on orgasm). Nevertheless, it seems that the strength of these contraction varies between different women and some reports describe a lack of uterine activity after orgasm [27–29].

Quantification of the effect intercourse has on the power generated by uterine contractions is challenging while amniotic membranes are intact. External tocodynamometry has long been the most common method for assessing uterine contractility during pregnancy and labor [30]. It is a noninvasive method that is based on mechanical measurement of abdominal wall stiffness by a transducer placed on the abdominal wall. This method mainly displays the presence of a contraction, but it cannot reliably display the effectiveness or intensity of contractions. It is also less reliable in detecting contractions in obese women because the accuracy of tocodynamometry is limited by the abdominal wall thickness as well as its position relative to the uterus. This technology is known to be unreliable in many cases and shows a high percentage of false-positive and false-negative results, which in turn hinders the efforts made to assess the effect different events may have on uterine contractility [31–33].

Much of the literature regarding sexual intercourse during low-risk and high-risk pregnancies is largely based on studies conducted decades ago; many had relatively small cohorts and suffered from information biases such as self-reporting bias.

12.2 Sexual Intercourse in Low-Risk Pregnancies

To date, there is no consensus regarding recommendations for sexual intercourse during a low-risk pregnancy. While nowadays sexual activity during pregnancy is generally considered safe [34], common practice dictates that when an "abnormal" event occurs in a pregnancy that was considered low-risk, recommendations often include abstinence from any sexual activity (known as pelvic rest); however, there is a paucity of studies to directly address this question.

Sexual intercourse during pregnancy, especially with advancing gestation, was traditionally considered unsafe and women were frequently discouraged from engaging in sexual activity in the third trimester [21]. It seems that even today, many couples still hold negative beliefs regarding sexual intercourse during pregnancy and its effect on the fetus and pregnancy itself [35].

A few studies conducted in the second half of the twentieth century suggested that coitus and orgasm could precipitate preterm labor. Javert [36] and Limner [37] suggested that coitus could cause abortions and even mental retardation, while Goodlin et al. [38] described in a paper published in 1971 under the title "Orgasm during late pregnancy: possible deleterious effects" that orgasms were more frequent in women who gave birth prematurely. On the contrary, other studies published around the same years came to different conclusions. Masters and Johnson reported that premature birth as a result of the uterine activity following coitus is unlikely and neither Pugh and Fernandez nor Klebanoff and others could find any association between intercourse and preterm labor and birth [21,39–42].

This topic has continued to intrigue researchers in recent years, mainly due to the large variations in opinions and the difficulty in understanding the direct effect of uterine contraction after coitus and possible adverse events during gestation.

12.2.1 Preterm Birth

As described previously, some reports suggested that coitus could cause powerful uterine contractions and precipitate labor. Evidence continues to be conflicting as to the association between sexual intercourse and preterm birth (see Chapter 16 for more details on preterm birth). One case–control study did not find an association between sexual activity in weeks 29–36 of gestation and increased risk for preterm birth, but did report a small increase in risk that was associated with the male superior position [43]. This study demonstrated a certain "protective" effect of sexual intercourse (odds ratio [OR] 0.34, 95% confidence interval [CI] 0.23–0.51), which could be tangential and result from the effect of sexual intercourse on women's general well-being. Kong et al. [5] sought to investigate whether sexual intercourse was associated with maternal and perinatal adverse outcomes. Except for a decreased rate of spontaneous onset of labor which the authors attributed to the small sample size and selection bias, no differences were found between women who engaged in sexual activity and women who did not.

Zhang et al. [44] in a case–control study on 1391 women who delivered prematurely found that sexual activity was an independent risk factor for preterm birth. It should be noted that data regarding coitus during pregnancy were obtained by a questionnaire after the woman had already given birth, and were therefore subject to information bias, especially in women who gave birth prematurely and were probably more meticulous about their sexual activity before delivery.

Multiple studies have proposed that inflammation caused by infective agents, some originating from the genital tract itself and ascending to the fetal membranes and uterus, could cause preterm birth [45,46]. It has therefore been postulated that coitus could elicit an ascending infection that might result in chorioamnionitis and subsequent preterm birth, especially in women suffering from bacterial vaginosis [47]. Read and Klebanoff [48] addressed this hypothesis as part of a large multicenter prospective Vaginal Infections and Prematurity Study Group, obtaining vaginal cultures from the participants at 23–26 weeks of gestation and questioning them regarding their coital frequency during the pregnancy. Similarly to other reports, this study found that frequent coital activity was associated with a decrease in preterm birth rates (OR 0.9, 95% CI 0.71–0.89), even when controlling for confounders. When evaluating the association between vaginal colonization, coital frequency, and preterm birth, the researchers found that *Mycoplasma hominis* and *Trichomonas vaginalis*, as well as bacterial vaginosis, increased the risk for delivering prematurely in women who engaged in sexual activity frequently.

12.2.2 Coitus at Term

Sexual intercourse is perceived in many cultures as a "natural" and safe way to hasten labor at term (see Chapter 6 for more details on sex in different cultures).

In 2010, the Cochrane Database of Systematic Reviews published a comprehensive review that aimed to investigate and establish the effects of sexual intercourse on cervical ripening or labor initiation, when compared with other methods of induction of labor, such as oral, vaginal, intravenous or extra-amniotic prostaglandins, intravenous oxytocin, extra-amniotic Foley catheter, amniotomy, acupuncture, and others [15]. The review concluded that the data were insufficient to draw any conclusions, which once again demonstrates the scarcity of the literature on this issue. Another systematic review and meta-analysis published in 2019 by Carbone et al. [49] analyzed 40 full-text articles, of them three were randomized controlled trials. The conclusion of this meta-analysis was that coitus in women with low-risk pregnancies did not increase the incidence of spontaneous onset of labor (see Chapter 22 for more details on induction of labor).

It is interesting to review one randomized controlled trial conducted by Omar et al. [50] that recruited women at 35–36 weeks of gestation who did not engage in coital activity in the 6 weeks prior to enrollment and randomized them to two groups. The study group was advised to engage in sexual intercourse frequently since it is safe and can hasten labor and the control group was not given any instructions except for documenting their coital frequency. The investigators found no difference in onset of labor between these two groups; additionally, in a post-hoc analysis that compared abstinent women with nonabstinent ones, there was no significant difference in induction of labor rates or in duration of pregnancy.

12.2.3 First-Trimester Pregnancy Loss

Pregnancy loss in the first trimester is common and usually caused by chromosomal anomalies in the fetus [51]. One of the presenting signs of an abortion is vaginal bleeding, albeit not all hemorrhages result in loss of the pregnancy [52](see Chapter 13 for more details on first-trimester bleeding). In these situations, women often seek medical advice regarding whether they should and can resume sexual activity after an episode of threatened abortion. Some women who experience vaginal bleeding in the first trimester are advised to abstain from coitus, probably due to concern about uterine contractions [53,54]. One population-based study found that sexual intercourse was associated with a decrease in the risk for pregnancy loss, unless there was an episode of vaginal bleeding during coitus [55]. In that case the OR was 2.14 (95% CI 1.46–3.13); however, the case group was very small ($n = 47$) and the control group was much larger ($n = 168$). To date, this is the only research paper that suggests any association between sexual intercourse and pregnancy loss but suffers from many limitations in its design (selection bias due to low response rate, absence of young women in the cohort, lack of data regarding chromosomal abnormalities in fetuses of women who miscarried, and more).

In summary, despite a paucity of studies in this field, the existing body of evidence implies that, generally, sexual activity in a low-risk pregnancy is safe and should not be discouraged. Moreover, Chen et al. [56] even suggested that women who engaged in sexual intercourse at least once a month had a stronger levator ani muscle compared to their abstinent counterparts. Clearly, much more high-quality research is needed in order to establish a set of recommendations that obstetric caregivers could offer to their patients.

12.3 Sexual Intercourse in High-Risk Pregnancies

As addressed in the following chapters, literature is sparse regarding the effect of sexual intercourse on complicated and high-risk pregnancies and recommendations are often given based on little to no evidence at all. MacPhedran [57] in her comprehensive review of the literature regarding the evidence for current restrictions of sexual activity in high-risk pregnancies addressed several conditions that complicate pregnancies.

12.3.1 Previous Preterm Birth

Preterm birth usually occurs spontaneously, following preterm uterine contractions, shortening of the cervix, or preterm prelabor rupture of the membranes (PPROM), and remains a leading cause of perinatal mortality and morbidity [45,58] (see Chapter 16 for more details on preterm birth). Even though the etiology of preterm birth is unknown, it is well established that prior preterm birth is a significant risk factor for recurrent preterm birth, and a woman with previous preterm birth has a risk of 30% for experiencing another preterm birth at her subsequent gestation [58,59].

As discussed previously, many studies have addressed the question of whether coitus may prompt preterm labor and birth in low-risk pregnancies, and conclude that it probably does not. To date, there is a lack of evidence regarding sexual intercourse as a risk factor for preterm birth in women with a prior preterm birth. A single study by Yost et al. [60] sought to address this question by performing a secondary analysis on a multicenter observational study of 187 women with singleton pregnancies who had a history of preterm birth at less than 32 weeks of gestation. The women were interviewed individually and questioned about their sexual history. The investigators found that sexual intercourse during pregnancy was not associated with an increased risk for another preterm birth in these women.

Mercer et al. [61] in a secondary analysis of the data collected as part of the National Institute of Child Health and Human Development (NICHD) Maternal–Fetal Medicine Units Network in the Preterm Prediction Study aimed to ascertain whether women with recurrent preterm births had different characteristics than women who gave birth at term. This study found that women with recurrent preterm births were more likely to experience uterine contractions at 22–24 weeks of gestation and to have been treated with tocolytic agents when compared with either term deliveries or women with preterm birth in the index pregnancy. Theoretically, coitus could trigger these uterine contractions and contribute to the risk of developing preterm birth in these high-risk women. In a prospective study of 30 parturients, half of whom had an episode of preterm birth in the index pregnancy, Brustman et al. [62] observed a period of 2–3 hours of postcoital contractions in these women compared with their low-risk counterparts. However, it is unclear whether these contractions are powerful enough to stimulate the process of preterm birth.

Clinical guidelines do not provide recommendations regarding engagement in sexual intercourse in women with a prior preterm birth (see Chapter 7 for more details on obstetric guidelines). The American College of Obstetricians and Gynecologists (ACOG) in their practice bulletin titled "Prediction and prevention of preterm birth" do not address this question whatsoever [63]. Medley et al. [64] published a systematic review of clinical practice guidelines related to preterm birth and its prevention that aimed to identify areas of international consensus in this field. This review also did not include any recommendations regarding coitus in women with a history of preterm birth.

12.3.2 Threatened Preterm Labor and Short Cervix

A short cervix is a significant risk factor for preterm birth, and is defined by a sonographically measured cervical length of less than 2.5 cm in the second trimester [65,66] (see Chapter 15 for more details on short cervix). The etiology of shortening of the cervix is multifactorial and probably involves several factors, so it is not always possible to identify the exact mechanism that led to this process. However, in many cases the clinical presentation is premature uterine contractions that eventually cause cervical dynamics [67].

Restriction of activity has been one of the measures taken in women with shortening of the cervix in order to reduce the risk for preterm birth, and pelvic rest often falls in line with this general restriction. Nevertheless, there is little evidence regarding the actual benefit of this restriction. Grobman et al. [68] performed a secondary analysis of data from the Short Cervix and Nulliparity trial, a randomized controlled trial that compared treatment with intramuscular 17α-hydroxyprogesterone caproate to placebo in nulliparous asymptomatic women with short cervices. As part of the follow-up meetings in the study, participants were asked on a weekly basis whether they had been recommended to restrict their daily activity (work related, work unrelated, or restriction in sexual activity). This secondary analysis found that 33.6% of the 646 participants were instructed to abstain from sexual activity, usually in combination with restriction of other types of daily activities. The women who were restricted from any physical activity had shorter cervices and were almost three times more likely to experience preterm birth. It should be noted that there was no separate analysis for women who were put on pelvic rest only. It is plausible that the women who were recommended to abstain from physical activity were women with a higher risk for preterm birth to begin with, but still these results raise the question regarding the need for pelvic rest in women without a history of preterm birth or other risk factors.

One of the proposed causes for shortening of the cervix is the process of inflammation, usually via an ascending infection from the vaginal flora [67]. The proinflammatory environment could potentially cause direct cervical change or invoke uterine contractions. Despite common belief, sexual intercourse probably does not increase the risk of infection. Kurki and Ylikorkala [69] prospectively examined healthy pregnant women and investigated whether there was an association between coitus, development of bacterial vaginosis, and subsequent preterm birth. Not only was there no association, but the study group has also reported that women who delivered preterm had less frequent sexual intercourse than women who delivered at term. On the other hand, in a study conducted on rodents, Robertson et al. [70] suggested that the presence of semen causes infiltration of endometrial stroma and uterine lumen with polymorphonuclear immune cells, probably as a response to secretion of proinflammatory cytokines from the uterine epithelium. In view of these data, it is theoretically plausible that coitus could invoke further shortening of the cervix and contribute to the risk for preterm birth.

12.3.3 Cervical Insufficiency and Cerclage

Cervical insufficiency is defined as painless cervical dilation and expulsion of the pregnancy at the second trimester with no apparent etiology; to this day, one of the treatment options for women with cervical insufficiency is transvaginal cerclage [71]. According to ACOG, the indications for placement of cerclage in singleton pregnancies are based on history (previous expulsion of the pregnancy at the second trimester without an apparent reason), physical examination (advanced cervical dilation without signs of placental abruption or signs of labor), or the population of women with a history of preterm birth before 34 weeks of gestation and a cervical length of less than 2.5 cm [72].

The above-mentioned ACOG practice bulletin states that pelvic rest has not been proven to be beneficial in women with cervical insufficiency; however, there is no guidance regarding the need for sexual abstinence in women after placement of cerclage. It seems that despite the lack of evidence-based guidelines, it is common practice to recommend sexual abstinence in this population, probably due to concerns that direct contact with the cervix or vaginal walls could induce uterine contractions and increase the risk for infection, even though the few studies that discuss this matter did not show an association between coitus and higher rates of infection [69,73–75].

12.3.4 Preterm Prelabor Rupture of the Membranes

PPROM is defined as rupture of the membranes before 37 weeks of gestation and is often associated with intra-amniotic infection [76] (see Chapter 16 for more details on PPROM). PPROM is further divided, according to week of gestation, into previable premature rupture of membranes (14–24 weeks), preterm PROM (24–34 weeks), and late preterm PROM (34–37 weeks) [77]. The gestational week correlates with the obstetric and neonatal outcomes of the pregnancy and therefore dictates the management. Overall, 50% of patients with PPROM will give birth within a week from the rupture; however, in some cases the leakage of amniotic fluid could stop, and their outcomes are usually more favorable [78,79].

A few studies conducted decades ago found a possible association between coitus and higher risk for PPROM. Ekwo et al. [80] found that sexual intercourse in the male superior position only was significantly associated with PPROM, while Naeye and Ross [47] reported that coitus was associated with chorioamnionitis, especially when the woman reached an orgasm. Additionally, it was found that digital vaginal examinations in women with PPROM may significantly decrease the latency period [81]. In light of the growing body of evidence, it is widely recommended that women with PPROM abstain from any vaginal penetration [78,82].

Since in many cases of PPROM every measure is taken to lengthen the latency period, even though there are few studies that address this matter, it seems reasonable to advise these women to restrict sexual activity of any kind.

12.3.5 Placenta Previa

Placenta previa is defined as a placenta that is entirely covering the os; it is associated with various adverse maternal and perinatal complications, most commonly antepartum vaginal bleeding [83](see Chapter 14 for more details on placenta previa). A placenta can be classified as "low-lying" if it is near but not overlying the cervical os [84]. The exact mechanism of the bleeding in placenta previa is unknown, but it is proposed that certain insults, such as uterine contractions and cervical dynamics, cause separation of the placenta from the decidua that results in vaginal bleeding.

No studies have directly investigated the topic of coitus in women with placenta previa. One retrospective report by Naeye [85] found an association between coitus and antepartum bleeding; however, it was not stated how many women suffered from placenta previa, and the focus of the study was mainly patients with placental abruption. Moreover, there is no possibility of determining causality in this study and therefore it is impossible to extrapolate that coitus may be the cause of vaginal bleeding in these cases.

It seems that the restriction of sexual activity in women with placenta previa is derived mainly from the notion that sexual intercourse resembles other activities that have been reported to cause harm. A study published in 1950 recommended avoidance of vaginal manipulation of the cervix out of concern that it causes bleeding [86]. Similarly, concerns were raised regarding the use of transvaginal probes and were rebutted [87,88]. We should bear in mind nonetheless that coitus could impact the lower uterine segment, cause mechanical stretching and contractions, and thereafter cause vaginal bleeding.

In accordance with these observations, guidelines published by the Society of Obstetricians and Gynaecologists of Canada (SOGC) regarding diagnosis and management of placenta previa recommend avoidance of sexual intercourse or insertion of foreign bodies in the vagina or rectum; however, the level of evidence of this recommendation is considered low [89].

12.3.6 Placental Abruption

Placental abruption complicates 0.4–1% of pregnancies and is a major cause of vaginal bleeding in the second and third trimesters of pregnancy, with possible catastrophic consequences for the mother and fetus [90,91] (see Chapter 14 for more details on placental abruption). Vaginal bleeding is one of the presenting symptoms of placental abruption, usually combined with abdominal pain, uterine tenderness, or tetanic contractions with nonreassuring fetal heart tracing [92].

Similarly to previous high-risk conditions, theoretically it is hazardous to engage in sexual activity that could invoke uterine contractions in the setting of acute placental abruption. Realistically, there are very few reports regarding this matter. As previously mentioned, a single study by Naeye [85] aimed to evaluate the association between coitus and antepartum bleeding, especially in cases suspected for placental abruption. The investigators found that coitus was indeed associated with the vaginal bleeding, independently of other risk factors. A case report from Nigeria described an incidence of intrauterine fetal demise following acute abruption after sexual intercourse; no other similar cases were found in the literature [93]. It is hard to assemble comprehensive recommendations from these sporadic studies and they probably should be tailored individually according to the extent of the vaginal bleeding and the maternal and fetal well-being. On the contrary, it seems that women with chronic and stable placental abruption who are under outpatient surveillance should not be placed under sexual activity restrictions [91].

12.3.7 Prior Cesarean Delivery

Women with one prior cesarean delivery are allowed and encouraged to opt for a trial of vaginal delivery and the rates of success are very high. However, these women have an increased risk of uterine rupture. The risk of uterine rupture after one cesarean delivery is 1% in cases of low transverse uterine incision and 4–9% in classic or T-shaped incision [94,95].

Several studies have found that induction of labor using prostaglandins, especially prostaglandin E1, increases the risk of uterine rupture when compared with either oxytocin or spontaneous onset of labor [96–98]. Bearing in mind that sexual intercourse could cause an increased level of prostaglandins raises questions about the safety of sexual intercourse in women with at least one prior cesarean delivery.

When scoping the literature, there are only a few case reports describing uterine rupture in women after cesarean deliveries, but no small- or large-scale descriptive studies have investigated this matter. One case report described a 34-year-old woman who presented with severe postcoital vaginal bleeding 4 months after an urgent cesarean delivery; angiography revealed that it was due to a uterine artery pseudoaneurysm [99]. Another case report described a 23-year-old woman with a previous cesarean delivery with a classical incision at 26 weeks of gestation due to placental abruption, which presented with uterine rupture at 15 weeks of gestation after intercourse that resulted in a hysterectomy. Pathological examination revealed placenta percreta and complete rupture of the uterus at the old scar site [100].

A few more similar case reports exist, but it is reasonable to assume that most of the women with a history of prior cesarean delivery engage in sexual intercourse during their next pregnancy, and had the risk for uterine rupture been significant these reports would not be as sporadic as they are today [101–103].

12.3.8 Multifetal Gestation

Preterm birth complicates twin gestations at a high and rising rate, and as in singleton pregnancies, sexual intercourse has been suspected as a possible trigger for this process [104] (see Chapter 17 for more details on twin pregnancies).

This question was first addressed in a study by Neilson and Mutambira [105] who performed a prospective study of 126 women with twin gestations who were questioned regarding their coital frequency. There were no differences in coital patterns between women who gave birth prematurely and women who gave birth at term. Stammler-Safar et al. [106] also addressed this topic in a prospective study of 50 women who filled out a questionnaire on their sexual behavior during pregnancy. Sexual intercourse was not found to be associated with preterm delivery in these women.

Both studies had relatively small sample sizes and only enrolled women with uncomplicated twin pregnancies, and therefore did not allow extrapolation of these results to all twin gestations. It is clear that further investigation is needed to establish proper guidelines for this population; nevertheless, it seems that there is no justification to restrict sexual activity in women with twin gestation with an uncomplicated pregnancy.

12.4 Summary of Sexual Intercourse in Low- and High-Risk Pregnancies

There are few data regarding the implications and safety of intercourse in low-and high-risk pregnancies. Evidence that has been published is usually of low quality, derived from nonrandomized studies with some of them addressing other issues. Randomized controlled trials are scarce if any.

This lack of evidence may derive from the inherent challenge of studying intercourse due to its intimate nature, in some cultures even taboo. Nevertheless, with intercourse being a healthy, important, and common practice, these issues deserve attention so that evidence-based recommendations may be given to women with low- and high-risk pregnancies.

In recent years, a novel device that measures electrical myometrial activity has been introduced and validated in several studies [107–109]. One interesting option for further evidence-based research would be to investigate the generated power of uterine contractions with relation to the different events during intercourse in order to provide quantification of the effect on uterine activity in low- and high-risk situations.

12.5 What Did Dr. Google Say?

A Google search for the term "sex in later pregnancy" comes up with some interesting results. The first result surprisingly targets not pregnant women but the future fathers. A website from Australia called Raisingchildren.net offers male partners of women carrying advanced pregnancies some advice regarding sexual practices, how to approach their partner, and how to handle abstinence [110]. Another website named Parents.com has an obstetrician deliver a crash course on some of the frequently asked questions about sex in later pregnancy with regard to different areas of concern, such as safety, positions, libido, risk of causing early labor, and oral and anal sex habits [111]. For official information, the UK National Health Service website provides couples with instructions and advice regarding situations when it would be best to avoid sexual relations in later pregnancy. The website is written is layman language, and offers visitors an option to sign up for a free newsletter with further advice [112]. Many other sites are hospital, commercial, or magazine-based and offer more non-peer-reviewed articles that address similar questions.

More official peer-reviewed information can be found on the March of Dimes website, with specific details regarding habits that should be avoided, contraindications to sex in pregnancy, venereal disease in pregnancy, and some advice regarding postpartum resumption of sexual activity [113].

To conclude, intercourse is an inseparable part of a parturient's normal activity, including during the advanced stages of pregnancy. As such, this practice and its implications for low- and high-risk pregnancies merits in-depth investigation to allow evidence-based robust recommendations.

References

1. M. Serati, S. Salvatore, G. Siesto, et al. Female sexual function during pregnancy and after childbirth. *J Sex Med* 2010;**7**:2782–90.

2. K. von Sydow. Sexuality during pregnancy and after childbirth: a metacontent analysis of 59 studies. *J Psychosom Res* 1999;**47**:27–49.

3. L. Sossah. Sexual behavior during pregnancy: a descriptive correlational study among pregnant women. *Eur J Med Res* 2014;**2**:16–27.

4. B. Erol, O. Sanli, D. Korkmaz, et al. A cross-sectional study of female sexual function and dysfunction during pregnancy. *J Sex Med* 2007;**4**:1381–7.

5. L. Kong, T. Li, L. Li. The impact of sexual intercourse during pregnancy on obstetric and neonatal outcomes: a cohort study in China. *J Obstet Gynaecol* 2019;**39**:455–60.

6. S. Chang, K. Chen, H. Lin, H. Yu. Comparison of overall sexual function, sexual intercourse/activity, sexual satisfaction, and sexual desire during the three trimesters of pregnancy and assessment of their determinants. *J Sex Med* 2011;**8**:2859–67.

7. D. A. Solberg, J. Butler, N. N. Wagner. Sexual behavior in pregnancy. *N Engl J Med* 1973;**288**:1098–103.

8. S. Jamali, L. Mosalanejad. Sexual dysfnction in Iranian pregnant women. *Iran J Reprod Med* 2013;**11**:479–86.

9. C. M. Glazener. Sexual function after childbirth: women's experiences, persistent morbidity and lack of professional recognition. *Br J Obstet Gynaecol* 1997;**104**:330–5.

10. M. D. Mitchell, A. P. Flint, J. Bibby, et al. Rapid increases in plasma prostaglandin concentrations after vaginal examination and amniotomy. *BMJ* 1977;**2**:1183–5.

11. J. J. Platz-Christensen, P. Pernevi, H. Bokström, N. Wiqvist. Prostaglandin E and F2α concentration in the cervical mucus and mechanism of cervical ripening. *Prostaglandins* 1997;**53**:253–61.

12. M. J. Novy, C. A. Ducsay, F. Z. Stanczyk. Plasma concentrations of prostaglandin F2α and prostaglandin E2 metabolites after transabdominal and transvaginal cervical cerclage. *Am J Obstet Gynecol* 1987;**156**:1543–52.

13. K. Gerozissis, P. Jouannet, J. C. Soufir, F. Dray. Origin of prostaglandins in human semen. *J Reprod Fertil* 1982;**65**:401–4.

14. R. W. Kelly. Prostaglandins in semen: their occurrence and possible physiological significance. *Int J Androl* 1978;**1**:188–200.

15. J. Kavanagh, A. J. Kelly, J. Thomas. Sexual intercourse for cervical ripening and induction of labour. *Cochrane Database Syst Rev* 2001;(2):CD003093.

16. J. Kavanagh, A. J. Kelly, J. Thomas. Breast stimulation for cervical ripening and induction of labour. *Cochrane Database Syst Rev* 2005;(3):CD003392.

17. I. F. Adewole, O. Franklin, A. A. Matiluko. Cervical ripening and induction of labour by breast stimulation. *Afr J Med Med Sci* 1993;**22**:81–5.

18. P. Curtis. Breast stimulation to augment labor: history, mystery, and culture. *Birth* 1999;**26**:123–6.

19. J. F. Huddleston, G. Sutliff, D. Robinson. Contraction stress test by intermittent nipple stimulation. *Obstet Gynecol* 1984;**63**:669–73.

20. J. K. W. Ferguson. A study of the motility of the intact uterus at term. *Surg Gynecol Obstet* 1941;**73**:359–66.

21. W. Masters, V. Johnson. *Human Sexual Response*. Boston: Little, Brown, 1966: 141–68.

22. N. Newton. The role of the oxytocin reflexes in three interpersonal reproductive acts: coitus, birth and breastfeeding. In L. Carenza, P. Pancheri, L. Zichella, eds. *Clinical Psychoneuroendocrinology in Reproduction*. New York: Academic Press, 1978: 411–18.

23. M. S. Carmichael, R. Humbert, J. Dixen, et al. Plasma oxytocin increases in the human sexual response. *J Clin Endocrinol Metab* 1987;**64**:27–31.

24. G. F. Pranzarone. Sexuoerotic stimulation and orgasmic response in the induction and management of parturition: clinical possibilities. In S. C. Satapathy, V. K. Prasad, B. P. Rani, S. K. Udgata, K. S. Raju, eds. *Proceedings of First International Conference on Orgasm*. Bombay: VRP Publishers, 1991.

25. R. C. Goodlin, W. Schmidt, D. C. Creevy. Uterine tension and fetal heart rate during maternal orgasm. *Obstet Gynecol* 1972;**39**:125–7.

26. S. Baxter. Labour and orgasm in primiparae. *J Psychosom Res* 1974;**18**:209–16.

27. B. Chayen, N. Tejani, U. L. Verma, G. Gordon. Fetal heart rate changes and uterine activity during coitus. *Acta Obstet Gynecol Scand* 1986;**65**:853–5.

28. C. M. Meston, R. J. Levin, M. L. Sipski, E. M. Hull, J. R. Heiman. Women's orgasm. *Annu Rev Sex Res* 2004;**15**:173–257.

29. R. King, J. Belsky, K. Mah, Y. Binik. Are there different types of female orgasm? *Arch Sex Behav* 2011;**40**:865–75.

30. W. R. Cohen. Clinical assessment of uterine contractions. *Int J Gynaecol Obstet* 2017;**139**:137–42.

31. R. B. Newman. Uterine contraction assessment. *Obstet Gynecol Clin North Am* 2005;**32**:341–67.

32. P. Bakker, P. H. J. Kurver, D. J. Kuik, H. P. Van Geijn. Elevated uterine activity

increases the risk of fetal acidosis at birth. *Am J Obstet Gynecol* 2007;**196**:313.e1–6.

33. H. Maul, W. L. Maner, G. Olson, G. R. Saade, R. E. Garfield. Non-invasive transabdominal uterine electromyography correlates with the strength of intrauterine pressure and is predictive of labor and delivery. *J Matern Fetal Neonatal Med* 2004;**15**:297–301.

34. National Institute for Health and Care Excellence. *Antenatal Care for Uncomplicated Pregnancies*. Clinical Guideline CG62. London: NICE, 2008. Last updated February 4, 2019. www.nice.org.uk/guidance/cg62 (accessed May 13, 2021).

35. M. C. Ribeiro, M. de Tubino Scanavino, M. L. S. do Amaral, A. L. de Moraes Horta, M. R. Torloni. Beliefs about sexual activity during pregnancy: a systematic review of the literature. *J Sex Marital Ther* 2017;**43**:822–32.

36. C. T. Javert. *Spontaneous and Habitual Abortion*. New York: McGraw-Hill, 1957.

37. R. R. Limner. *Sex and the Unborn Child: Damage to the Fetus Resulting from Sexual Intercourse during Pregnancy*. New York: Julian Press, 1969.

38. R. C. Goodlin, D. W. Keller, M. Raffin. Orgasm during late pregnancy: possible deleterious effects. *Obstet Gynecol* 1971;**38**:916–20.

39. W. E. Pugh, F. L. Fernandez. Coitus in late pregnancy: a follow-up study of the effects of coitus on late pregnancy, delivery, and the puerperium. *Obstet Gynecol* 1953;**2**:636–42.

40. M. Klebanoff, R. Nugent, G. Rhoads. Coitus during pregnancy: is it safe? *Lancet* 1984;**324**:914–17.

41. J. Mills, S. Harlap, E. Harley. Should coitus late in pregnancy be discouraged? *Lancet* 1981;**318**:136–8.

42. A. L. Herbst. Coitus and the fetus. *N Engl J Med* 1979;**301**:1235–6.

43. A. E. Sayle, D. A. Savitz, J. M. Thorp Jr., I. Hertz-Picciotto, A. J. Wilcox. Sexual activity during late pregnancy and risk of preterm delivery. *Obstet Gynecol* 2001;**97**:283–9.

44. Y. P. Zhang, X. H. Liu, S. H. Gao, et al. Risk factors for preterm birth in five maternal and child health hospitals in Beijing. *PLoS ONE* 2012;**7**:e52780.

45. R. L. Goldenberg, J. F. Culhane, J. D. Iams, R. Romero. Epidemiology and causes of preterm birth. *Lancet* 2008;**371**:75–84.

46. R. Romero, S. K. Dey, S. J. Fisher. Preterm labor: one syndrome, many causes. *Science* 2014;**345**:760–5.

47. R. L. Naeye, S. Ross. Coitus and chorioamnionitis: a prospective study. *Early Hum Dev* 1982;**6**:91–7.

48. J. S. Read, M. A. Klebanoff. Sexual intercourse during pregnancy and preterm delivery: effects of vaginal microorganisms. *Am J Obstet Gynecol* 1993;**168**:514–19.

49. L. Carbone, V. De Vivo, G. Saccone, et al. Sexual intercourse for induction of spontaneous onset of labor: a systematic review and meta-analysis of randomized controlled trials. *J Sex Med* 2019;**16**:1787–95.

50. N. S. Omar, P. C. Tan, N. Sabir, E. S. Yusop, S. Z. Omar. Coitus to expedite the onset of labour: a randomised trial. *BJOG* 2013;**120**:338–45.

51. H. B. Ford, D. J. Schust. Recurrent pregnancy loss: etiology, diagnosis, and therapy. *Rev Obstet Gynecol* 2009;**2**:76–83.

52. J. L. Weiss, F. D. Malone, J. Vidaver, et al. Threatened abortion: a risk factor for poor pregnancy outcome, a population-based screening study. *Am J Obstet Gynecol* 2004;**190**:745–50.

53. G. Chamberlain. ABC of antenatal care: vaginal bleeding in early pregnancy – I. *BMJ* 1991;**302**:1141–3.

54. J. C. Tien, T. Y. T. Tan. Non-surgical interventions for threatened and recurrent miscarriages. *Singapore Med J* 2007;**48**:1074–90.

55. N. Maconochie, P. Doyle, S. Prior, R. Simmons. Risk factors for first trimester miscarriage: results from a UK-population-based case–control study. *BJOG* 2007;**114**:170–86.

56. L. Chen, M. Jin, D. Luo, et al. Association between sexual intercourse frequency and pelvic floor muscle morphology in pregnant women. *Int Urogynecol J* 2020;**31**:1933–41.

57. S. E. MacPhedran. Sexual activity recommendations in high-risk pregnancies: what is the evidence? *Sex Med Rev* 2018;**6**:343–57.

58. C. Phillips, Z. Velji, C. Hanly, A. Metcalfe. Risk of recurrent spontaneous preterm birth: a systematic review and meta-analysis. *BMJ Open* 2017;**7**:e015402.

59. S. Mazaki-Tovi, R. Romero, J. P. Kusanovic, et al. Recurrent preterm birth. *Semin Perinatol* 2007;**31**:142–58.

60. N. P. Yost, J. Owen, V. Berghella, et al. Effect of coitus on recurrent preterm birth. *Obstet Gynecol* 2006;**107**:793–7.

61. B. M. Mercer, C. A. Macpherson, R. L. Goldenberg, et al. Are women with recurrent spontaneous preterm births different from those without such history? *Am J Obstet Gynecol* 2006;**194**:1176–84.

62. L. Brustman, M. Raptoulis, O. Langer, A. Anyaegbunam, I. Merkatz. Changes in the pattern of uterine contractility in relationship to coitus during pregnancies at low and high risk for preterm labor. *Obstet Gynecol* 1989;**73**:166–8.

63. American College of Obstetricians and Gynecologists Committee on Practice Bulletins – Obstetrics. Practice bulletin no. 130: prediction and prevention of preterm birth. *Obstet Gynecol* 2012;**120**:964–73.

64. N. Medley, B. Poljak, S. Mammarella, Z. Alfirevic. Clinical guidelines for prevention and management of preterm birth: a systematic review. *BJOG* 2018;**125**:1361–9.

65. W. W. Andrews, R. Copper, J. C. Hauth, et al. Second-trimester cervical ultrasound: associations with increased risk for recurrent early spontaneous delivery. *Obstet Gynecol* 2000;**95**:222–6.

66. J. D. Iams, R. L. Goldenberg, P. J. Meis, et al. The length of the cervix and the risk of spontaneous premature delivery. *N Engl J Med* 1996;**334**:567–73.

67. E. O. Jones, Z.-Q. Liew, O. A. Rust. The short cervix: a critical analysis of diagnosis and treatment. *Obstet Gynecol Clin North Am* 2020;**47**:545–67.

68. W. A. Grobman, S. A. Gilbert, J. D. Iams, et al. Activity restriction among women with a short cervix. *Obstet Gynecol* 2013;**121**:1181–6.

69. T. Kurki, O. Ylikorkala. Coitus during pregnancy is not related to bacterial vaginosis or preterm birth. *Am J Obstet Gynecol* 1993;**169**:1130–4.

70. S. A. Robertson, V. J. Mau, K. P. Tremellen, R. F. Seamark. Role of high molecular weight seminal vesicle proteins in eliciting the uterine inflammatory response to semen in mice. *Reproduction* 1996;**107**:265–77.

71. R. Brown, R. Gagnon, M.-F. Delisle, et al. Cervical insufficiency and cervical cerclage. *J Obstet Gynaecol Can* 2013;**35**:1115–27.

72. American College of Obstetricians and Gynecologists. Practice bulletin no. 142: cerclage for the management of cervical insufficiency. *Obstet Gynecol* 2014;**123**:372–9.

73. Z. Alfirevic, J. Owen, E. Carreras Moratonas, et al. Vaginal progesterone, cerclage or cervical pessary for preventing preterm birth in asymptomatic singleton pregnant women with a history of preterm birth and a sonographic short cervix. *Ultrasound Obstet Gynecol* 2013;**41**:146–51.

74. J. Owen, G. Hankins, J. D. Iams, et al. Multicenter randomized trial of cerclage for preterm birth prevention in high-risk women with shortened midtrimester cervical length. *Am J Obstet Gynecol* 2009;**201**:375.e1–8.

75. Y. Çakıroğlu, Ş. Çalışkan, E. Doğer, et al. Do the interactions between coital frequency, cervical length, and urogenital infection affect obstetric outcomes? *Turk J Obstet Gynecol* 2015;**12**:66–70.

76. S. Kenyon, M. Boulvain, J. Neilson. Antibiotics for preterm premature

rupture of membranes. *Cochrane Database Syst Rev* 2001;(12):CD001058.

77. American College of Obstetricians and Gynecologists Committee on Practice Bulletins – Obstetrics. Practice bulletin no. 172: premature rupture of membranes. *Obstet Gynecol* 2016;**128**: e165–77.

78. B. M. Mercer. Preterm premature rupture of the membranes. *Obstet Gynecol* 2003;**101**:178–93.

79. J. W. Johnson, R. S. Egerman, J. Moorhead. Cases with ruptured membranes that "reseal." *Am J Obstet Gynecol* 1990;**163**:1024–30.

80. E. E. Ekwo, C. A. Gosselink, R. Woolson, A. Moawad, C. R. Long. Coitus late in pregnancy: risk of preterm rupture of amniotic sac membranes. *Am J Obstet Gynecol* 1993;**168**:22–31.

81. R. J. Nadišauskienė, D. Vaitkienė. Effects of digital vaginal examinations on latency period in preterm premature rupture of membranes (PROM-P). In *VIth Baltic Sea Conference on Obstetrics and Gynecology: Abstracts, July 31 to August 2 1997.* Kiel, Germany, 1997.

82. B. M. Mercer. Preterm premature rupture of the membranes: diagnosis and management. *Clin Perinatol* 2004;**31**:765–82.

83. R. M. Silver. Abnormal placentation: placenta previa, vasa previa, and placenta accreta. *Obstet Gynecol* 2015;**126**:654–68.

84. U. M. Reddy, A. Z. Abuhamad, D. Levine, G. R. Saade, Participants FIWI. Fetal imaging: executive summary of a joint Eunice Kennedy Shriver National Institute of Child Health and Human Development, Society for Maternal–Fetal medicine, American Institute of Ultrasound in Medicine, American College of Obstetricians and Gynecologists, American College of Radiology, Society for Pediatric Radiology, and Society of Radiologists in Ultrasound Fetal Imaging Workshop. *Am J Obstet Gynecol* 2014;**210**:387–97.

85. R. L. Naeye. Coitus and antepartum haemorrhage. *Br J Obstet Gynaecol* 1981;**88**:765–70.

86. H. W. Johnson. The management of placenta previa: a review of 201 cases with emphasis on conservatism. *Am J Obstet Gynecol* 1950;**59**:1236–42.

87. I. E. Timor-Tritsch, R. A. Yunis. Confirming the safety of transvaginal sonography in patients suspected of placenta previa. *Obstet Gynecol* 1993;**81**:742–4.

88. W. C. Mabie. Placenta previa. *Clin Perinatol* 1992;**19**:425–35.

89. V. Jain, H. Bos, E. Bujold. Guideline no. 402: diagnosis and management of placenta previa. *J Obstet Gynaecol Can* 2020;**42**:906–17.e1.

90. T. Boisramé, N. Sananès, G. Fritz, et al. Placental abruption: risk factors, management and maternal–fetal prognosis. Cohort study over 10 years. *Eur J Obstet Gynecol Reprod Biol* 2014;**179**:100–4.

91. Y. Oyelese, C. V. Ananth. Placental abruption. *Obstet Gynecol* 2006;**108**:1005–16.

92. C. V. Ananth, J. A. Lavery, A. M. Vintzileos, et al. Severe placental abruption: clinical definition and associations with maternal complications. *Am J Obstet Gynecol* 2016;**214**:272.e1–9.

93. M. E. Aziken. Abruptio placenta following sexual intercourse: case report. *Niger Postgrad Med J* 2003;**10**:113–14.

94. R. W. Naef III, M. A. Ray, S. P. Chauhan, et al. Trial of labor after cesarean delivery with a lower-segment, vertical uterine incision: is it safe? *Am J Obstet Gynecol* 1995;**172**:1666–74.

95. S. P. Chauhan, J. N. Martin Jr., C. E. Henrichs, J. C. Morrison, E. F. Magann. Maternal and perinatal complications with uterine rupture in 142,075 patients who attempted vaginal birth after cesarean delivery: a review of the literature. *Am J Obstet Gynecol* 2003;**189**:408–17.

96. American College of Obstetricians and Gynecologists. Practice bulletin no. 205: vaginal birth after cesarean delivery. *Obstet Gynecol* 2019;**133**:e110–27.

97. M. Lydon-Rochelle, V. L. Holt, T. R. Easterling, D. P. Martin. Risk of uterine rupture during labor among women with a prior cesarean delivery. *N Engl J Med* 2001;**345**:3–8.

98. G. A. Dekker, A. Chan, C. G. Luke, et al. Risk of uterine rupture in Australian women attempting vaginal birth after one prior caesarean section: a retrospective population-based cohort study. *BJOG* 2010;**117**:1358–65.

99. K. Chummun, N. Kroon, G. Flannelly, D. Brophy. Severe postcoital bleeding from a uterine artery pseudoaneurysm 4 months after cesarean delivery. *Obstet Gynecol* 2015;**126**:638–41.

100. L. K. Endres, K. Barnhart. Spontaneous second trimester uterine rupture after classical cesarean. *Obstet Gynecol* 2000;**96**:806–8.

101. T.-L. Tan, S. Kolhe, A. Shafik. Spontaneous uterine rupture following intercourse in a scarred uterus. *J Obstet Gynaecol* 2005;**25**:392.

102. H.-F. Tsai, H.-L. Song, W.-C. Chen, et al. Delayed uterine rupture occurred 4 weeks after cesarean section following sexual intercourse: a case report and literature review. *Taiwan J Obstet Gynecol* 2013;**52**:411–14.

103. A. Nassar, I. Usta, A. Finianos, H. Kaspar. Spontaneous uterine rupture following intercourse. *Acta Obstet Gynecol Scand* 2004;**83**:114–15.

104. J. A. Martin, B. E. Hamilton, M. J. Osterman, S. C. Curtin, T. J. Matthews. Births: final data for 2013. *Natl Vital Stat Rep* 2015;**64**:1–65.

105. J. P. Neilson, M. Mutambira. Coitus, twin pregnancy, and preterm labor. *Am J Obstet Gynecol* 1989;**160**:416–18.

106. M. Stammler-Safar, J. Ott, S. Weber, E. Krampl. Sexual behaviour of women with twin pregnancies. *Twin Res Hum Genet* 2010;**13**:383–8.

107. G. Haran, M. Elbaz, M. D. Fejgin, T. Biron-Shental. A comparison of surface acquired uterine electromyography and intrauterine pressure catheter to assess uterine activity. *Am J Obstet Gynecol* 2012;**206**:412.e1–5.

108. B. C. Jacod, E. M. Graatsma, E. Van Hagen, G. H. Visser. A validation of electrohysterography for uterine activity monitoring during labour. *J Matern Fetal Neonatal Med* 2010;**23**:17–22.

109. R. E. Garfield, W. L. Maner, L. B. MacKay, D. Schlembach, G. R. Saade. Comparing uterine electromyography activity of antepartum patients versus term labor patients. *Am J Obstet Gynecol* 2005;**193**:23–9.

110. Sex in late pregnancy: men. https://raisingchildren.net.au/pregnancy/dads-guide-to-pregnancy/late-pregnancy/sex-in-late-pregnancy

111. A crash course in having sex during your third trimester. www.parents.com/pregnancy/my-life/sex-relationship/a-crash-course-in-having-sex-during-your-third-trimester/

112. Sex in pregnancy. www.nhs.uk/pregnancy/keeping-well/sex/

113. Sex during pregnancy. www.marchofdimes.org/pregnancy/sex-during-pregnancy.aspx

Chapter 13

Sex with Bleeding in the First Trimester

Hugo Madar, Aurélien Mattuizzi, Hanane Bouchghoul, and Loïc Sentilhes

13.1 Introduction

Bleeding in the first trimester of pregnancy involves blood loss from the vagina between weeks 4 and 12 of gestation. This complication is relatively frequent and affects between 10 and 15% of pregnancies [1,2]. Bleeding in the first trimester is mainly considered to increase the risk of spontaneous miscarriage, premature birth, and low birthweight [3,4]. However, these risks may be overestimated because of the recall and information biases inherent to the retrospective nature of most studies that have assessed pregnancy outcomes after bleeding in the first trimester of pregnancy. Such first-trimester bleeding calls for diagnostic rigor to avoid overlooking, for example, an ectopic pregnancy or an impending miscarriage. To our knowledge, no study has specifically evaluated the impact of sexual intercourse when there is bleeding during the first trimester of pregnancy. Therefore, in this chapter we explore the suspected or proven effects of sexual intercourse as a function of the different etiologies of first-trimester bleeding.

13.2 Changes in Sexual Behavior in Early Pregnancy

The frequency of sexual intercourse decreases throughout pregnancy, and mainly after the second trimester [5–7]. Hormonal and physical changes during pregnancy alter self-esteem, psychological behavior, and sense of attractiveness, which are the main reasons for the decline in intercourse during pregnancy (see Chapter 3 for more details on changes during pregnancy). However, it should be borne in mind that sexual behavior is multifactorial and subject to cultural influences, which explains the significant variability in published surveys [5,7] (see Chapters 5 and 6 for more details on demographics and sex in other cultures). This decrease in sexual activity is small in the first trimester, with an interest in sex that is slightly diminished in women and unchanged in men. However, in nearly 20% of cases, there is an increased frequency of erotic dreams in women during pregnancy [7]. As for sexual behavior in general in the first trimester of pregnancy, there is no decrease in tenderness or touching, while the results concerning masturbation, anal sex, and oral sex are discordant. However, there is no significant change in sexual behavior apart from a decrease in vaginal intercourse [5,7].

Interestingly, while 76–79% of women report being sexually satisfied before pregnancy, only 59% do so in the first trimester of pregnancy [7]. This difference may be explained by fear of miscarriage and by awareness of pregnancy [5]. Furthermore, other factors such as nausea and vomiting and asthenia, which are frequently noted in the first trimester of pregnancy, could lead to decreased libido. In addition to a decline in the frequency of sex from the first trimester of pregnancy, there is also a significant decrease in Female Sexual Function Index (FSFI), which explores sexual satisfaction in five domains: desire, lubrication, orgasm, pain, and satisfaction [8]. All these changes in sexual activity in the first trimester of pregnancy occur in the absence of complications. Modified sexual activity in the first trimester is significantly associated with the following determinants: a history of infertility, discomfort during sex, high educational level, and previous miscarriage [8]. When bleeding occurs, it is legitimate to think that fear of miscarriage is preponderant and reduces sexual activity further.

13.3 Sexual Intercourse and the Risk of Miscarriage

Bleeding during the first trimester of pregnancy is regularly associated with spontaneous miscarriage, and either precedes the miscarriage or is a symptom of impending miscarriage [9]. The risk of miscarriage is greater when bleeding is severe or associated with pelvic pain [9]. A population-based case–control study published in 2007 found a protective effect of vaginal sex on the risk of miscarriage in the first trimester (adjusted odds ratio [aOR] 0.78, 95% confidence interval [CI] 0.62–0.98) and when sex did not cause bleeding (aOR 0.67, 95% CI 0.52–0.84) [10]. Conversely, the risk of early miscarriage was doubled when bleeding occurred during sex (aOR 1.96, 95% CI 1.31–2.92) [10]. Nevertheless, the effect of sex on the risk of miscarriage could not be dissociated from the effect of bleeding in this study. It is highly likely that this additional risk is explained by the presence of bleeding strongly associated with the risk of miscarriage and not by sex in the first trimester of pregnancy, which seems to be protective. Unfortunately, no other studies have specifically investigated the supposed deleterious role in early miscarriage of vaginal sex plus bleeding in the first trimester. Based on these results alone, it is probably unwarranted to advise against sex during the first trimester of pregnancy in the event of bleeding, because of the low level of evidence and the lack of demonstration of causality. Conversely, there is no argument suggesting that in the absence of bleeding during intercourse, sex is a risk factor for miscarriage since it even seems to be protective. However, practitioners cannot satisfactorily answer parents' questions due to the scarcity of studies that have specifically investigated sexual activity and the risk of miscarriage early in pregnancy. A recent review of the literature on miscarriage published in *The Lancet* in 2021 does not mention the impact of sex during the first trimester on the risk of miscarriage, highlighting the lack of scientific data on this subject [11–13]. These crucial questions are not always addressed by researchers and clinicians, although they are in theory answerable. Hence, practitioners' excessive modesty and hesitancy to talk about sexuality in consultations with patients, and the reluctance of researchers to suggest innovative research topics concerning the sexuality of pregnant women, prevent the delivery of potentially helpful sexual advice to women [14].

13.4 Sex and Very Early Unexplained Bleeding

A prospective study in 221 women wishing to become pregnant explored the outcome of unexplained bleeding during the first 8 weeks of pregnancy [15]. Of 151 women who became clinically pregnant (at least 6 weeks of gestation) during the period of follow-up, 14 (9%) presented bleeding during the start of pregnancy, two of whom unfortunately had a miscarriage. In comparison, in the 13 miscarriages among the 137 women who did not have bleeding in the first trimester of pregnancy, the relative risk of miscarriage estimated after unexplained bleeding very early in the first trimester was 1.5 (95% CI

0.4–6.0), though no conclusion was possible because of the small number of subjects [15]. Nevertheless, in this prospective study, the daily diaries kept by the women revealed no association between sexual intercourse in the first trimester of pregnancy and the occurrence of unexplained bleeding [15].

Implantation has been described as the cause of bleeding very early in pregnancy [16]. Surprisingly, a prospective observational study in 743 women found a significant decrease in fecundability in women who had peri-implantation intercourse on more than two consecutive days, in comparison with women who had no intercourse during this peri-implantation window, after adjusting for the frequency of intercourse during the fertile window (periovulatory period) [17]. The hypothesis behind these results is that increased myometrial activity during intercourse with uterine contractions on orgasm reduces the implantation rate [17]. However, these results should be interpreted with caution because of numerous biases linked to the observational nature of the study and because they have not been confirmed by other authors. Therefore, this isolated finding should not raise fears about intercourse during implantation among couples seeking pregnancy.

13.5 Sex and Ectopic Pregnancy

Ectopic pregnancies, the classic form of which is tubal pregnancy, are a frequent cause of bleeding during the first trimester of pregnancy [18]. No published study has investigated the risk associated with intercourse in the case of ectopic pregnancy. The clinical presentation of ectopic pregnancies mainly associates mild dark intermenstrual bleeding with pelvic pain in a setting of delayed menstruation or pregnancy of unknown location. A pelvic examination can reveal an adnexal mass painful to the touch. Moreover, hemoperitoneum is frequently associated and can cause sharp pain in the pelvic region. Also, it is reasonable to think that pain generated during intercourse associated with vaginal bleeding in a setting of delayed menstruation or pregnancy of unknown location should point to a diagnosis of ectopic pregnancy. A prompt emergency work-up could lead to the diagnosis with an assay of plasma human chorionic gonadotropin and endovaginal ultrasound. There is no suggestion that sexual activity after fertilization increases or reduces the risk of ectopic pregnancy. Instead, ectopic pregnancy is linked to the patient's age, assisted conception, a history of ectopic pregnancy, smoking, previous pelvic surgery, and *Chlamydia trachomatis* infection of the upper genital tract [18].

13.6 Sex and Vaginal or Cervical Bleeding

Bleeding after sex during pregnancy is frequently reported. There is no question of abnormal placental insertion or the threat of premature delivery in the first trimester of pregnancy. Consequently, cervical or vaginal bleeding is probably associated with the physiological changes that accompany pregnancy [19].

A cervical ectropion causes slight bleeding, and a speculum examination highlights the ectropion, which bleeds upon contact. In this case, intercourse is generally painless, as is pelvic examination during the gynecological exam that reveals a closed cervix. Bleeding concomitant with intercourse, a known cervical ectropion, and the absence of pain are reassuring. Nevertheless, any suspected cervical or vaginal lesion should prompt a Pap smear test, perhaps combined with colposcopy and screening for human papillomavirus. Screening for cervical cancer is possible during the first trimester.

Vaginal or cervical bleeding worsened or produced by intercourse can also be caused by infections such as cervicitis or vaginal mycosis and by trauma such as vaginal lesions or ulcers. The risk of sexually transmitted infection is increased in unprotected sex and a setting of bleeding. This risk should not be overlooked in a situation suggestive of sexually transmitted disease (e.g. multiple partners, absence of screening, previous sexually transmitted disease) to enable appropriate medical management.

13.7 What Did Dr. Google Say?

In order to discover the online information available to the patient regarding sex and bleeding in the first trimester, we conducted an Internet search with a combination of the terms "sex," "sexual intercourse," "pregnancy," "bleeding," and "first trimester." The available information is consistent with the contents of this chapter, and is for the most part reassuring. The website www.healthline.com is the first one referenced and is the most detailed, explaining that "it's safe to have sex during all three trimesters" and that patients "may experience some new side effects such as vaginal spotting or bleeding after having sex . . . that is quite common (15 to 25 percent of women will experience bleeding during the first 12 weeks of pregnancy) with no need to worry." This website refers to a reliable source, the "Frequently Asked Questions" section of the website of the American College of Obstetricians and Gynecologists (ACOG) (www.acog.org/womens-health/faqs/bleeding-during-pregnancy). The various websites warn if the amount of blood is more than light spotting and, according to the ACOG, heavy bleeding after sex is not normal and should be addressed immediately. Concerning the risk of miscarriage in the first trimester, we found on the Healthonline.com website this information directly addressed to the patients, with which we agree: "sex doesn't cause you to miscarry, if you notice heavy bleeding after penetration, your pregnancy may be at risk of ending. Heavy vaginal bleeding that fills a pad every hour or lasts for several days is the most common sign of a miscarriage. Call your doctor right away if you're experiencing these symptoms." We encourage patients to consult only reliable sources of information, such as the official ACOG website, and to be especially wary of discussion forums where the available information is generally not relevant.

16.8 Conclusion

The literature lacks data on sexual activity and bleeding in the first trimester of pregnancy. To our knowledge, no study has specifically evaluated the impact of sexual intercourse in this setting. The sexuality of couples varies considerably, and a reduction in vaginal sex is expected at the start of pregnancy because of the physical and psychological changes that occur during pregnancy. It does not appear that sex, in whatever form, affects the progress of the pregnancy. There is an increased risk of first-trimester miscarriage when vaginal sex results in bleeding.

In contrast, this association between miscarriage and bleeding is statistically significant, but there is no indication that intercourse plays a harmful role. Bleeding in the first trimester of pregnancy, whether induced or preceded by intercourse, should prompt a gynecological examination combined with pelvic ultrasound to check that the pregnancy is progressing normally and is intrauterine. The lack of data in the scientific literature on the sexuality of women is indicative of the modesty of both pregnancy care teams and researchers and of a certain reluctance to study this question, albeit also fundamental, at the start of pregnancy. Sexuality is rarely addressed during care because of the inhibitions of women and their practitioners. Yet, it is an integral part of the well-being of couples and in the framework of overall care it is essential that obstetricians and gynecologists, whose work touches on the intimate relations between couples, provide women with advice based on robust data in the scientific literature without relying on beliefs or adopting a paternalistic attitude.

References

1. C. V. Ananth, D. A. Savitz. Vaginal bleeding and adverse reproductive outcomes: a meta-analysis. *Paediatr Perinat Epidemiol* 1994;**8**:62–78.

2. C. Everett. Incidence and outcome of bleeding before the 20th week of pregnancy: a prospective study from general practice. *BMJ* 1997;**315**:32–4.

3. R. Hasan, D. D. Baird, A. H. Herring, et al. Association between first-trimester vaginal bleeding and miscarriage. *Obstet Gynecol* 2009;**114**:860–7.

4. J. A. Lykke, K. L. Dideriksen, O. Lidegaard, J. Langhoff-Roos. First-trimester vaginal bleeding and complications later in pregnancy. *Obstet Gynecol* 2010;**115**:935–44.

5. S. Jawed-Wessel, E. Sevick. The impact of pregnancy and childbirth on sexual behaviors: a systematic review. *J Sex Res* 2017;**54**:411–23.

6. C. E. Johnson. Sexual health during pregnancy and the postpartum. *J Sex Med* 2011;**8**:1267–84.

7. K. von Sydow. Sexuality during pregnancy and after childbirth: a metacontent analysis of 59 studies. *J Psychosom Res* 1999;**47**:27–49.

8. S. R. Chang, K. H. Chen, H. H. Lin, H. J. Yu. Comparison of overall sexual function, sexual intercourse/activity, sexual satisfaction, and sexual desire during the three trimesters of pregnancy and assessment of their determinants. *J Sex Med* 2011;**8**:2859–67.

9. C. R. Gracia, M. D. Sammel, J. Chittams, et al. Risk factors for spontaneous abortion in early symptomatic first-trimester pregnancies. *Obstet Gynecol* 2005;**106**:993–9.

10. N. Maconochie, P. Doyle, S. Prior, R. Simmons. Risk factors for first trimester miscarriage: results from a UK-population-based case-control study. *BJOG* 2007;**114**:170–86.

11. S. Quenby, I. D. Gallos, R. K. Dhillon-Smith, et al. Miscarriage matters: the epidemiological, physical, psychological, and economic costs of early pregnancy loss. *Lancet* 2021;**397**:1658–67.

12. A. Coomarasamy, I. D. Gallos, A. Papadopoulou, et al. Sporadic miscarriage: evidence to provide effective care. *Lancet* 2021;**397**:1668–74.

13. A. Coomarasamy, R. K. Dhillon-Smith, A. Papadopoulou, et al. Recurrent miscarriage: evidence to accelerate action. *Lancet* 2021;**397**:1675–82.

14. A. Moscrop. Can sex during pregnancy cause a miscarriage? A concise history of not knowing. *Br J Gen Pract* 2012;**62**: e308–10.

15. E. W. Harville, A. J. Wilcox, D. D. Baird, C. R. Weinberg. Vaginal bleeding in very early pregnancy. *Hum Reprod* 2003;**18**:1944–7.

16. H. Speert, A. F. Guttmacher. Frequency and significance of bleeding in early pregnancy. *JAMA* 1954;**155**:712–15.

17. A. Z. Steiner, D. A. Pritchard, S. L. Young, A. H. Herring. Peri-implantation intercourse lowers fecundability. *Fertil Steril* 2014;**102**:178–82.

18. B. E. Seeber, K. T. Barnhart. Suspected ectopic pregnancy. *Obstet Gynecol* 2006;**107**:399–413.

19. S. Badir, E. Mazza, R. Zimmermann, M. Bajka. Cervical softening occurs early in pregnancy: characterization of cervical stiffness in 100 healthy women using the aspiration technique. *Prenat Diagn* 2013;**33**:737–41.

Chapter

14

Sex with Bleeding in the Second and Third Trimesters

Hisham T. Nasief, Duaa M. Bahkali, and Lawrence W. Oppenheimer

14.1 Introduction

This chapter tackles the issue of what advice to give pregnant women who are at risk of bleeding or who have experienced vaginal bleeding (antepartum hemorrhage) during pregnancy, either remote from or as a result of intercourse. This is a common concern raised by women in pregnancy. Historically, the standard advice in any of these situations has been to refrain from sexual intercourse. In the vast majority of cases, bleeding after sex in pregnancy is unlikely to be serious or to have any impact on the fetus. We examine the causes of bleeding and the risk in relation to sexual intercourse.

An extensive literature review was performed but there is very limited published information on which any recommendations can be grounded. The incidence of antepartum hemorrhage is about 19 per 1000 births when women reported no recent sex compared with 30 per 1000 when there had been recent sex [1]. We have summarized the available evidence and augmented this with commonsense advice and consensus opinion from other authors.

The causes of bleeding in pregnancy (antepartum hemorrhage) are divided into three categories:

1. Local causes from the cervix and vagina.
2. Placental abruptio (bleeding due to separation of a normally situated placenta).
3. Placenta previa (bleeding from a placenta that is lying close to or over the internal cervical os).

Bleeding can also be related to second-trimester pregnancy loss and preterm labor (see Chapters 16 and 26 for more details on preterm birth and stillbirth).

14.2 Local Causes/Trauma

In a nonpregnant woman, bleeding after intercourse (postcoital bleeding) is relatively common and the overall incidence is up to 9%. It is age-related and the annual incidence is 12.6%, 7.2%, and 4.8% for ages 18–24 years, 24–34 years, and 35–44 years, respectively [1,2]. During pregnancy, the external surface of the cervix within the vagina (external cervical os) undergoes some cellular changes due to the influence of increased hormones in pregnancy, particularly estrogen. This results in softening of the cervix in preparation for childbirth, with increased friability and vascularity of the surface epithelium. This is referred to as cervical erosion or ectropion and is a normal process visible on the cervix; it is exacerbated by pregnancy and can lead to bleeding if it is disturbed by, for example, vaginal examination or intercourse. While clinical examination may demonstrate that the bleeding is coming from the cervix, in pregnancy it can be difficult to differentiate this from abruption. Careful clinical assessment including an ultrasound examination is indicated. Only an ultrasound can exclude a low-lying placenta or placenta previa and will also provide reassurance on fetal health.

14.2.1 Recommendations

If a local cause of bleeding is suspected, it is very unlikely that it would be heavy or cause any actual damage, or that it would have any adverse effect on the fetus [3]. There is no reason to abstain from any sexual activity once the bleeding has had time to settle.

If cervical erosion is seen, the avoidance of deep penetration by the penis, which might result in contact with the cervix, is advisable, although in one case report no actual contact with the cervix was observed during sex in pregnancy [4].

Recurrent hemorrhage is an indication for reassessment, particularly as one cannot rule out abruption with certainty.

14.3 Placental Abruption

Placental abruption is the term used to describe separation of the placenta from its implantation site in the uterus before delivery, with an incidence of around 1% [5]. Approximately 50% of placental abruptions occur before 36 weeks of gestation, often resulting in preterm birth. In a severe case there can be fetal death and maternal morbidity. When vaginal bleeding is persistent and recurrent, the risk of a more severe abruption is increased. However, mild abruption is a much more common presentation with slight vaginal bleeding and a healthy fetus. The sensitivity of ultrasound to detect abruption is low, and the scan is often normal even in the presence of significant bleeding. Risk factors for placental abruption include multiparity, advanced maternal age, smoking, hypertensive disorders, chorioamnionitis, and preterm rupture of membranes [6]. During sexual activity systolic blood pressure was demonstrated to be increased from the baseline and might be a factor in placental abruption in a pregnancy with preexisting hypertension [7]. Most abruptions are thought to start with rupture of a decidual arteriole, which leads to retroplacental hemorrhage. This might explain why the hemorrhages increase in frequency when women smoke cigarettes or develop gestational hypertension, since both smoking and hypertension damage arterioles.

It has been reported that coitus within 48 hours preceding delivery is significantly correlated with placental abruption, with coitus occurring in 21% of those with abruption compared with 3% in the group with no abruption [8]. In the largest prospective study of coitus and antepartum hemorrhage, the frequency of hemorrhage was around one-third higher in women who reported coitus versus those with no coitus since the last antenatal visit before admission [9]. Coitus was found to be associated with antepartum hemorrhage, independent of other risk factors that predispose to bleeding. A strong association has been found between coitus and deciduo-chorioamnionitis, which is a significant risk factor for abruption [10]. Hemorrhage may be due to blood vessel damage caused by the inflammation in the decidua. There are two case reports in the third trimester of placental abruption and intrauterine fetal death after orgasmic coitus. One involved a 38-year-old grand multiparous woman at 29 weeks of gestation, known to have gestational hypertension and taking nifedipine, who started to have abdominal pain and vaginal bleeding 2 hours after orgasmic coitus leading to severe abruption [11]. In another case report with similar features, fetal death occurred in a 29-year-old multiparous woman at 38 weeks of gestation immediately after orgasmic coitus [12]. Case reports suggested that nipple stimulation or breastfeeding could have led to oxytocin release stimulating uterine contractions resulting in placental abruption, particularly when there were preexisting risk factors for placental abruption [13,14].

These reports are anecdotal and the paucity of information about abruption caused by coitus suggests that it is probably a rare phenomenon. Although practicing sex is safe during pregnancy, especially in a low-risk cohort, the data are limited regarding high-risk pregnancies [15].

14.3.1 Recommendations

14.3.1.1 Risk Factors for Abruption

In women who have minor risk factors for abruption and no history of bleeding, there is no reason to avoid sexual intercourse, although in the presence of significantly raised blood pressure, the further increase in blood pressure caused by sex could be detrimental.

14.3.1.2 Mild Abruption or Unexplained Bleeding

The most common situation is when a pregnant woman has experienced a minor degree of vaginal bleeding, attributed to a small abruption that has settled down. In the second half of pregnancy, patients are often admitted to the hospital for a period of observation, but once the bleeding has stopped they may be sent home and managed as an outpatient. Sexual stimulation and penetrative acts with or without the presence of orgasm need not be limited unless frequent, intense, or painful uterine contractions occur. Any further significant bleeding is an indication to cease sexual activity.

Any sexual activity that results in bleeding should be avoided.

14.4 Placenta Previa

Placenta previa is the term used to describe a placenta that is implanted low down in the uterus close to or over the cervix, instead of the usual location at the fundus of the uterus. Placenta previa may be suspected based on the presence of vaginal bleeding and an unstable fetal lie in the third trimester, but because of the ubiquitous use of ultrasound it is usually diagnosed as an asymptomatic finding in early pregnancy. If a low placenta is suspected on routine ultrasound, the exact location of the edge of the placenta in relation to the internal cervical os can be measured by examining the lower uterus and cervix using transvaginal ultrasound and a specialized probe. A simplified classification has been recommended: (1) placenta previa, where the placenta is covering the cervical os; (2) low-lying placenta, where the placental edge is within 2 cm of the cervical os; and (3) normal placental location, with the placental edge more than 2 cm from the cervical os (no increase in risk of antepartum hemorrhage or cesarean delivery) [16]. However, at the time of the routine anatomy scan at around 20 weeks, the diagnosis is provisional only as in many cases the placental position changes with growth of the uterus. It is recommended that a repeat scan be performed at 32 weeks or more to confirm the diagnosis. When an overlap of around 20 mm is noted at 18–23 weeks of gestation, placenta previa will persist in approximately less than half of cases.

The principal risk of placenta previa is maternal hemorrhage rather than fetal blood from the uterine side of the placenta where it is exposed by the close proximity to the cervix. A low placenta gives rise to hemorrhage in 0.5% of all pregnancies [17].

The risk of hemorrhage is related to the proximity to the internal cervical os, as described previously. Other factors, such as the thickness of the placental edge, also affect the risk. In general, the greater the degree of encroachment to, or overlap of, the cervix, the greater the risk of hemorrhage. When there is placenta previa (overlap of the cervix) and a placental edge thickness greater than 1 cm, the risk of hemorrhage after 20 weeks of gestation was 88% [16]. All cases of placenta previa are managed by cesarean section either electively close to term or, infrequently, as a result of preterm vaginal bleeding. Most cases of bleeding with previa can be managed expectantly and do not result in preterm delivery. When the placenta is low-lying but does not cover the cervix, the incidence of bleeding was reported to be 29% when the edge was within 10 mm of the cervix and 3% when it was within 11–20 mm [18]. Other risk factors for more severe bleeding include women with a history of bleeding in early pregnancy and prior cesarean section, particularly where there is ultrasound evidence of a morbidly adherent placenta.

There is general agreement to avoid any digital manipulation or cervical examination in placenta previa. It is clear from historical experience that touching a placenta previa through a partially dilated cervix can result in severe hemorrhage. This concern has been extrapolated to vaginal penetration in sexual intercourse. However, it is very unlikely that penetration of the cervix can occur during sex. A study using magnetic resonance imaging (MRI) showed that the penis might be in direct contact with the anterior fornix in the missionary position or the posterior fornix with the rear-entry position but not inside the cervix [19]. There is also evidence of the safety of using a vaginal ultrasound probe. A study examining the angle of the cervix related to the transducer concluded that transvaginal ultrasound was safe because the probe does not enter the cervical canal, and the use of vaginal sonography appears to be safe even when performed in the presence of vaginal bleeding [20].

Bleeding with placenta previa often occurs in the absence of contractions. However, 20% of patients who present with bleeding from placenta previa also report uterine contractions. It is unclear if bleeding from the placenta previa causes contractions or if uterine contractions are the cause of the bleeding. The risk of hemorrhage leading to delivery may be associated with cervical shortening and uterine contractility. In women with a cervix less than 3 cm long, there was evidence of contractions in 70%, and 79% required delivery because of hemorrhage. Conversely, when the cervix was greater than 3 cm, only 21% demonstrated contractions and only 36% had an episode of bleeding [21].

Opinions on the safety of sexual intercourse with placenta previa vary widely. The presence of placenta previa influences sexual practice because of fear of bleeding and associated adverse events. There is no conclusive evidence to support bedrest, reduced activity, or avoidance of intercourse [22]. The risk of bleeding or more catastrophic events with sexual activity in pregnancies complicated by a previa is based on extrapolation of nonsexual acts. The 25th edition of *Williams Obstetrics* [17] continues to provide the time-worn advice of "pelvic rest" following bleeding due to placenta previa. One guideline recommends avoidance of vaginal or anal sexual activity and insertion of any foreign object into the anus/rectum or the vagina, such as a tampon [16]. An opinion on the UpToDate website states the following [23]:

> We advise women with placenta previa after 20 weeks of gestation (earlier if they have experienced vaginal bleeding) to avoid any sexual activity that may lead to orgasm. The

rationale is that this activity, especially if orgasm occurs, may be associated with transient uterine contractions, which, in turn, may provoke bleeding. Additionally, there is concern that vaginal intercourse (or putting any object deep into the vagina) might cause direct trauma to the previa, resulting in bleeding. There are no published studies that either support or refute this recommendation.

14.4.1 Recommendations

Where placenta previa is suspected prior to approximately 20 weeks, in the absence of bleeding or until the placental location has been confirmed by a later ultrasound scan, gentle coitus is acceptable although women should be warned of the possibility of bleeding. Given the lack of any clear data regarding sexual intercourse and placental previa, it seems logical to individualize recommendations based on the background risk of hemorrhage according to the above classification of placenta previa.

14.4.1.1 Normal Placental Location

Where the edge of the placenta lies greater than 2 cm from the cervical os, the risk of bleeding is approximately the same as in a normal pregnancy and sexual activity of any kind need not be restricted.

14.4.1.2 Low-Lying Placenta

Where the placenta edge is within 2 cm of the internal cervical os, the risk of bleeding during the pregnancy rises with proximity to the os but the risk of severe hemorrhage is low. In a woman who has not bled, gentle vaginal intercourse including orgasm may be acceptable. If contractions or bleeding does occur, it would be safest to avoid any further penetrative sex.

14.4.1.3 Placenta Previa

Where there is true placenta previa with the placental edge overlapping the cervical os, gentle sex may be permissible but the avoidance of orgasmic sex or any activity that results in contractions is preferable.

Where there has been an initial episode of bleeding that has settled (sentinel bleed), sexual activity need not be restricted if the cervix remains greater than 3 cm in length, with the exception of higher-risk cases where the placental edge is thick or there is a significant degree of overlap.

There is no evidence to support or refute the safety of nonpenetrative sexual activity with or without orgasm or anal penetration. If it does not result in patient-perceived uterine contractions, such activity need not be restricted after the sentinel bleeding episode.

14.5 What Did Dr. Google Say?

The information available to patients on the Internet was consulted. Using a web search engine, the terms "bleeding," "sex," "second trimester," or "third trimester" were used to obtain information for the second half of pregnancy while avoiding sites that discussed mainly first-trimester bleeding (discussed in the previous chapter). The terms "abruption" and "placenta previa" were later added to search for the specific conditions discussed in this chapter.

In an article at www.healthline.com commenting on bleeding after sex during pregnancy, the most frequent causes of bleeding in pregnancy are discussed (implantation bleeding, cervical ectropion), but placental abruption and placenta previa are also mentioned with both conditions explained briefly: "sex isn't a cause of placenta previa, but penetration can cause bleeding" [24]. Another article at www.parents.com discusses causes of bleeding, noting that most of the cases are related to the physiological changes of pregnancy, but also mentioning placenta previa and abruption [25].

In general, most sites recommend seeking medical attention in cases of heavy bleeding, notifying a healthcare provider of light bleeding during clinical visits [26,27]. Some will also mention that sex should be avoided in any case until the bleeding ceases.

Patients should trust sites that contain articles written by health professionals and quoting and referencing medical articles in order to obtain the most accurate information.

14.6 Conclusions

There are very few published studies regarding sexual activity and bleeding in pregnancy on which to base any recommendations. The suggestions in this chapter are the opinions of the authors and others (Level III evidence). Advice should be tailored to the patient's individual circumstances, comorbidities, and fears and concerns of both her and her partner. Any bleeding during pregnancy can be alarming and many pregnant women prefer to avoid sex altogether following even minor complications.

References

1. C. M. Tarney, J. Han. Postcoital bleeding: a review on etiology, diagnosis, and management. *Obstet Gynecol Int* 2014;**2014**:192087.

2. M. Shapley, K. Jordan, P. R. Croft. An epidemiological survey of symptoms of menstrual loss in the community. *Br J Gen Pract* 2004;**54**:359–63.

3. P. M. Casey, M. E. Long, M. L. Marnach. Abnormal cervical appearance: what to do, when to worry? *Mayo Clin Proc* 2011;**86**:147–50.

4. O. Buisson, P. Foldes, E. Jannini, S. Mimoun. Coitus as revealed by ultrasound in one volunteer couple. *J Sex Med* 2010;**7**:2750–4.

5. C. V. Ananth, J. A. Lavery, A. M. Vintzileos, et al. Severe placental abruption: clinical definition and associations with maternal complications. *Am J Obstet Gynecol* 2016;**214**:272.e1–9.

6. M. Tikkanen. Placental abruption: epidemiology, risk factors and consequences. *Acta Obstet Gynecol Scand* 2011;**90**:140–9.

7. S. T. Palmeri, J. B. Kostis, L. Casazza, et al. Heart rate and blood pressure response in adult men and women during exercise and sexual activity. *Am J Cardiol* 2007;**100**:1795–801.

8. A. L. Brink, H. J. Odendaal. Risk factors for abruptio placentae. *S Afr Med J* 1987;**72**:250–2.

9. R. L. Naeye. Coitus and antepartum haemorrhage. *Br J Obstet Gynaecol* 1981;**88**:765–70.

10. R. L. Naeye. Coitus and associated amniotic-fluid infections. *N Engl J Med* 1979;**301**:1198–200.

11. M. Zsoldos, M. Vezér, H. Pusztafalvi, et al. Orgasmic coitus triggered stillbirth via placental abruption: a case report. *Arch Case Rep* 2019;**3**:56–8.

12. M. E. Aziken. Abruptio placenta following sexual intercourse: case report. *Niger Postgrad Med J* 2003;**10**:113–14.

13. R. N. Taylor, J. R. Green. Abruptio placentae following nipple stimulation. *Am J Perinatol* 1987;**4**:94–7.

14. S. Eckford, J. Westgate. Breast-feeding and placental abruption. *J Obstet Gynaecol* 1997;**17**:164–5.

15. C. Jones, C. Chan, D. Farine. Sex in pregnancy. *Can Med Assoc J* 2011;**183**:815–18.

16. V. Jain, H. Bos, E. Bujold. Guideline No. 402. Diagnosis and management of placenta previa. *J Obstet Gynaecol Can* 2020;**42**:906–17.

17. F. Cunningham, K. J. Levono, S. L. Bloom, et al., eds. Obstetrical hemorrhage. In *Williams Obstetrics*, 25th ed. New York: McGraw-Hill, 2018.

18. P. Vergani, S. Ornaghi, I. Pozzi, et al. Placenta previa: distance to internal os and mode of delivery. *Am J Obstet Gynecol* 2009;**201**:266.e1–5.

19. A. Faix, J. F. Lapray, O. Callede, A. Maubon, K. Lanfrey. Magnetic resonance imaging (MRI) of sexual intercourse: second experience in missionary position and initial experience in posterior position. *J Sex Marital Ther* 2002;**28**:63–76.

20. I. E. Timor-Tritsch, R. A. Yunis. Confirming the safety of transvaginal sonography in patients suspected of placenta previa. *Obstet Gynecol* 1993;**81**:742–4.

21. I. A. Stafford, J. S. Dashe, S. A. Shivvers, et al. Ultrasonographic cervical length and risk of hemorrhage in pregnancies with placenta previa. *Obstet Gynecol* 2010;**116**:595–600.

22. K. P. Rao, V. Belogolovkin, J. Yankowitz, J. A. Spinnato II. Abnormal placentation: evidence-based diagnosis and management of placenta previa, placenta accreta, and vasa previa. *Obstet Gynecol Surv* 2012;**67**:503–19.

23. C. J. Lockwood, K. Russo-Stieglitz. Placenta previa: management. www .uptodate.com/contents/placenta-previa-management (accessed April 2, 2021).

24. S. Lindberg. Is bleeding after sex while pregnant cause for concern? www .healthline.com/health/pregnancy/ bleeding-after-sex-during-pregnancy#serious-causes (accessed September 17, 2021).

25. N. Harris. Bleeding after sex while pregnant: should I worry? www.parents .com/pregnancy/my-life/sex-relationship/ bleeding-after-sex-while-pregnant-should-i-worry/ (accessed September 17, 2021).

26. Emma's Diary. Is it normal to bleed after sex during pregnancy? www.emmasdiary .co.uk/wellbeing/prenatal/is-bleeding-after-sex-during-pregnancy-normal (accessed September 17, 2021).

27. M. Kuna. Bleeding after sex during pregnancy. Is it normal? www .babydoppler.com/blog/bleeding-after-sex-during-pregnancy-is-it-normal/ (accessed September 17, 2021).

Short Cervix and Sex

Yara Maia Villar de Carvalho, Francisco Marcelo Carvalho, Beatriz Maria Villar de Carvalho, and Eduardo Borges da Fonseca

15.1 Introduction

Spontaneous preterm birth (PTB) refers to a delivery that occurs between weeks 20 and 37 of pregnancy because of preterm labor (PTL, 40–50%), preterm prelabor rupture of membranes (PPROM, 20–30%), or short cervical length at mid-trimester. The three most common risk factors for PTB are prior history of preterm delivery, twin pregnancy, and short cervix at mid-trimester ultrasound [1–3]. Several studies have demonstrated that short cervical length is the most powerful predictor for PTB in the index pregnancy for both singleton and twin pregnancies [4–6].

15.1.1 Short Sonographic Cervical Length: A Powerful Predictor of Preterm Delivery

Cervical endovaginal scan is the best method for assessing cervical length [4,6–9]. The shorter the sonographic cervical length in the mid-trimester, the higher the risk of spontaneous PTL and delivery [6].

A short cervical length indicates that the measured length of the cervix is shorter than expected for the current gestational age. Contemporary clinical practice assumes that the cutoff value should be between 20 and 25 mm [4,6–9].

A sonographic short cervix (Figure 15.1), defined as a length of less than 25 mm during mid-gestation, is the most powerful predictor of PTB [6,9]. However, compared with using a cutoff cervical length of less than 25 mm, a customized cervical length assessment by maternal characteristics, such as prior history of spontaneous PTB and gestational age at sonographic examination, identifies more women at risk of spontaneous PTB and also improves the distinction between patients at risk for impending PTB in those who have an episode of PTL [6].

15.1.2 Singleton Asymptomatic Pregnancies

In a population-based prospective multicenter study in 39 284 women with singleton pregnancies attending for routine hospital antenatal care, the median cervical length was 36 mm. In addition, the cervix measured ≤30 mm, ≤25 mm, ≤20 mm, and ≤15 mm in 18.6%, 8.1%, 3.4%, and 1.0% of pregnancies, respectively [10].

15.1.3 Twin Asymptomatic Pregnancies

In 1163 twin pregnancies attending for routine antenatal care, the rate of delivery before 32 weeks was inversely related to cervical length, being 66% for 10 mm, 24% for 20 mm,

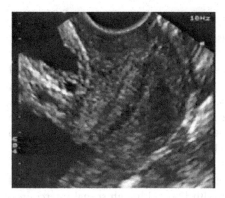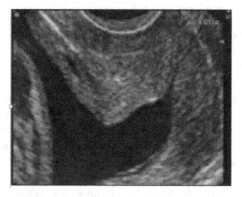

Figure 15.1 Sonographic appearance of normal cervix (left) and short cervix (right) with transvaginal ultrasound.

12% for 25 mm, and less than 1% for 40 mm [11]. The median cervical length was 35 mm and the length was 25 mm or less in about 16% of women, 20 mm or less in 8%, and 15 mm or less in 5% [11].

15.1.4 Symptomatic Pregnancies

In pregnant women presenting with premature uterine contractions, sonographic measurement of cervical length at evaluation can help to distinguish between those women who do and those who do not deliver within the subsequent 7 days. In the combined data from three sonographic studies in a total of 532 singleton pregnancies presenting with threatened PTL at 24–36 weeks, delivery within 7 days occurred in 49% of those with a cervical length of less than 15 mm and in 1.2% of those with a cervical length of 15 mm or more [12–14]. Tsoi et al. [15] evaluated 510 pregnancies with threatened PTL, and the PTB rate within 48 hours and 7 days was 4.1% (21/510) and 8.4% (43/510), respectively. In such a population, there was an indirect relationship between cervical length and PTB within both 48 hours and 7 days. For those 171 pregnant women having a measured cervix of 20 mm or less, 21 delivered prematurely within 48 hours (12.3%) and 42 (24.6%) within 7 days. Therefore, the majority (75.4%) of those who had a very short cervical length (≤20 mm) did not deliver within 7 days [15].

This chapter aims to identify the scientific evidence to address the recommendations regarding sexual intercourse in those pregnant women with a short cervical length at mid-trimester or with an arrested episode of PTL.

15.2 Sexual Activity and Orgasm as Triggers of Spontaneous Preterm Delivery

Sexual intercourse by itself is not a demonstrated risk factor for PTB, and therefore abstinence after pregnancy has been achieved has no role in strategies for prevention of PTB [1,2,16,17]. In addition, most sexual positions and noncoital activities (oral sex, masturbation, etc.) during late pregnancy are not clearly associated with adverse pregnancy outcomes [17,18].

15.2.1 Sexual Intercourse

Sexual intercourse (or coitus or copulation) is sexual activity typically involving the insertion and thrusting of the penis into the vagina for sexual pleasure, reproduction, or both [19]. This is also known as vaginal intercourse or vaginal sex [20]. Other forms of penetrative sexual intercourse include anal sex (penetration of the anus by the penis), oral sex (penetration of the mouth by the penis or oral penetration of the female genitalia), fingering (sexual penetration by the fingers), and penetration using a dildo (especially a strap-on dildo) [21]. These activities involve physical intimacy between two or more individuals and are usually used among humans solely for physical or emotional pleasure and can contribute to human bonding [22].

There are different views on what constitutes sexual intercourse or other sexual activity, which can impact on views on sexual health [23]. Although sexual intercourse, particularly the term coitus, generally denotes penile–vaginal penetration and the possibility of creating offspring, it also commonly denotes penetrative oral sex and penile–anal sex, especially the latter [19,24]. It usually encompasses sexual penetration, while nonpenetrative sex has been labeled "outercourse," but nonpenetrative sex may also be considered sexual intercourse [25,26]. Sex, often a shorthand for sexual intercourse, can mean any form of sexual activity [23].

15.2.2 Orgasm

Orgasm or sexual climax is the sudden discharge of accumulated sexual excitement during the sexual response cycle, resulting in rhythmic muscular contractions in the pelvic region characterized by sexual pleasure [27,28] (see Chapter 4 for more details on orgasm). For both males and females, orgasms are controlled by the involuntary or autonomic nervous system. They are usually associated with involuntary actions, including muscular spasms in multiple areas of the body, a general euphoric sensation and, frequently, body movements and vocalizations [28].

The period after orgasm, known as the refractory period, is typically a relaxing experience, attributed to the release of the neurohormones oxytocin and prolactin as well as endorphins [29].

Human orgasms usually result from physical sexual stimulation of the penis in males (typically accompanying ejaculation) and of the clitoris in females [28,30,31]. Sexual stimulation can be by self-practice or with a sex partner (penetrative sex, nonpenetrative sex, or other sexual activity).

The health effects surrounding the human orgasm are diverse. There are many physiological responses during sexual activity, including a relaxed state created by prolactin, as well as changes in the central nervous system such as a temporary decrease in the metabolic activity of large parts of the cerebral cortex while there is no change or increased metabolic activity in the limbic (i.e. "bordering") areas of the brain [32].

15.3 Is Sexual Activity in a Patient with a Short Cervix Safe?

There is inadequate empirical evidence for making recommendations to couples about the safety of sexual activity during pregnancy. Many studies had methodological problems and yielded conflicting results [33–37]. Only a few studies were controlled for potential confounders [37–40]. Many studies have assessed sexual activity for preterm cases and term controls at different gestational ages [39,41–43]. Such comparisons are biased because the frequency of sexual activity declines throughout pregnancy, particularly in the last weeks [34,44,45]. And, to the best of our knowledge, there are no studies in women with mid-trimester short cervix or in those with a short cervix after arrested PTL.

Sayle et al. [46] examined the association between sexual intercourse and orgasm in late pregnancy and preterm delivery using information on sexual activity obtained through standardized interviews conducted at similar gestational ages for 187 cases who delivered prematurely and 409 controls. They did not find evidence that sexual activity in late pregnancy increased a woman's risk of PTB between 29 and 36 weeks. Previous studies that also compared sexual activity at similar gestational ages for cases and controls also tended to find a reduced risk of preterm delivery with sexual activity [37,38,40,47,48].

Indeed, among women in the Collaborative Perinatal Project, a higher frequency of intercourse in late pregnancy was significantly associated with longer gestation [38]. In a prospective study of 13 285 women, PTB was less common among women who had intercourse at least once per week at 23–26 weeks (odds ratio [OR] 0.85, 95% confidence interval [CI] 0.75, 0.95) [40]. There is one report that found a positive relationship between intercourse and risk of preterm delivery among 18 women with idiopathic PTL compared with 111 women delivering at term who were interviewed at comparable gestational ages [49].

Most studies that evaluated sexual activity focused on intercourse. Some have considered the effects of orgasm but usually only in the context of intercourse. An old study by Masters and Johnson in 1960 [50] suggested that in nonpregnant women, orgasms resulting from masturbation were associated with stronger uterine contractions than orgasms resulting from sexual intercourse.

Sayle et al. [46] found that orgasm during late pregnancy was associated with reduced risk of PTB regardless of whether women reported having intercourse during the same period. Few studies have reported that orgasm with last coitus was associated with a reduced risk of PTB [43,49]. A study by Perkins [41] found a reduced risk of PTB associated with orgasm with or without intercourse. In contrast, Goodlin et al. [42]-reported that twice as many cases of PTB as controls had orgasm after 32 weeks, and Ekwo et al. [39] reported that orgasm was associated with preterm PROM (OR 1.9, 95% CI 1.0, 3.9), but that study compared orgasm in the 4 weeks before delivery for preterm cases and term controls, which likely overestimated any association because frequency of orgasm would likely decline with advancing gestation.

There is consensus that digital vaginal examination and vaginal intercourse should be avoided to reduce the risk of intrauterine infection in cases of PPROM [17,18]. Therefore, many physicians discourage sexual intercourse without distinction among vaginal, anal, or oral sexual activity after PPROM. However, in a case–control study of PPROM with controls matched by gestational age, the OR for intercourse within 7 days before delivery or interview was 0.5 (95% CI 0.4, 0.7) [47].

Infection might modify the effect of sexual activity on risk of PTB. Sayle et al. [46] found no association between sexual activity and PTB according to bacterial vaginosis status. However, Read and Klebanoff [40] found that frequent intercourse among pregnant women with bacterial vaginosis was associated with increased risk of PTB, whereas among those without bacterial vaginosis, frequent intercourse was associated with a reduced risk of PTB.

Extrapolating the data from these studies, we can conclude that there is no absolute contraindication for sexual intercourse in asymptomatic pregnant women with a mid-trimester short cervix, or for those with a short cervix after an arrested episode of PTL. Nevertheless, taking into account that the first-line treatment for such cases is vaginal progesterone, we advise patients with arrested PTL or with mid-trimester short cervical length to consider avoiding vaginal intercourse, or any sexual intercourse, if they experience an increased frequency or intensity of contractions afterwards [51–55].

There is no strong evidence that sexual activity affects the risk of PTB or onset of labor in healthy individuals (see Chapters 16 and 22 for more details on preterm birth and labor induction). However, it is theoretically possible that a small subgroup of susceptible women, especially those with a very short cervix (≤5–10 mm) with or without bulging membranes, may develop PTL with sexual intercourse because both the prostaglandins in semen and the orgasm increase myometrial activity [19,46,56,57].

15.4 What Did Dr. Google Say?

When introducing the terms "short cervix" and "sex" in a web search engine, different results arise along with general information regarding the recommendations of pelvic rest and sex during pregnancy.

Some results include articles written by medical professionals. In www.verywellfamily.com, for example, the specific situation of a shortened cervix is reviewed [58]. No recommendations are given after briefly explaining what a short cervix is, apart from discussing pelvic rest with a healthcare provider. At the website of the International Society for Sexual Medicine, a brief summary of a medical article states "sexual activity is safe as long as there is no bleeding, increases in uterine contractions, or worsening cervical length" in patients with a short cervix [59]. Another article that reviews the diagnosis, management, and prognosis of short cervix in pregnancy notes that bedrest may be recommended, as well as avoiding sex [60].

Journalists or other nonmedical professionals are the authors of other hits. At https://maternity-matters.com.au, again it redirects patients to seek medical advice, but states that in patients with a short cervix or a cerclage "sex, even orgasm via masturbation, is *not* recommended" [61]. Other sites explain that sex may be restricted, as well as bedrest recommended, addressing the prostaglandin content of semen [62].

References

1. E. B. da Fonseca, R. Damiao, D. A. Moreira. Preterm birth prevention. *Best Pract Res Clin Obstet Gynaecol* 2020;**69**:40–9.

2. R. Romero, S. K. Dey, S. J. Fisher. Preterm labor: one syndrome, many causes. *Science* 2014;**345**:760–5.

3. J. P. Vogel, S. Chawanpaiboon, A. B. Moller, et al. The global epidemiology of preterm birth. *Best Pract Res Clin Obstet Gynaecol* 2018;**52**:3–12.

4. V. C. Heath, T. R. Southall, A. P. Souka, A. Elisseou, K. H. Nicolaides. Cervical length at 23 weeks of gestation: prediction of spontaneous preterm delivery. *Ultrasound Obstet Gynecol* 1998;**12**:312–17.

5. V. C. Heath, T. R. Southall, A. P. Souka, A. Novakov, K. H. Nicolaides. Cervical length at 23 weeks of gestation: relation to demographic characteristics and previous obstetric history. *Ultrasound Obstet Gynecol* 1998;**12**:304–11.

6. D. W. Gudicha, R. Romero, D. Kabiri, et al. Personalized assessment of cervical length improves prediction of spontaneous preterm birth: a standard and a percentile calculator. *Am J Obstet Gynecol* 2021;**224**:288.e1–17.

7. J. D. Iams, R. L. Goldenberg, P. J. Meis, et al. The length of the cervix and the risk of spontaneous premature delivery. *N Engl J Med* 1996;**334**:567–72.

8. S. S. Hassan, R. Romero, S. M. Berry, et al. Patients with an ultrasonographic cervical length ≤15 mm have nearly a 50% risk of early spontaneous preterm delivery. *Am J Obstet Gynecol* 2000;**182**:1458–67.

9. R. Romero. Prevention of spontaneous preterm birth: the role of sonographic cervical length in identifying patients who may benefit from progesterone treatment. *Ultrasound Obstet Gynecol* 2007;**30**:675–86.

10. M. S. To, C. A. Skentou, P. Royston, C. K. Yu, K. H. Nicolaides. Prediction of patient-specific risk of early preterm delivery using maternal history and sonographic measurement of cervical length: a population-based prospective study. *Ultrasound Obstet Gynecol* 2006;**27**:362–7.

11. M. S. To, E. B. Fonseca, F. S. Molina, A. M. Cacho, K. H. Nicolaides. Maternal characteristics and cervical length in the prediction of spontaneous early preterm delivery in twins. *Am J Obstet Gynecol* 2006;**194**:1360–5.

12. E. Tsoi, S. Akmal, S. Rane, C. Otigbah, K. H. Nicolaides. Ultrasound assessment of cervical length in threatened preterm labor. *Ultrasound Obstet Gynecol* 2003;**21**:552–5.

13. I. Fuchs, E. Tsoi, W. Henrich, J. W. Dudenhausen, K. H. Nicolaides. Sonographic measurement of cervical length in twin pregnancies in threatened preterm labor. *Ultrasound Obstet Gynecol* 2004;**23**:42–5.

14. E. Tsoi, L. Geerts, B. Jeffery, H. J. Odendaal, K. H. Nicolaides. Sonographic cervical length in threatened preterm labor in a South African population. *Ultrasound Obstet Gynecol* 2004;**24**:644–6.

15. E. Tsoi, I. B. Fuchs, S. Rane, L. Geerts, K. H. Nicolaides. Sonographic measurement of cervical length in threatened preterm labor in singleton pregnancies with intact membranes. *Ultrasound Obstet Gynecol* 2005;**25**:353–6.

16. H. Lipworth, L. Hiersch, D. Farine, J. F. R. Barrett, N. Melamed. Current practice of maternal–fetal medicine specialists regarding the prevention and management of preterm birth in twin gestations. *J Obstet Gynaecol Can* 2021;**43**:831–8.

17. E. Maisonneuve. [Lifestyle recommendations for prevention of spontaneous preterm birth in asymptomatic pregnant women]. *J Gynecol Obstet Biol Reprod (Paris)* 2016;**45**:1231–46.

18. S. Hernandez-Diaz, C. E. Boeke, A. T. Romans, et al. Triggers of spontaneous preterm delivery: why today? *Paediatr Perinat Epidemiol* 2014;**28**:79–87.

19. R. M. Lerner, L. Steinberg, eds. *Handbook of Adolescent Psychology*. Hoboken, NJ: John Wiley & Sons, 2004: 193–6.

20. J. L. Carroll. *Sexuality Now: Embracing Diversity*. Boston: Cengage Learning, 2018: 289.

21. Sexual intercourse. https://en.wikipedia.org/wiki/Sexual_intercourse

22. L. Freberg. *Discovering Biological Psychology*. Boston: Cengage Learning, 2009: 308–10.

23. World Health Organization, Department of Reproductive Health and Research. *Defining Sexual Health: Report of a Technical Consultation on Sexual Health 28–31 January 2002, Geneva*. Geneva: World Health Organization, 2006.

24. N. W. Denney, D. Quadagno. *Human Sexuality*. St. Louis, MO: Mosby-Year Book, 1988: 273.

25. D. Hales. *An Invitation to Health: Live It Now! Brief Edition*. Boston: Cengage Learning, 2015: 251.

26. A. P. Kahn, J. Fawcett. *The Encyclopedia of Mental Health*. New York: Infobase Publishing, 2008: 111.

27. P. Winn. *Dictionary of Biological Psychology*. London: Routledge, 2003: 1189.

28. M. Rosenthal. *Human Sexuality: From Cells to Society*. Boston: Cengage Learning, 2012.

29. M. S. Exton, T. H. Kruger, M. Koch, et al. Coitus-induced orgasm stimulates prolactin secretion in healthy subjects. *Psychoneuroendocrinology* 2001;**26**:287–94.

30. W. Weiten, D. S. Dunn, E. Y. Hammer. *Psychology Applied to Modern Life: Adjustment in the 21st Century*. Boston: Cengage Learning, 2011: 386.

31. H. E. O'Connell, K. V. Sanjeevan, J. M. Hutson. Anatomy of the clitoris. *J Urol* 2005;**174**:1189–95.

32. J. R. Georgiadis, A. A. Reinders, A. M. Paans, R. Renken, R. Kortekaas. Men versus women on sexual brain function: prominent differences during tactile genital stimulation, but not during orgasm. *Hum Brain Mapp* 2009;**30**:3089–101.

33. G. S. Berkowitz, E. Papiernik. Epidemiology of preterm birth. *Epidemiol Rev* 1993;**15**:414–43.

34. D. A. Solberg, J. Butler, N. N. Wagner. Sexual behavior in pregnancy. *N Engl J Med* 1973;**288**:1098–103.

35. N. N. Wagner, J. C. Butler, J. P. Sanders. Prematurity and orgasmic coitus during pregnancy: data on a small sample. *Fertil Steril* 1976;**27**:911–15.

36. J. P. Neilson, M. Mutambira. Coitus, twin pregnancy, and preterm labor. *Am J Obstet Gynecol* 1989;**160**:416–18.

37. J. L. Mills, S. Harlap, E. E. Harley. Should coitus late in pregnancy be discouraged? *Lancet* 1981;**318**:136–8.

38. M. A. Klebanoff, R. P. Nugent, G. G. Rhoads. Coitus during pregnancy: is it safe? *Lancet* 1984;**324**:914–17.

39. E. E. Ekwo, C. A. Gosselink, R. Woolson, A. Moawad, C. R. Long. Coitus late in pregnancy: risk of preterm rupture of amniotic sac membranes. *Am J Obstet Gynecol* 1993;**168**:22–31.

40. J. S. Read, M. A. Klebanoff. Sexual intercourse during pregnancy and preterm delivery: effects of vaginal microorganisms. *Am J Obstet Gynecol* 1993;**168**:514–19.

41. R. P. Perkins. Sexual behavior and response in relation to complications of pregnancy. *Am J Obstet Gynecol* 1979;**134**:498–505.

42. R. C. Goodlin, D. W. Keller, M. Raffin. Orgasm during late pregnancy. Possible deleterious effects. *Obstet Gynecol* 1971;**38**:916–20.

43. P. A. Georgakopoulos, D. Dodos, D. Mechleris. Sexuality in pregnancy and premature labour. *Br J Obstet Gynaecol* 1984;**91**:891–3.

44. N. M. Morris. The frequency of sexual intercourse during pregnancy. *Arch Sex Behav* 1975;**4**:501–7.

45. K. Reamy, S. E. White, W. C. Daniell, E. S. Le Vine. Sexuality and pregnancy. A prospective study. *J Reprod Med* 1982;**27**:321–7.

46. A. E. Sayle, D. A. Savitz, J. M. Thorp Jr., I. Hertz-Picciotto, A. J. Wilcox. Sexual activity during late pregnancy and risk of preterm delivery. *Obstet Gynecol* 2001;**97**:283–9.

47. J. H. Harger, A. W. Hsing, R. E. Tuomala, et al. Risk factors for preterm premature rupture of fetal membranes: a multicenter case-control study. *Am J Obstet Gynecol* 1990;**163**:130–7.

48. T. Kurki, O. Ylikorkala. Coitus during pregnancy is not related to bacterial vaginosis or preterm birth. *Am J Obstet Gynecol* 1993;**169**:1130–4.

49. W. F. Rayburn, E. A. Wilson. Coital activity and premature delivery. *Am J Obstet Gynecol* 1980;**137**:972–4.

50. W. H. Masters, V. E. Johnson. *Human Sexual Response*. Boston: Little, Brown, 1966.

51. R. Romero, A. Conde-Agudelo, E. Da Fonseca, et al. Vaginal progesterone for preventing preterm birth and adverse perinatal outcomes in singleton gestations

with a short cervix: a meta-analysis of individual patient data. *Am J Obstet Gynecol* 2018;**218**:161–80.

52. A. Conde-Agudelo, R. Romero, E. Da Fonseca, et al. Vaginal progesterone is as effective as cervical cerclage to prevent preterm birth in women with a singleton gestation, previous spontaneous preterm birth, and a short cervix: updated indirect comparison meta-analysis. *Am J Obstet Gynecol* 2018;**219**:10–25.

53. R. Romero, A. Conde-Agudelo, W. El-Refaie, et al. Vaginal progesterone decreases preterm birth and neonatal morbidity and mortality in women with a twin gestation and a short cervix: an updated meta-analysis of individual patient data. *Ultrasound Obstet Gynecol* 2017;**49**:303–14.

54. G. C. Di Renzo, V. Tosto, V. Tsibizova. Progesterone: history, facts, and artifacts. *Best Pract Res Clin Obstet Gynaecol* 2020;**69**:2–12.

55. A. Rehal, Z. Benko, C. De Paco Matallana, et al. Early vaginal progesterone versus placebo in twin pregnancies for the prevention of spontaneous preterm birth: a randomized, double-blind trial. *Am J Obstet Gynecol* 2021;**224**:86.e1–19.

56. R. C. Goodlin, W. Schmidt, D. C. Creevy. Uterine tension and fetal heart rate during maternal orgasm. *Obstet Gynecol* 1972;**39**:125–7.

57. S. Sahmay, T. Atasu, I. Karacan. The effect of intrauterine insemination on uterine activity. *Int J Fertil* 1990;**35**:310–14.

58. R. E. Weiss. Pelvic rest and sex during pregnancy. 2021. www.verywellfamily .com/pelvic-rest-reasons-you-can-t-have-sex-in-pregnancy-4111084 (accessed September 15, 2021).

59. Medical Professionals of the ISSM's Communication Committee. Review discusses safety of sexual activity during high-risk pregnancy. 2021. https://issm .info/sexual-health-headlines/review-discusses-safety-of-sexual-activity-during-high-risk-pregnancy (accessed September 15, 2021).

60. J. Jondle. Diagnosing and treating a short cervix during pregnancy. 2019. www.healthline.com/health/pregnancy/short-cervix (accessed September 15, 2021).

61. W. Burton. Relax, it is (almost always) ok to enjoy sex during pregnancy. 2019. https://maternity-matters.com.au/brisbane-pregnancy-and-babies/2019/04/07/sex-in-pregnancy (accessed September 15, 2021).

62. What to expect when diagnosed with a short cervix during pregnancy. 2018. https://fitmombirthgeek.com/short-cervix-during-pregnancy/ (accessed September 15, 2021).

Chapter

Preterm Birth and Sex

Julia Burd and Vincenzo Berghella

16.1 Physiology

There is a physiological basis for concern for preterm birth (PTB) with sex. As described in preceding chapters, the female orgasm is associated with the release of prostaglandins and oxytocin, known stimulators of labor (see Chapter 4 for more details on orgasm). Moreover, semen contains prostaglandins that could act to ripen the cervix through both direct contact with the cervical mucosa and absorption of these prostaglandins into the maternal circulation. Finally, cervical manipulation is associated with endogenous release of prostaglandins. Commonly referred to as the eponymous Ferguson reflex, in 1941 Dr. Ferguson demonstrated that pressure applied to the cervix or vagina is associated with oxytocin release and uterine contractions [1].

We aim to review the studies on the effects of these physiological principles in the preterm period, as well as other causes of PTB associated with sexual activity.

16.2 Sexually Transmitted Infections Are Associated with Preterm Birth

Beyond known detrimental effects to the woman and the neonate, sexually transmitted infections (STIs) have been noted to greatly increase the risk of preterm birth (see Chapter 21 for more details on STIs). A Cochrane review has demonstrated an increased risk of PTB associated with *Chlamydia trachomatis*, with an odds ratio (OR) of 2.28 [2]. Similarly, untreated genital herpes in the first or second trimester has been demonstrated to double the risk of PTB in case–control studies (OR 2.23). Treatment of the herpes virus has been noted to decrease this risk of PTB [3].

Trichomonas spp. has been demonstrated to increase the risk of PTB in patients who have frequent intercourse but does not increase the risk of PTB when intercourse is infrequent when studied between 23 and 26 weeks [4]. Similarly, in patients who resumed sexual activity after effective treatment of *Trichomonas*, there was no increase in the risk of PTB or decrease in the treatment effect [5].

Often confused for an STI by patients, bacterial vaginosis is a risk factor for PTB and this risk is generally not mitigated by treatment of the organism [6]. Resumption of sexual activity after treatment of bacterial vaginosis does not increase the risk of PTB [5].

In summary, STIs are associated with PTB and should be avoided; when diagnosed, they should be adequately treated in pregnancy.

16.3 Prepregnancy Sexual Exposure to Paternal Sperm Decreases the Development of Preeclampsia

The development of preeclampsia is a major contributor to PTB. Aggregating data from 7125 pregnant patients across seven studies, a meta-analysis examined the rate of development of preeclampsia based on maternal exposure to paternal sperm. Sperm exposure was defined as an absence of barrier contraception prior to conception and sexual cohabitation or oral sex. The authors found that while overall those who, before conception, had a higher exposure to paternal sperm had a similar risk of PTB (774/5512, 14% in the exposed group vs. 220/1619, 13.6% in the control group; OR 1.04, 95% confidence interval [CI] 0.88–1.22), when only primiparous patients were considered there was a statistically significant decrease in PTB with sperm exposure (643/3946, 16.1% vs. 170/725, 23.4%; OR 0.63, 95% CI 0.52–0.76). Similarly, those with greater than 12 months of sexual cohabitation demonstrated a statistically significant decreases in the rate of development of preeclampsia. These data contribute to the hypothesis that there is an immunological role for exposure to sperm in creating maternal tolerance for the fetus prior to implantation [7]. In fact, a prospective trial demonstrated that for every month of sexual cohabitation prior to conception, there was a 4% decrease in the development of gestational hypertension [8].

In summary, sexual cohabitation without barrier contraception for 12 months prior to conception is associated with a decrease in the risk of preeclampsia in the subsequent pregnancy, and therefore probably a decrease in the risk of PTB.

16.4 Sexual Intercourse Seems to Be Associated with a Decrease in Preterm Birth in the General Population

The eight nonrandomized trials and the secondary analysis of two randomized controlled trials reviewed here assessed the risk of PTB and preterm premature rupture of membranes (PPROM) with sexual activity in pregnancy in the general population (patients without risk factors for preterm birth). These studies are outlined in Table 16.1. Overall, the data are weak, largely based on retrospective studies. These data are at risk for recall bias, given that patients who deliver preterm are more likely to try to pinpoint a cause for their PTB. Moreover, those who have frequent sexual intercourse in pregnancy are more likely to have fewer medical complications and be overall healthier. Nonetheless, many studies report a possible decrease in PTB associated with sexual intercourse [4,5,9].

In summary, cessation or decrease of sexual activity in pregnancy in low-risk individuals for the prevention of PTB cannot be recommended [4,9–15]. In fact, sexual activity should be encouraged, as it has often been associated with a decrease in PTB. This may also be because healthier women with healthier relationships engage in sexual activity more often than less healthy counterparts in less healthy relationships.

16.5 Foreplay, Orgasms, Oral Sex, and Preterm Birth

16.5.1 Nipple Stimulation

Nipple stimulation has been used to complete contraction stress tests and can produce contractions with similar patterns and intensity to those produced by oxytocin in

Table 16.1. Selected studies of low-risk patients (e.g. no prior PTB) that compared patients who then had a preterm birth and those who did not and assessed sexual activity in pregnancy

Reference	Study design	Study groups	Number of included patients	Outcome of interest
Sexual activity may improve pregnancy outcomes				
Harger et al. (1990) [11]	Case–control with structured interviews	Cases: PPROM. Controls: matched patients with intact membranes at time of interview	341 cases, 253 controls	Fewer cases than controls had had sexual intercourse in the last week before. No difference in frequency of oral sex, coitarche, number of prior partners, or STIs
Read and Klebanoff (1993) [4]	Multicenter prospective study with genital cultures collected at 23–26 weeks	Prospective cohort of women seeking prenatal care, studied as preterm vs. term deliveries	Preterm deliveries: 1527. Term deliveries: 9849	Frequent intercourse ($\geq$1 event per week) at 23–26 weeks reduced risk of PTB in patients without *Trichomonas vaginalis*, *Mycoplasma hominis*, or bacterial vaginosis. No statistically significant difference in PTB in patients with these infections
Sayle et al. (2001) [9]	Prospective study	Prospective cohort of women recruited at prenatal visits and queried about sexual activity before and during pregnancy	Preterm delivery: 187 (29–36 weeks). Term delivery: 490 randomly selected patients	Unadjusted statistics: lower risk of PTB with sex in late pregnancy (>6 months) (OR 0.34, 95% CI 0.23, 0.51). Decreased risk of PTB with female orgasms. Notable that cases of PTB were more likely to have poorer health with medical reasons for decreased sexual activity
Berghella et al. (2002) [5]	Secondary analysis of two RCTs	Experimental group: treated for BV or *T. vaginalis*	BV treatment group: 966	Patients who had intercourse between second and third doses of metronidazole for BV had a lower risk of PTB than those who abstained (10% vs. 16%, RR 0.6, 95% CI 0.4–0.9). Increased frequency of intercourse also associated with lower risk of PTB

Sexual activity may be associated with preterm birth

Ekwo et al. (1993) [10]	Case–control with structured interviews	Cases: PPROM, PTL, or term PROM Control: delivery ≥39 weeks with labor before ROM	588 cases, 588 controls	Male superior position associated with PPROM (OR 2.4, 95% CI 1.16–4.97) and PTD without PPROM (OR 1.82, 95% CI 1.02–3.25) after controlling for covariates
Petridou et al. (2001) [13]	Case–control study	Cases: PPROM/PTL <33 weeks, PPROM/PTL 33–35 weeks Controls: deliveries 36–37 weeks	Cases: 92 at <33 weeks, 95 at 33–35 weeks Controls: 58	Coitus within last 2 weeks of pregnancy is associated with increased risk of prematurity (OR 3.21, 95% CI 1.45–7.09 for <33 weeks; OR 2.20, 95% CI 1.03–4.70 for 33–35 weeks). Coitus is the only triggering effect of prematurity found in this study
Zhang et al. (2012) [15]	Case–control study of patients with preterm or term birth interviewed within 48 hours of delivery about sexual activity in pregnancy	Cases: 1391 Controls: 1391	In a logistic regression, sexual activity in pregnancy was an independent risk factor for PTB (OR 1.67, 95% CI 1.28–2.19)

No difference in rate of preterm birth with sexual activity

Hernández-Diaz et al. (2014) [12]	Case–crossover examining 72 hours before event (cases) or interview (controls)	Cases: PPROM or PTL Control: matched patients at prenatal appointments	Cases: 50 PPROM, 50 PTL Controls: 158	Risk of PTB with sexual activity within 24 hours of event does not reach statistical significance (OR 6.0, 95% CI 0.7, 69.8)
Purisch et al. (2014) [14]	Prospective cohort study, queried on sexual habits	Prospective cohort of women with singleton pregnancies <24 weeks' gestation	Total patients: 509 PTB: 81 PPROM: 5	No statistically significant difference in the rate of PTB or PPROM with frequent (≥2 events/week) vs. infrequent (≥1 event/week) sexual intercourse

BV, bacterial vaginosis; CI, confidence interval; OR, odds ratio; PPROM, preterm premature rupture of membranes; PTB, preterm birth; PTL, preterm labor; RCT, randomized controlled trial; ROM, rupture of membranes; RR, relative risk; STI, sexually transmitted infection.

pregnancy (see Chapter 23 for more details on nipple stimulation). However, a Cochrane review demonstrated insufficient data for nipple stimulation as an effective mechanism of induction of labor at term. As contraction stress tests (CSTs) have been deemed safe in high-risk pregnancies in the preterm period and the average duration of foreplay in pregnancy is 7 minutes, less than the duration of a CST, data indicate that nipple stimulation is not harmful in pregnancy and not associated with a significant increase in PTB [1].

In summary, based on available data, pregnant patients do not need to avoid nipple stimulation.

16.5.2 Female Orgasms

Female orgasms were associated with lower rates of PTB in a cohort study. Sayle et al. [9] reported a decrease in PTB in patients who had an orgasm in the previous 2 weeks (cases with orgasms 34/183, 18.6% vs. controls 166/405, 40.99%; OR 0.25, 95% CI 0.07, 0.89). This study notably makes the point that those who had preterm deliveries were generally less "healthy" than matched controls, with more frequent recommendations to limit physical activity, potentially including intercourse or masturbation.

In summary, based on limited available data, female orgasms do not increase the risk of PTB and may decrease this risk.

16.5.3 Oral Sex

One case–control study on oral sex in pregnancy examined 97 cases of miscarriage and compared them with matched controls. Those who maintained the pregnancy had a statistically higher rate of oral sex in pregnancy. The authors postulate that oral sex allows for immunomodulation to the partner and therefore the pregnancy [16].

There are six reports of PTB in the setting of chorioamnionitis secondary to *Eikenella corrodens*, a bacterium typically found within dental plaque and gastrointestinal mucosa. Oral sex is considered a possible risk factor for this infection [17].

In summary, based on limited data, patients should not be discouraged from engaging in oral sex.

16.6 Patients at Increased Risk of Preterm Delivery

16.6.1 Patients with a History of Preterm Delivery

There are limited data of the effect of coitus on those with a prior pregnancy affected by PTB. Yost et al. [18] examined 165 patients with a prior spontaneous PTB at less than 32 weeks' gestation with a subsequent pregnancy. They found no statistically significant increase in PTB with coitus. Additionally, the number of sexual partners in pregnancy did not increase the risk of PTB. The authors did not find a significant difference in the rate of spontaneous PTB in those who had "infrequent intercourse" in early pregnancy (28%) compared with those who had "some intercourse" (38%; $p = 0.35$).

In summary, based on limited data, patients with a prior PTB should not be advised to abstain from intercourse in pregnancy.

16.6.2 Twins

See Chapter 17 for more details on twin pregnancies. In summary, available studies on twins and PTB indicate no increased risk of PTB in the setting of sexual activity in a twin pregnancy [19,20].

16.6.3 Short Cervix

See Chapter 15 for more details on short cervix. In brief, there is theoretical concern that trauma to the cervix/vagina in the setting of an already weakened cervix could increase PTB. A study by Grobman et al. [21], a secondary analysis of a randomized controlled trial for 17α-hydroxyprogesterone caproate for PTB prevention, surveyed patients weekly about their activity restrictions, including pelvic rest. They found that PTB was more likely in those placed on pelvic rest (37% vs. 17% risk of delivery at <37 weeks; p <0.001). However, these data must be assessed cautiously as, when the demographics were examined, patients who were placed on activity restriction were more likely to have cervical funneling, intra-amniotic debris, and shorter cervices, all known risk factors for delivery.

In summary, based on limited available data, it is not possible to make definitive recommendations on intercourse in the setting of short cervix.

16.6.4 Cerclage

There are no available trials examining the effect of sexual intercourse on rate of PTB in the setting of cerclage. Expert opinion encourages pelvic rest [1]. Authors at UpToDate emphasize the risk of infection with a cerclage in place. They recommend total pelvic rest for 1 week, then use of condoms to minimize risk of infection during the remainder of the pregnancy [22].

In summary, based on limited available data, the theoretical risks of intercourse should be discussed with patients with cerclage in place to make the best decision for their pregnancy. Other risk factors for PTB, including indication for cerclage, should be considered. Generally, patients with a history-indicated cerclage do not need to avoid intercourse given their longer cervical length.

16.6.5 Preterm Premature Rupture of Membranes

There are no available trials on sexual activity in those who have already had PPROM. Based on data indicating a decreased latency of pregnancy with digital cervical exams in the setting of PPROM [23], vaginal penetration in the setting of PPROM is strongly discouraged. Similarly, there are no data on masturbation or orgasm in the setting of PPROM. Given the tenuous nature of patients with PPROM, the risk of release of oxytocin and prostaglandins as previously described carries a risk of triggering contractions and should likely be avoided.

In summary, in patients with preexisting PPROM, vaginal penetration should be avoided. While data are weaker for orgasm without penetration, theoretically risks exist of which patients should be informed.

16.7 What Did Dr. Google Say?

Overall, the quality of articles available on the Internet is high. Various blogs and news sites emphasize that data are mixed and poor in quality. They recommend a conversation with the patient's healthcare provider about the best practice in their situation. The following websites are recommended:

www.nytimes.com/article/sex-during-pregnancy.html

www.babycenter.com/pregnancy/relationships/sex-during-pregnancy-overview_390

www.psychologytoday.com/us/blog/all-about-sex/201707/sex-during-late-pregnancy-risk-premature-delivery

References

1. S. E. MacPhedran. Sexual activity recommendations in high-risk pregnancies: what is the evidence? *Sex Med Rev* 2018;**6**:343–57.

2. A. Ahmadi, R. Ramazanzadeh, K. Sayehmiri, F. Sayehmiri, N. Amirmozafari. Association of *Chlamydia trachomatis* infections with preterm delivery: a systematic review and meta-analysis. *BMC Pregnancy Childbirth* 2018;**18**:240.

3. D.-K. Li, M. A. Raebel, T. C. Cheetham, et al. Genital herpes and its treatment in relation to preterm delivery. *Am J Epidemiol* 2014;**180**:1109–17.

4. J. S. Read, M. A. Klebanoff. Sexual intercourse during pregnancy and preterm delivery: effects of vaginal microorganisms. *Am J Obstet Gynecol* 1993;**168**:514–19.

5. V. Berghella, M. Klebanoff, C. McPherson, et al. Sexual intercourse association with asymptomatic bacterial vaginosis and *Trichomonas vaginalis* treatment in relationship to preterm birth. *Am J Obstet Gynecol* 2002;**187**:1277–82.

6. J. C. Carey, M. A. Klebanoff, J. C. Hauth, et al. Metronidazole to prevent preterm delivery in pregnant women with asymptomatic bacterial vaginosis. *N Engl J Med* 2000;**342**:534–40.

7. D. Di Mascio, G. Saccone, F. Bellussi, A. Vitagliano, V. Berghella. Type of paternal sperm exposure before pregnancy and the risk of preeclampsia: a systematic review. *Eur J Obstet Gynecol Reprod Biol* 2020;**251**:246–53.

8. O. Olayemi, D. Strobino, C. Aimakhu, et al. Influence of duration of sexual cohabitation on the risk of hypertension in nulliparous parturients in Ibadan: a cohort study. *Aust NZ J Obstet Gynaecol* 2010;**50**:40–4.

9. A. E. Sayle, D. A. Savitz, J. M. Thorp, I. Hertz-Picciotto, A. J. Wilcox. Sexual activity during late pregnancy and risk of preterm delivery. *Obstet Gynecol* 2001;**97**:283–9.

10. E. Ekwo, R. Woolson, C. R. Long, A. Moawad. Coitus late in pregnancy: risk of preterm rupture of amniotic sac membranes. *Am J Obstet Gynecol* 1993;**168**:22–31.

11. J. H. Harger, A. W. Hsing, R. E. Tuomala, et al. Risk factors for preterm premature rupture of fetal membranes: a multicenter case-control study. *Am J Obstet Gynecol* 1990;**163**:130–7.

12. S. Hernández-Díaz, C. E. Boeke, A. T. Romans, et al. Triggers of spontaneous preterm delivery: why today? *Paediatr Perinat Epidemiol* 2014;**28**:79–87.

13. E. Petridou, H. Salvanos, A. Skalkidou, et al. Are there common triggers of preterm deliveries? *BJOG* 2001;**108**:598–604.

14. S. Purisch, J. Brandt, S. Srinivas, J. Bastek. 829: Is frequency of sexual intercourse during pregnancy associated with preterm birth? *Am J Obstet Gynecol* 2014;**210**(1 Suppl):S403.

15. Y. P. Zhang, X. H. Liu, S. H. Gao, et al. Risk factors for preterm birth in five maternal and child health hospitals in Beijing. *PLoS ONE* 2012;7:e52780.

16. T. Meuleman, N. Baden, G. W. Haasnoot, et al. Oral sex is associated with reduced incidence of recurrent miscarriage. *J Reprod Immunol* 2019;**133**:1–6.

17. F. Garnier, G. Masson, A. Bedu, et al. Maternofetal infections due to *Eikenella corrodens*. *J Med Microbiol* 2009;**58**:273–5.

18. N. P. Yost, J. Owen, V. Berghella, et al. Effect of coitus on recurrent preterm birth. *Obstet Gynecol* 2006;**107**:793–7.

19. J. P. Neilson, M. Mutambira. Coitus, twin pregnancy, and preterm labor. *Am J Obstet Gynecol* 1989;**160**:416–18.

20. M. Stammler-Safar, J. Ott, S. Weber, E. Krampl. Sexual behaviour of women with twin pregnancies. *Twin Res Hum Genet* 2010;**13**:383–8.

21. W. A. Grobman, S. A. Gilbert, J. D. Iams, et al. Activity restriction among women with a short cervix. *Obstet Gynecol* 2013;**121**:1181–6.

22. E. R. Norwitz. Transvaginal cervical cerclage. 2020. www.uptodate.com/contents/transvaginal-cervical-cerclage (accessed April 24, 2021).

23. J. M. Alexander, B. M. Mercer, M. Miodovnik, et al. The impact of digital cervical examination on expectantly managed preterm rupture of membranes. *Am J Obstet Gynecol* 2000;**183**:1003–7.

Chapter 17

Multiple Pregnancies and Sex

Hayley Lipworth, Jon F. R. Barrett, and Nir Melamed

17.1 Introduction

Across the globe, but mainly in high- and middle-income countries, the incidence of twin pregnancies has increased, primarily due to assisted reproductive technologies (ARTs). In the USA between 1980 and 2009, the National Center for Health Statistics reported that twinning rates rose by more than 200% among individuals aged 40 and over, and in 2009 one in every 30 infants born was a twin [1]. This increase in multiple births is considered an important public health issue as twin and triplet pregnancies have been associated with an increased risk for adverse maternal and neonatal outcomes; in particular, preterm birth (PTB) is the leading cause of mortality and a major cause of neonatal morbidity in this population. Although twins account for only 1–3% of pregnancies in the USA, they account for over 17% of all PTBs, with more than half of twins born prior to 37 weeks [2]. In addition, there is a significant overrepresentation of twins in neonatal intensive care units (NICUs): one study of 14 033 neonates found that 15% of singletons are admitted to the NICU, compared with almost 48% of twins and 78% of higher-order multiples [3]. These infants are at higher risk of adverse outcomes, such as cerebral palsy and other neurodevelopmental disabilities, short-term morbidity, and neonatal mortality. Thus, prevention of PTB is a major goal of antenatal care in twin pregnancies.

17.1.1 Prediction and Prevention of PTB

Prediction of PTB in twin pregnancy is a debated topic. Some of the common methods include transvaginal sonographic cervical length (CL) measurements, fetal fibronectin, digital examination, and home uterine monitoring. Regarding CL measurements, a systematic review and meta-analysis found that transvaginal sonographic CL at 20–24 weeks' gestation is a good predictor of spontaneous PTB in asymptomatic women with twin pregnancies [4]. In addition, more recent studies have shown that the integration of serial CL measurements can improve the detection of PTB in twins [5]. Many major societies have published guidelines on the management of twin gestations, with conflicting recommendations on the use of CL for the prediction of PTB [6]. Some societies recommend CL measurements for asymptomatic twin pregnancies, and others do not [7–10]. The argument against CL screening is the conflicting evidence regarding the efficacy of preventive interventions in women with twins and a short cervix. In contrast, others believe the use of CL can aid in the identification of women with twin pregnancies who are at an even higher risk for PTB, and who may benefit from referral to a tertiary center, closer monitoring, and timely administration of antenatal corticosteroids [11].

Determining effective strategies to prevent PTB has been a considerable focus in twin pregnancy research. Progesterone, cerclage, pessary, tocolysis, bedrest, and nutrition/gestational weight gain interventions have been examined, with conflicting results [12–14].

The increased risk for PTB in twins may have some pregnant individuals and providers concerned that intercourse may prompt preterm labor or delivery; this anxiety may be heightened in a pregnancy where ARTs were used to conceive the pregnancy as is the case in many twin pregnancies. The safety concerns may be greater in women with twins who are thought to be at increased risk of PTB, such as those with a short or dilated cervix. This chapter discusses select important issues about sexual activity and twin pregnancy, with special attention paid to PTB and shortened cervix.

17.2 Rationale for the Concerns Surrounding Sex in Twin Pregnancies

17.2.1 Prostaglandins in Seminal Fluid

Prostaglandins (PGs) have been shown to increase in the amniotic fluid, placenta, myometrium, and blood at the start of labor, and have also been shown to induce labor and stimulate activity in the myometrium [15]. The seminal fluid contains high concentrations of PGs and human ejaculate has been shown to weaken chorionic membranes [16]. The logical concern is that introduction of semen into the vagina may promote cervical ripening and initiation of labor. A 2001 Cochrane review of sexual intercourse for cervical ripening and induction of labor found only one study of 28 women that specifically studied the potential effects of semen on timing of delivery [17]. The study assessed the impact of coitus with vaginal deposit of semen over three nights compared with abstinence, with the primary outcome being change of Bishop score [18]. The authors found no differences in the Bishop score between the two groups (average change in the coitus group was 1.0, compared with 0.5 in the abstinence group; p <0.05). There was also no difference in the number of participants who delivered within three days of the intervention (46% vs. 47%; relative risk [RR] 0.99, 95% confidence interval [CI] 0.45–2.20) [18]. One limitation of this study is the lack of details regarding the method of randomization and concealment. There have since been other studies on this topic. One such study was a randomized controlled trial of 1137 women with a singleton pregnancy at 35 weeks that evaluated the effect of discussing coitus as a method to expedite labor and avoid induction, versus the suggestion that coitus is safe [19]. Consented participants had a one-on-one counseling session with a medically qualified researcher, and the intervention group were told that vaginal intercourse at term could be used as a method to safely expedite labor. Control group members were told sexual intercourse is safe but its effect on labor is uncertain. There was no further intervention. All participants were given a diary to record the timing and number of episodes of intercourse. This study reported no association between intercourse and onset of labor, but conclusions are limited as there was no certainty about contact with semen, and many participants did not return their coitus diaries, so much of the data were collected over the phone and relied on recall of participants. Researchers from another study conducted in 2006 asked participants with term singleton pregnancies whether they had engaged in intercourse during the previous week and compared delivery outcomes between those with and those without exposure to intercourse [20]. Women were also asked if a condom was used. No relationship was found between coitus at term and onset of labor [20]. Each of these studies had limitations, such as the assumption of introduction of semen into the vagina during coitus with/without condom use, and the data being collected a week before labor rather than immediately before labor. Thus, the effect of semen cannot be accurately determined. None of these studies included women with twin pregnancies, and thus the impact of intercourse and semen on the risk of PTB in this population remains uncertain.

17.2.2 Mechanical Stimulation

Another concern related to coitus in twin pregnancies is mechanical stimulation of the cervix or lower uterine segment. Stimulation of the lower uterine segment does result in local release of PGs [21]. There are no studies that have examined endogenous PG levels after intercourse, nor are there studies comparing condom use to coitus without a condom (which may aid in separating mechanical stimulation causing release of PGs, or PGs from semen). In addition, the cervix and lower uterine segment in low-risk pregnancies seems to be able to tolerate the impact of penetration during coitus [22]. Once again, no studies on mechanical stimulation have been performed on individuals with twin pregnancies.

17.2.3 Impact of Female Orgasm

Researchers have observed similarities between the uterine contractions and release of oxytocin during female orgasm and the pattern of uterine contractions in labor [23]. This has raised concerns that female orgasm may elicit contractions and stimulate preterm labor. Much of the literature in this area is conflicting, dated, and limited by study design and methodological flaws. In a case–control study from 1971, researchers interviewed 50 women who experienced PTB and 50 who delivered at term and reported an association between orgasm and PTB [24]. However, the interpretation of this study is limited by the fact that the groups were not matched for risk factors for PTB, such as previous PTB, low weight gain, or use of lysergic acid diethylamide (LSD) [24]. A second study from 1979 investigated 155 women who experienced a singleton PTB, and reported no significant association between orgasm and proximity to onset of labor [25]. In fact, the author reported that at all stages of pregnancy there was either no association between orgasm and PTB, or an association with a *decreased* risk of PTB [25]. Other studies have since reported similar findings on the safety of orgasm in pregnancy [22,26,27]. A study completed in 2001 examined sexual activity and orgasm in late pregnancy and the risk for PTB [22]. Women with singleton pregnancies were interviewed about their sexual activity before and during their pregnancy. Interestingly, both intercourse and female orgasm during late pregnancy were associated with a reduction in the risk of PTB [22]. One point made by the authors of this study was the fact that within those who delivered at term, the frequency of coitus decreased as pregnancies progressed, so there may be a bias in comparing them with those individuals who delivered preterm (who may have been more sexually active at the time of their early delivery). This is thus an incorrect comparison to make and the authors adjusted their analyses accordingly. Yet even without this adjustment, they still found that sexual activity was associated with a reduced risk of PTB. It is important to note that even strong uterine contractions as a result of orgasm are likely not as strong or sufficiently long-lasting to induce labor [28]. Similar studies on female orgasm in twin pregnancies are lacking.

17.3 Safety of Sex in Twin Pregnancies: Available Evidence

17.3.1 Uncomplicated Twin Pregnancies

Evidence on the safety of sex in uncomplicated twin pregnancies is limited and is completely lacking for higher-order multiples [6,29,30].

Two studies addressed the association of sexual activity with PTB in twin pregnancies. A prospective study of 124 participants published in 1989 by Nielson and Mutambira [30] examined sexual behavior and PTB in twin pregnancies. Through questioning, the authors recorded the frequency of coitus during the week prior to delivery. Participants were divided into groups according to whether coitus had occurred in the previous week. There was no evidence that coitus occurring in the third trimester was associated with the risk of PTB. The proportion of participants who reported having intercourse more than once per week was 35% at 28–29 weeks, 13% at 30–31 weeks, 20% at 32–33 weeks, 14% at 34–35 weeks, and only 4% at 36 weeks' gestation. Even within this subgroup, no evidence of an association between coitus and PTB was identified [30]. This study is limited by a small sample size, recruitment from only one tertiary referral center, and by the lack of detailed information about sexual acts related to presence or absence of orgasm or ejaculation within the vagina. In addition, this study was conducted over 30 years ago and may not apply to the current practice for the screening and prevention of PTB in twins.

The second study was a prospective cohort study of 50 participants published by Stammler-Safar et al. in 2010 [29]. The authors investigated the sexual behavior of individuals pregnant with twins through a questionnaire examining both changes in sexual activities and whether a higher frequency of sexual intercourse was associated with increased risks for PTB and other complications. Overall 42% (21/50) of participants had an uncomplicated pregnancy, and all 50 delivered via cesarean section. Approximately half (51.7%) experienced PTB, and 12 of 29 (24.0%) delivered prior to 34 weeks. There was no significant association between the frequency of coitus during early and late pregnancy and the risk of PTB [29]. This study was not powered to examine the influence of intercourse within 48 hours of delivery. There was also a potential selection bias as 35% of candidates refused to participate in the study. Overall, these studies do not support a relationship between sexual behavior and PTB in uncomplicated twin pregnancies.

17.3.2 Complicated Twin Pregnancies

17.3.2.1 Short Cervix

The safety of sex has been mainly questioned in the context of twin pregnancies identified to be at high risk of PTB, such as in cases of short cervix. Short cervix, often defined as a cervical length of less than 25 mm, is a risk factor for PTB in both singleton and twin pregnancies [4] (see Chapter 15 for more details on short cervix). Therefore, care providers often recommend limiting or restricting sexual activity during pregnancy in patients with a short cervix over concerns that intercourse may further increase the risk of PTB in this high-risk population.

In singleton pregnancies, a recent literature review on sexual activity restrictions in high-risk pregnancies identified only one study on women with a short cervix. In that study, a secondary analysis of a randomized controlled trial of hydroxyprogesterone caproate for the prevention of PTB in nulliparous patients with singleton gestations, the authors investigated "activity restriction" in women with a short cervix, where activity restriction was defined as reductions in pelvic (prohibition of sexual activity), work, or nonwork activity [31]. The authors found that PTB at less than 37 weeks was significantly more common among those who were advised to restrict activity (37% vs. 17%; odds ratio [OR] 2.91, 95% CI 2.0–4.21, p <0.001). Even after controlling for demographic and sonographic differences between those with and without restricted activity, PTB prior to 37 weeks was still more common in those on activity restriction (adjusted OR 2.37, 95% CI 1.60–3.53). Results were similar for the outcome of PTB at less than 34 weeks (adjusted OR 2.28, 95% CI 1.36–3.80) [31]. The main limitation of this study was a potential selection bias, as individuals placed on activity restriction may have been perceived by their provider as being at greater risk of PTB.

In a 2017 literature review, it was suggested that based on the limited available data, individuals with a short cervix need not be discouraged from sexual activity of any type unless they have experienced a prior PTB or are experiencing bleeding, increased baseline uterine contraction frequency/intensity, or worsening of cervical length [28].

We were unable to identify any studies on the safety of sex in twins with a short cervix. As a result, unanswered questions still abound regarding abstention from sexual activity in those patients with twins who are at especially high risk of PTB, the effects of PGs in semen on cervical length, the intensity of uterine contractions with orgasm on a compromised cervix, and sexual activity in the case of cervical cerclage.

17.4 Current Recommendations

The major obstetric and medical societies are united in recommending against activity restriction in unselected twin pregnancies [9,32,33]. It is important to note that none of the guidelines cited specifically refer to sexual activity. The literature review by MacPhedran [28] provides the author's recommendations for multiple pregnancies, stating that sexual activity should not be discouraged in twin pregnancies unless complicated by other obstetric risk factors; recommendations should also be individualized based on obstetric history and patient needs. We have recently examined the management of twin pregnancies in Canada, including healthcare provider recommendations on sexual activity [6]. This study included 95 maternal–fetal medicine specialists (MFMs), of whom a majority (59/95, 62.1%) have been practicing for over 10 years and 90.5% (86/95) work in a tertiary referral center. Only 22.1% (21/95) of surveyed MFMs reported recommending restriction of activity level to their twin-bearing patients, and 96.7% (87/90) of MFMs recommend against avoidance of sexual activity [6]. In other areas of this survey, there was considerable variation among MFM specialists in their recommendations of how to manage a twin pregnancy; however, in the case of sexual activity the responses were strongly aligned. While there are no data to guide the recommendations for women with a short cervix, the approach we take in our twins clinic is to recommend against sexual intercourse in this population, especially in cases with severe or early-onset cervical shortening.

17.5 What Did Dr. Google Say?

A Google search related to intercourse and twins yields a variety of results. Many of these hits are related to "how to get pregnant with twins," detailing positions "most suited for conceiving twins." However, a variety of non-peer-reviewed resources on the safety of intercourse in twin pregnancies are also available. WebMD published an article in 2019 [34] about discomfort related to sex during twin pregnancy, suggesting that the pregnant woman avoids lying on her back during sex after the fourth month of pregnancy, trying different positions to reduce pressure, and using personal lubricant for discomfort due to dryness. The article recommends calling a doctor if the pregnant woman notices symptoms such as pain, bleeding, discharge after intercourse, or contractions that continue after sex [34]. Another article on WebMD discusses libido changes during twin pregnancy and suggests similar behavioral and positional changes [35]. BabyMed.com (a website developed by Dr. Amos Grunebaum, Professor of Obstetrics and Gynecology at the Zucker School of Medicine) published an article entitled "Having twins: should I avoid orgasms?" [36]. In this article, Dr. Grunebaum explains on a general level why preterm birth and twin pregnancies are associated and that some twin pregnancies are at higher risk for preterm birth. Dr. Grunebaum advises that orgasms are safe for most pregnancies, but that individuals pregnant with twins should talk with their physicians about their own risk factors and the impact of orgasm on their pregnancy [36]. Finally, the UK National Health Service (NHS) website advises that it is safe to have sex during pregnancy unless your doctor or midwife has told you otherwise, and that your midwife or doctor may advise you to avoid sex if "you're having twins, or have previously had early labours, and are in the later stages of pregnancy" [37]. The placement of the "and" in this sentence has generated confusion on some pregnancy message boards, such as that of TwinsTrust.org, a charity aimed at educating and supporting families of multiples in the UK [38]. On this website, the moderators mention that though the NHS advice may seem to say that you should avoid sex while pregnant with twins, it actually states that you should avoid sex if pregnant with twins *and* are in the later stages of pregnancy [37,38]. One midwife on TwinsTrust.org thus advises that if you are fit and well with a healthy twin pregnancy, sex which is comfortable and pain-free is safe [38].

17.6 Conclusion

There is a paucity of literature on the risks of sexual activity in unselected and high-risk twin pregnancies. We suggest that sexual activity of any type should not be discouraged in twin gestations without other obstetric risk factors such as short cervix. Recommendations should be individualized bearing in mind patient history, comorbidities, and emotional needs. No studies have been performed in higher-order multiples. Further research is necessary to make specific recommendations in this population.

References

1. J. Martin, B. Hamilton, M. Osterman. Three decades of twin births in the United States, 1980–2009. NCHS Data Brief No. 80, January 2012. www.cdc.gov/nchs/products/databriefs/db80.htm (accessed December 16, 2020).

2. D. B. Fell, K. Joseph. Temporal trends in the frequency of twins and higher-order multiple births in Canada and the United

States. *BMC Pregnancy Childbirth* 2012;**12**:103.

3. T. L. Callahan, J. E. Hall, S. L. Ettner, et al. The economic impact of multiple-gestation pregnancies and the contribution of assisted-reproduction techniques to their incidence. *N Engl J Med* 1994;**331**:244–9.

4. A. Conde-Agudelo, R. Romero, S. S. Hassan, L. Yeo. Transvaginal sonographic cervical length for the prediction of spontaneous preterm birth in twin pregnancies: a systematic review and metaanalysis. *Am J Obstet Gynecol* 2010;**203**:128.e1–12.

5. N. Melamed, A. Pittini, L. Hiersch, et al. Do serial measurements of cervical length improve the prediction of preterm birth in asymptomatic women with twin gestations? *Am J Obstet Gynecol* 2016;**215**:616.e1–14.

6. H. Lipworth, L. Hiersch, D. Farine, J. F. R. Barrett, N. Melamed. Current practice of maternal–fetal medicine specialists regarding the prevention and management of preterm birth in twin gestations. *J Obstet Gynaecol Can* 2021;**43**:831–8.

7. C. P. Howson, M. V. Kinney, J. E. Lawn. *Born Too Soon: The Global Action Report on Preterm Birth*. Geneva: World Health Organization, 2012. www.who.int/pmnch/media/news/2012/201204%5Fborntoosoon-report.pdf (accessed June 5, 2020).

8. FIGO Working Group on Good Clinical Practice in Maternal–Fetal Medicine. Good clinical practice advice: management of twin pregnancy. *Int J Gynecol Obstet* 2019;**144**:330–7.

9. J. Barrett, A. Bocking. SOGC consensus statement: management of twin pregnancies (Part 1). *J Obstet Gynaecol Can* 2000;**22**:519–29.

10. Society for Maternal–Fetal Medicine (SMFM), J. McIntosh, H. Feltovich, V. Berghella, T. Manuck. The role of routine cervical length screening in selected high-risk and low-risk women for preterm birth prevention. *Am J Obstet Gynecol* 2016;**215**:B2–7.

11. Society for Maternal–Fetal Medicine Committee on Practice Bulletins – Obstetrics. Practice bulletin no. 169: multifetal gestations: twin, triplet, and higher-order multifetal pregnancies. *Obstet Gynecol* 2016;**128**:e131–46.

12. A. Jarde, O. Lutsiv, C. Park, et al. Preterm birth prevention in twin pregnancies with progesterone, pessary, or cerclage: a systematic review and meta-analysis. *BJOG* 2017;**124**:1163–73.

13. K. da Silva Lopes, Y. Takemoto, E. Ota, S. Tanigaki, R. Mori. Bed rest with and without hospitalisation in multiple pregnancy for improving perinatal outcomes. *Cochrane Database Syst Rev* 2017;(3):CD012031.

14. W. Yamasmit, S. Chaithongwongwatthana, J. E. Tolosa, et al. Prophylactic oral betamimetics for reducing preterm birth in women with a twin pregnancy. *Cochrane Database Syst Rev* 2015;(12):CD004733.

15. D. M. Olson. The role of prostaglandins in the initiation of parturition. *Best Pract Res Clin Obstet Gynaecol* 2003;**17**:717–30.

16. O. H. Harmanli, R. J. Wapner, J. F. Lontz. Human ejaculate. Effects on the biomechanical properties of the human chorioamniotic membranes. *J Reprod Med* 1998;**43**:779–82.

17. J. Kavanagh, A. J. Kelly, J. Thomas. Sexual intercourse for cervical ripening and induction of labour. *Cochrane Database Syst Rev* 2001;(2):CD003093.

18. E. Bendvold. Coitus and induction of labour. *Tidsskr Jordmodre* 1990;**96**:6–8.

19. N. S. Omar, P. C. Tan, N. Sabir, E. S. Yusop, S. Z. Omar. Coitus to expedite the onset of labour: a randomised trial. *BJOG* 2013;**120**:338–45.

20. J. Schaffir. Sexual intercourse at term and onset of labor. *Obstet Gynecol* 2006;**107**:1310–14.

21. J. J. Platz-Christensen, P. Pernevi, H. Bokström, N. Wiqvist. Prostaglandin E and F2α concentration in the cervical mucus and mechanism of cervical ripening. *Prostaglandins* 1997;**53**:253–61.

22. A. E. Sayle, D. A. Savitz, J. M. Thorp, I. Hertz-Picciotto, A. J. Wilcox. Sexual activity during late pregnancy and risk of preterm delivery. *Obstet Gynecol* 2001;**97**:283–9.

23. G. Pranzarone. Sexuoerotic stimulation and orgasmic response in the induction and management of parturition: clinical possibilities. In P. Kothari, R. Patel, eds. *Proceedings of First International Conference on Orgasm.* Bombay: VRP Publishers, 1991: 105–19.

24. R. C. Goodlin, D. W. Keller, M. Raffin M. Orgasm during late pregnancy. Possible deleterious effects. *Obstet Gynecol* 1971;**38**:916–20.

25. R. P. Perkins. Sexual behavior and response in relation to complications of pregnancy. *Am J Obstet Gynecol* 1979;**134**:498–505.

26. W. F. Rayburn, E. A. Wilson. Coital activity and premature delivery. *Am J Obstet Gynecol* 1980;**137**:972–4.

27. P. A. Georgakopoulos, D. Dodos, D. Mechleris. Sexuality in pregnancy and premature labour. *Br J Obstet Gynaecol* 1984;**91**:891–3.

28. S. E. MacPhedran. Sexual activity recommendations in high-risk pregnancies: what is the evidence? *Sex Med Rev* 2018;**6**:343–57.

29. M. Stammler-Safar, J. Ott, S. Weber, E. Krampl. Sexual behaviour of women with twin pregnancies. *Twin Res Hum Genet* 2010;**13**:383–8.

30. J. P. Neilson, M. Mutambira. Coitus, twin pregnancy, and preterm labor. *Am J Obstet Gynecol* 1989;**160**:416–18.

31. W. A. Grobman, S. A. Gilbert, J. D. Iams, et al. Activity restriction among women with a short cervix. *Obstet Gynecol* 2013;**121**:1181–6.

32. World Health Organization. *WHO Recommendations on Antenatal Care for a Positive Pregnancy Experience.* Geneva: World Health Organization, 2016.

33. American College of Obstetricians and Gynecologists Committee on Practice Bulletins – Obstetrics, Society for Maternal–Fetal Medicine, ACOG Joint Editorial Committee. ACOG Practice bulletin no. 56: multiple gestation: complicated twin, triplet, and high-order multifetal pregnancy. *Obstet Gynecol* 2004;**104**:869–83.

34. R. B. Taylor. Sex discomforts with twins. 2021. www.webmd.com/baby/sex-discomforts-twins (accessed February 8, 2021).

35. R. B. Taylor. Libido changes with twins. 2021. www.webmd.com/baby/libido-changes-twins (accessed February 8, 2021).

36. A. Grunebaum. Having twins: should I avoid orgasms? 2020. www.babymed.com/having-twins-should-i-avoid-orgasms (accessed February 8, 2021).

37. National Health Service. Sex in pregnancy. 2020. www.nhs.uk/pregnancy/keeping-well/sex/ (accessed February 8, 2021).

38. Twins Trust. Pregnancy. https://twinstrust.org/group/pregnancy/discussion.html?id=6DF75CC6-FAD0-442E-BA62724DD3CD3035 (accessed May 29, 2022).

18

Special Pregnancies and Sex

Evangelia Vlachodimitropoulou Koumoutsea
and Cynthia Maxwell

18.1 Hemodynamic Changes with Phases of Sexual Arousal and Orgasm

The female body undergoes a number of changes during pregnancy that affect sexual desire, arousal, and orgasm (see Chapters 3 and 4 for more details on physiology and orgasm). Some of the earliest changes reflecting pregnancy occur in the breasts. Tumescence develops in the areolae as an early indication of conception. The breasts rapidly increase in size during the first trimester and the onset of tenderness along the sides of the breasts and the rapid size increase are the particular trademarks of the newly pregnant woman. When a first-time mother responds to sexual stimuli in the first trimester, there is an obvious 20–25% increase in breast size in response to sexual tension. By the third trimester breast volume has increased by approximately one-third. High levels of sexual tension frequently do not cause further obvious increase in breast size at this stage of pregnancy.

Pregnancy also markedly increases blood flow in the pelvis, which is then even further increased secondary to sexual stimulation. In the first trimester, there is great variation reported in levels of eroticism and effectiveness of sexual performance, ranging from voluntary rejection of all physical forms of sexual activity to significant increase in sexual interest and elevated demand for increased rate of performance. Reduced sexual tensions and effectiveness often coincide with nausea and vomiting, chronic fatigue, and fear of injury to the fetus or miscarriage. During the second trimester sexual patterns generally reflect a marked increase in sexual desire and effectiveness of performance. Women are not only interested in sexual encounters but also often find themselves planning for sexual encounters, having fantasies and erotic dreams. A significant improvement in basic sexuality beyond their concept of previously established norms of performance when not pregnant is reported. Barriers to sexual pleasure include worsening irritability, abdominal fullness, pelvic tension, and backache of increasing severity, factors which occasionally contribute to a gradual loss of interest in sexual activity toward the end of the third trimester.

Pregnancy has been noted to increase general sensitivity to the overall effects of orgasm, with an increase in contractile intensity compared with that outside of pregnancy. Orgasmic contractions of the uterus have been recorded during the second and third trimesters consistently and have been reported as subjectively more intense sensations. During the second trimester it may take 10–15 minutes after orgasm for the increased labial and vaginal swelling to resolve. The normal resolution phase can be further delayed by positions such as the missionary, which further contributes to blood flow congestion secondary to compression. Residual pelvic blood flow congestion from the second- and third-trimester uterus may account for the high levels of maintained sexual tensions frequently described.

18.2 Gastrointestinal Conditions: Inflammatory Bowel Disease and Perianal/Perineal Disease

Changes in gastrointestinal motility during pregnancy include decreased gastric peristalsis, delayed gastric emptying, and reduced gastric motility, leading to the common symptom of constipation. A major fear of many people with inflammatory bowel disease (IBD) is having an "accident" during sex; emptying bowels before sex is advised to help increase confidence. A number of antidiarrheal drugs, such as loperamide, that are used prior to intercourse are not recommended for general use in pregnancy and consultation with a physician is advised. The reduced gut motility during pregnancy and choosing a moment when the bowel is less active will help to ensure continence. Scarring of the skin, abscesses, or fistulas can result in pain in the genital area and a water-based lubricant is advised prior to vaginal penetrative sex. If there is significant stricturing (narrowing) of the anus or an abscess or fistula around the anal area, then penetrative anal sex should be avoided. If steroids are being used as part of treatment, they can influence sexual satisfaction by causing mood changes such as depression and weight gain and by affecting sleep. In pregnancy, steroids are sometimes given as rectal suppositories, usually at night-time, and intercourse is advised prior to their administration.

Surgery for IBD can often involve removal of part of the bowel and may result in an ileostomy or colostomy draining into a stoma or an internal ileoanal pouch. Having a stoma bag should not be a barrier to an active sex life. However, with the expanding size of the abdomen the individual should make sure that the stoma is attached securely, and the bag should be emptied prior to intercourse. Different sizes of bags are available and the bag can be swapped for a smaller one during sex. There are also other bags that can be folded and safely secured to a smaller size, and fabric pouch covers to prevent the pouch from rubbing on skin or making a rustling noise. Another option is to wear a stoma wrap with an inner pocket. The wrap will conceal and hold the pouch close to the torso. There are also various clothing accessories such as bellybands, cummerbunds, and crotchless underwear that help conceal the pouch during intimacy. Women with an internal ileoanal pouch, otherwise known as a J-pouch, report baseline or increased frequency of intercourse postoperatively, with some experiencing an increased quality of orgasm [1]. Vaginal sex is encouraged, although anal penetration is often considered risky. As the functioning of the J-pouch is heavily dependent on the integrity of the anal sphincter, a conversation with a surgeon who knows the details of each individual's anatomy will provide further advice on this topic.

18.3 Cardiac Conditions

Pregnancy results in a physiological increase of about 40% in the total amount of blood pumped out of the heart (cardiac output), as well as an increase in the heart rate, which will add extra strain on the heart. The ability to tolerate pregnancy will depend on lung pressures, cardiac function, presence of reduced oxygen saturation, or history of arrhythmias or a heart attack and heart failure. If a woman can walk at a reasonable speed

(3 miles per hour) on level ground or climb 20 stairs relatively easily, then the exertion of sex is unlikely to affect her heart condition. However, if the condition is categorized as Class IV on the New York Heart Association classification, or if a procedure has been undertaken within the last 2 weeks, the woman is at high risk of complications during sexual activity. It should be noted that the risk of experiencing a cardiac event during sex is extremely low. Fewer than 1% of all heart attacks occur during sexual activity in the nonpregnant population, with a greater chance of experiencing a shark bite or being hit by lightning.

Sexual health concerns are common in patients with all types of cardiac disease, including coronary artery disease, heart attack, heart failure, and valvular and rhythm disorders, and in those with implantable cardioverter-defibrillators. Symptoms of cardiovascular disease, such as chest pain, shortness of breath, and fatigue, can worsen during pregnancy and the exertion may interfere with sexual performance and enjoyment. Cardiovascular disease and its treatments change the way blood circulates throughout the body and may reduce the amount of blood supplied to distant areas of the body, including the genital region. This can cause added difficulties with sexual arousal in women in and outside of pregnancy.

Certain positions or practices may be more comfortable, depending on exercise tolerance and physical limitations. Extra support with pillows can improve comfort, and erotic devices are generally safe for cardiac patients and those with implantable cardioverter-defibrillators. Women who are receiving blood thinners (e.g. for mechanical heart valves) or who are on aspirin plus other blood clot-preventing medications should take care to adopt positions that do not put pressure on joints in order to avoid hemorrhage, and partners should be gentle to avoid bruising or skin injury.

18.4 Pulmonary Conditions

Pregnancy causes a significant increase in oxygen demand, with three-quarters of women experiencing physiological breathlessness. This is commonest in the third trimester but may start at any point in gestation. Asthma is the commonest chronic medical illness that complicates pregnancy, affecting up to 7% of women of childbearing age. Asthma may improve, deteriorate, or remain unchanged during pregnancy. Women with only mild disease are unlikely to experience issues, whereas those with severe asthma are at greater risk of deterioration, particularly during late pregnancy. Deterioration is commonly associated with a reduction or cessation of medication due to fear of harm; however, the continuation of prescriptions including inhalers and tablets (e.g. steroids) is strongly advised. Furthermore, it is important to treat gastroesophageal reflux occurring in pregnancy as it can exacerbate asthma.

Having intercourse is similar to exercising, increasing further a woman's heart rate and breathing rate, which are already physiologically elevated due to pregnancy. This type of activity will only trigger symptoms of asthma, such as breathlessness, coughing, wheezing, and chest tightness, if asthma is not well controlled. It is advised to stop sexual activity if this occurs, use a reliever inhaler, and rest until one feels better. Medical attention should be sought if symptoms do not resolve. Positions where the chest is not weighed down, such as "spooning" and "woman on top," are advised. These principles also apply to other types of lung disease, where the added pregnancy element will worsen respiratory symptoms and energy levels. Prior to intercourse, it should be ensured that the area is free of irritants such as dust, pet hair, smoke, or fragrances, and a fan providing a cool breeze on the face should be considered to ease shortness of breath during sex. Taking reliever inhalers prophylactically 15 minutes prior to intercourse can also help prevent symptoms. To get rid of any unpleasant aftertaste, the mouth can be rinsed with mouthwash after inhaler use. Some shortness of breath during sex is expected but slowing down at any point or taking a break is perfectly acceptable.

18.5 Epilepsy, Idiopathic Intracranial Hypertension, Shunts, and Stroke

In most women, pregnancy does not affect their epilepsy nor their frequency of seizures, and those who have been seizure-free for many years are unlikely to note deterioration. Women with poorly controlled epilepsy are more likely to notice an increased seizure frequency. Deterioration can be attributed to poor compliance with anticonvulsants, nausea and vomiting, poorer gastrointestinal absorption, decreased drug levels due to increased blood volume, and lack of sleep, which can lower the seizure threshold. Epilepsy can lower sexual desire and increase dryness and vaginal spasms in women, making intercourse painful at times. Prior to having sex during pregnancy, a woman with epilepsy needs to ensure that she is well rested and well hydrated and uses a water-based lubricant if required. There is often a fear of having a seizure during sex due to the extra weight of pregnancy and increasing shortness of breath, particularly if seizures are triggered by physical activity, excitement, or fast breathing. Reassuringly, having a seizure during sex is no more likely than having one at any other time, and orgasm-induced seizures are very rare [2].

In certain medical conditions such as idiopathic intracranial hypertension and hydrocephalus, a shunt may be inserted in the brain to help drain extra fluid, usually into the abdomen, helping improve symptoms such as headache. Outside of pregnancy, shunt insertion is known to lead to an improvement in sexual function due to symptom reduction. There are no restrictions to having sex with a shunt in situ, following healing, and it is not problematic to lie on the side of the head with the shunt. Partners should be informed not to touch any palpable valves on the woman's scalp. If headaches or nausea and vomiting are experienced, a medical opinion should be sought as ventriculoperitoneal shunts can malfunction during pregnancy, particularly in the third trimester. Shunt complications are related to increased accumulation of water, increased intracranial cerebrospinal fluid volume, and increased pressure in the abdomen as a result of the growing uterus, and complications are not caused by sexual activity.

A stroke can change how an individual's body feels and functions and how one feels about oneself. It can affect a woman's emotional and intimate physical relationship with her partner, whether the event happened prior to or during pregnancy. However, intercourse following a stroke should not be avoided due to fear that it can trigger another event, as there is no evidence to support this. It is recommended that following a stroke the individual communicates with their partner about feelings of embarrassment or lack of desire, as talking openly about these issues will help deal with sexual problems and improve emotional well-being. Changes in emotion and mood can include anger, irritability, and depression, which will reduce an individual's interest in sex. If these are persistent, medical attention should be sought.

A stroke can cause numerous physical changes, such as weakness, muscle stiffness, and fatigue, all of which can be worsened by the advancing pregnancy, and impact sexual activity. Fatigue is likely to worsen during the day, and intercourse during the morning or when the woman has more energy is advised. If there is muscle weakness and balance issues, time should be taken to explore how the enlarged abdomen affects this and find comfortable positions using aids such as large pillows. It is advised that a woman lies on her weak side to leave the stronger arm free and adopts positions requiring less balance, such as the "missionary position" with the woman underneath or the "spooning" position where both individuals are laying on their side facing in the same direction.

Changes in sensation such as numbness can make the skin less sensitive to touch or cause painful sensations. If sensations have greatly changed, masturbation can help learn once again how the body responds to physical stimulation, and also by experimenting with one's partner with touching, kissing, cuddling, and massage in unaffected areas. Furthermore, lubricants should be used to reduce pain and improve enjoyment. A stroke may have caused continence issues, in which case the bladder should be emptied prior to intercourse and the bedding should be protected with a waterproof sheet and towels. If there is a catheter in place, the woman should be trained on how to remove and replace it or how to clamp it and remove the bag during sex.

18.6 Autoimmune and Connective Tissue Diseases

Autoimmune and connective tissue diseases are more common in women than men, with an actual prevalence of up to 15 times higher in females for systemic lupus erythematosus (SLE) and four times for rheumatoid arthritis (RA). These diseases are not only found in the elderly but also affect the younger population and the signs and symptoms can vary in severity, for example within the menstrual cycle and during pregnancy. Within pregnancy, variations are attributed to an alteration in maternal immunity, leading to a relative immunosuppressed state so as to protect the fetus from attack by the mother's immune system. Also, estrogen, which increases during pregnancy, may worsen autoimmune diseases. Nevertheless, about one-third of women will notice improvement, but only a smaller percentage of those will achieve complete disease remission. Rheumatoid arthritis occurs at an average age of 40 years, and in this population 25% of patients will have substantial disability with worsening symptoms of changes in bones and joints and morning stiffness in pregnancy. Other diseases, such as SLE and Sjögren's syndrome, which are also common in women of childbearing age, are multisystem disorders that attack numerous organ systems, such as kidneys, skin, and brain.

In the nonpregnant population, patients with inflammatory diseases such as RA are at a significantly increased risk of sexual dysfunction, attributed to pain, reduced sexual desire, fatigue, and mobility restrictions [3]. Restricting medications such as nonsteroidal anti-inflammatory drugs (NSAIDs) because of pregnancy can cause poorer pain control and further reduce sexual desire. Immunosuppressive treatments, such as azathioprine, mycophenolate, and rituximab, are often continued during pregnancy and may increase the risk of infection, so protection against sexually transmitted infections is advised. Disease complications may include thrombocytopenia, such as in antiphospholipid syndrome, and intercourse should be undertaken with care if the platelet count is as low as 50×10^9/L or if the woman is receiving blood-thinning medication, for example due to a history of blood clots or a blood clot in pregnancy. Furthermore, steroid treatment, often used in pregnancy to manage disease symptoms, can cause skin fragility and poor healing. Care should be taken to adopt positions that do not put pressure on joints in order to avoid hemorrhage, and partners should be gentle to avoid bruising or skin injury. Furthermore, lubrication to reduce friction is advised. From a psychological aspect, a number of disorders such as SLE may be associated with an increased risk of miscarriage or preterm delivery, and the thought of sexual intercourse may lead to the fear of compromising the current pregnancy.

18.7 Chemotherapy

Because more women are postponing childbearing to later in life, there is an increasing number experiencing cancer and many may receive chemotherapy during pregnancy. The immune system is suppressed in pregnancy and to a much greater extent following chemotherapy. It is essential to avoid an infection during chemotherapy treatment. Certain treatments cause low blood counts that will further increase this risk. Women should be given the following advice to prevent infection:

- Urine should be passed prior to intercourse.
- Sexually transmitted infections such as HIV can be prevented by using a condom or dental dam.
- If toys are used, they should be washed with hot soapy water every time prior to use.
- Yeast infections should be watched for and a healthcare provider contacted if vaginal discharge, itching, or irritation is experienced. Steroid therapy, antibiotics, and pregnancy put the woman at increased risk.
- Any sexual activity that could expose the mouth to feces should be avoided.
- Sex that involves penetration, anal or vaginal, should be avoided while blood counts are low (platelet count $<50 \times 10^9$/L or white cell count $<1.5 \times 10^9$/L). This includes insertion of fingers, vibrators, or other toys into the vagina or anus.

18.8 Bleeding Disorders

Changes in the coagulation system mean that a number of bleeding disorders will improve during pregnancy. The concentration of clotting factors such as factor VIII and X, fibrinogen, and von Willebrand factor may increase by up to 50% by the third trimester, in preparation for blood loss in labor. Women will therefore often find an improvement in their bleeding condition.

Sexual activity can be relatively safe; however, it may resemble strenuous exercise and can cause a bleed in any part of the body or in a muscle/joint. Limited movement or pain in the joints will mean that some positions are more comfortable than others. Women are likely to experience bruising during sex, but muscle bleeds such as in the forearm or joint bleeds are rarer events. However, bleeding within joints may be exacerbated by the added pregnancy weight, and some positions may be more difficult to achieve. Intercourse in the context of joint bleeds can be very painful, and women must therefore stop or change position and not wait until a severe injury occurs. Pillows should be used to help relieve pressure points, and any routine treatments administered prior to intercourse.

Because some bleeding disorders are more severe than others, partners need to be gentle and not too heavy-handed during intimate moments to avoid bruising. Any activity that can draw blood to the skin's surface, like biting or nibbling for example, could potentially cause complications. A break in the skin may bleed for a prolonged period, result in pain, or become infected. Furthermore, lip or tongue studs can scratch, so partners should be asked to remove them.

Love bites can be very noticeable in the context of bleeding disorders. Bruises may be large or develop into large and painful hematomas. Kissing on the lips may also cause bruising. If this is experienced, the partner should be encouraged to kiss other erogenous areas such as the neck, hands, breasts, or other parts of the body.

Vaginal bleeding is not uncommon (even for women without bleeding disorders). However, if a bleeding disorder is present, ensure the partner's nails are tidy to avoid cuts of the vagina or rectum. Lubrication can be helpful to reduce friction.

18.9 Considerations for Patients with Obesity

Fatness can be viewed as a multisystem disorder that increases risk during pregnancy. Obesity is often thought to have a negative effect on a nonpregnant woman's sexual function, with reduced arousal, lubrication, orgasm, and satisfaction; however, sexual function in pregnancy in this group is less well understood [4]. A study of sexual function in 105 overweight women with a body mass index (BMI) above 25 found that BMI significantly reduced sexual function compared with normal-weight women, especially in the third trimester. Given the importance of intimacy in a relationship, this knowledge should empower physicians to encourage obese women to lose weight prior to embarking on a pregnancy [5].

Obese pregnant women report increasing shortness of breath with advancing gestation, particularly on lying flat. This is most likely exacerbated by uterine and adipose compression of blood flow in the abdomen and increasing pressure from adipose and breast tissue on the chest wall. Interestingly, partners of obese pregnant women have reported compromised cleanliness in the urogenital area compared with the prepregnancy state that has suppressed their sexual desire, and hence meticulous hygiene is recommended.

During intimacy, numerous pillows should be available and the mattress firm and springy. Memory foam mattresses should be avoided as obese women may sink down instead of bouncing back up during exertion. Furthermore, a water-based lubricant is encouraged due to the adiposity around the vagina (in the mons pubis and labia), making it harder to achieve penetration. The "spooning" position is best avoided, as the buttocks will often get in the way. The missionary position can be modified to accommodate the woman's enlarged abdomen and thighs by adding a pillow under her bottom, and she can use her hands from the sides to pull up her knees and thighs toward her chest. Furthermore, the woman-on-top position can be improved by leaning forward and placing the hands firmly on the bed rather than sitting up. Finally, the "doggie" is a favorite sex position for obese women and gives the partner plenty of room and also keeps the enlarged belly out of the way.

18.10 Considerations for Differently Abled Persons

18.10.1 Spinal Cord Injury

A spinal cord injury certainly does not mean a woman cannot become pregnant and the injury is not the end of a fulfilling sex life. The added weight of pregnancy requires some attention to a few practical matters, but women should endeavor to seek new sensations and opportunities. In preparation for intercourse, a woman is encouraged to empty her bladder to avoid accidents or interruptions. Being pregnant often exacerbates bladder symptoms and causes urinary frequency due to the effect of added pressure. Furthermore, plenty of pillows should be available to allow a comfortable position, along with Velcro restraints or supports. Women with spinal cord injuries may experience less vaginal lubrication and having a partner perform oral sex may help achieve penetration. Using a water-based lubricant is another option.

Individuals should take some time to explore areas of the body where sensation is still intact. The entire body should be explored including the head, hair, face, neck, chest, abdomen, back, buttocks, hands, and feet. Aids such as lotions, oils, feathers, and vibrators are also encouraged. Stimulation of the genitals, together with sensual touching in a sensitive area, may help to achieve orgasm. A gentle suction device can increase the ability of the clitoris to respond and achieve orgasm. Achieving an orgasm will often take a little longer and sensation may feel different compared to prior to the injury. An injury at or above vertebra T6 can sometimes lead to autonomic dysreflexia, which usually manifests as feeling flushed or a pounding headache, and these signs should be watched for. If they occur, all activity should cease and medical advice sought immediately as blood pressure can become dangerously high and, coupled with a low heart rate, could lead to a stroke, seizure, or cardiac arrest.

18.10.2 Knee or Hip Replacements

Once recovered from a joint replacement operation, patients report an improvement in libido and intercourse duration, which likely reflects a reduction in pain and improvement in general well-being. With knee replacements, positions that are uncomfortable, cause pain, and involve kneeling or deep knee bending should be avoided. Following a knee replacement, it takes a few weeks to regain balance and with the pregnancy shifting the center of gravity forward, the woman must take care to ensure that she feels stable prior to sexual activity. The weight of the growing uterus also accentuates the curvature of the spine and adds extra load on joints. In women with hip replacements, intercourse can be trickier due to the wide range of hip flexion, rotation, and extension often required. Pillows and towels should be used to prop the woman or her partner to a comfortable height. Relaxation is always advised, as stress will make the body stiffer. There is a role for stretching for 20–30 minutes prior to intercourse, as rehabilitation exercises will allow for improved strength, flexibility, and body preparation. The following three positions are considered safe: the missionary, where the woman assumes the bottom position and keeps her legs straight using pillows for support; sitting in a chair, where the man sits on a firm chair with his feet flat on the floor and the woman sits on his lap; and the standing position, if balance has been regained. Positions that pose a risk of injury and joint dislocation should be avoided and include "doggy style" with the woman on her hands and knees and the partner behind, and woman crouched on top, where the woman is on top with her legs bent and leaning forward on the man's chest.

18.11 Pandemic Viruses, Bodily Fluid, and Respiratory Precautions

Viral or bacterial infections will often compromise pregnant women more due to the changes that the immune system undergoes and can have serious lifelong consequences for the mother and fetus, including death. Being pregnant during a pandemic poses many added challenges, and emotional and physical connections are pivotal for an individual's overall well-being during such times. It should be remembered that the woman herself is her own safest sex partner. Women may choose to take advantage and become further acquainted with their own bodies and have solo fun. If meeting someone, new women should at a minimum do their own screening in terms of infection symptoms and potential exposures prior to embarking on indoor adventures. To minimize the spread of infections, both partners should wash their full body with soap and water. Hands should be washed for a minimum of 20 seconds and sex toys should also be thoroughly sanitized as per manufacturer's instructions. Heavy breathing during sex can create droplets that may increase the risk of transmission of airborne organisms. Avoiding kissing and saliva exchange is advised as well as wearing a facemask or covering. Couples are encouraged to be creative with physical barriers preventing face-to-face contact, and the use of condoms, lubricants, and dental dams can minimize chances of infection spread through saliva, semen, feces, blood, or bodily fluids. We advise being creative in order to maintain one's mental sanity during challenging times and to keep the pregnant woman and her unborn baby safe!

18.12 What Did Dr. Google Say?

Many medical conditions that impact pregnancy are described in this chapter. For the sake of concretion, the information that patients may access when performing an Internet search of only some of them will be reviewed in this last section as in other chapters.

When searching online for information regarding IBD and sex during pregnancy, free medical articles appear as first hits, some of them actually mentioning sexual health (not specifically during pregnancy), such as the *British Medical Journal* [6]. Dyspareunia and vaginal candidiasis are noted to be more frequent in patients with IBD. Some symptoms of IBD such as fatigue, tiredness, or abdominal pain that affect sexual desire and frequency are usually mentioned [7,8]. As for many issues referred to in this book, explicit information about sexuality during pregnancy is lacking.

With regard to epilepsy, almost all of the patient available information addresses the issue of family planning and contraception due to the association of antiepileptic drugs and birth defects, with no reference to sex during pregnancy [9,10].

The same picture is obtained when searching for lupus or rheumatoid arthritis during pregnancy. Symptoms of the diseases, issues with family planning, and impact on sexuality outside of pregnancy are all that can be found using an internet search engine.

Unfortunately, although accurate information on medical conditions and how they affect pregnancy can easily be found using an internet search engine, answers to questions patients may have about sexuality during pregnancy are not available.

18.13 Conclusion

Because of screening, medical interventions, and sophisticated medicines, millions of women live active sex lives in and outside of their pregnancies. Although a chronic disease adds physical and emotional strain to a couple's intimate activities, we advocate that sexual activity and function are major quality-of-life issues and advise perseverance and enjoyment. We hope we have provided some useful tips for safe sex.

References

1. B. Damgaard, A. Wettergren, P. Kirkegaard. Social and sexual function following ileal pouch–anal anastomosis. *Dis Colon Rectum* 1995;**38**:286–9.

2. C. Ozkara, S. Ozdemir, A. Yilmaz, et al. Orgasm-induced seizures: a study of six patients. *Epilepsia* 2006;**47**:2193–7.

3. S. Zhao, E. Li, J. Wang, et al. Rheumatoid arthritis and risk of sexual dysfunction: a systematic review and metaanalysis. *J Rheumatol* 2018;**45**:1375–82.

4. K. Esposito, M. Ciotola, F. Giugliano, et al. Association of body weight with sexual function in women. *Int J Impot Res* 2007;**19**:353–7.

5. M. C. Ribeiro, M. U. Nakamura, M. R. Torloni, et al. Maternal overweight and sexual function in pregnancy. *Acta Obstet Gynecol Scand* 2016;**95**:45–51.

6. E. M. Alstead. Inflammatory bowel disease in pregnancy. *Postgrad Med J* 2002;**78**:23–6. https://pmj.bmj.com/content/78/915/23 (accessed August 23, 2021).

7. D. Volek. Inflammatory bowel disease and female reproduction. www.premiermedicalhv.com/news/inflammatory-bowel-disease-and-female-reproduction/ (accessed August 23, 2021).

8. Living with Crohn's or Colitis: Reproductive Health. https://crohnsandcolitis.org.uk/info-support/information-about-crohns-and-colitis/all-information-about-crohns-and-colitis/living-with-crohns-or-colitis/reproductive-health (accessed August 23, 2021).

9. Relationships and sexuality. Epilepsy Foundation, 2014. https://epilepsyfoundation.org.au/managing-epilepsy/social-and-family-life/relationships-and-sexuality/ (accessed August 23, 2021).

10. Epilepsy: sex and reproduction. Sick Kids, 2010. www.aboutkidshealth.ca/Article?contentid=2122&language=English (accessed August 23, 2021).

11. R. Khurana. Systemic lupus erythematosus and pregnancy. 2020. https://emedicine.medscape.com/article/335055-overview (accessed August 23, 2021).

12. K. Ludlam. Lupus and pregnancy: tips for living with lupus while pregnant. 2011. www.webmd.com/lupus/features/lupus-pregnancy-pregnant (accessed August 23, 2021).

Air Embolism Related to Sex in Pregnancy and the Postpartum

Chapter **19**

Dina Mohamed, Mohamed Momtaz, and Dan Farine

19.1 Historical Background

Air embolism is a form of acute embolism resulting from vaginal insufflation [1]. Heid was the first to report such a condition in 1936, when a 16-year-old primigravida died during sexual intercourse with her fiancé. Postmortem examination revealed an obvious air embolism with a huge amount of air in the retroplacental area, vena cava, heart, and pulmonary artery. As the fiancé was later charged with criminal abortion, he admitted that he had blown air into her vagina while she was sitting on a chair during intercourse [1].

In 1981, Ragan reported three cases of air embolism during pregnancy. In each case, it was shown that forcible blowing of air into the vagina during sexual intercourse was the most probable cause. Other causes of air embolism may include vaginal douching with a bulb syringe or effervescent fluid, powder insufflation as a treatment for vaginal infections, and attempts at criminal abortion. According to Ragan, data from Ohio and Indiana show that approximately 1% of maternal deaths are due to air embolism (antepartum, intrapartum, and postpartum) [2].

Publications from the late 1980s report a total of 16 cases suffering from air embolism as a result of vaginal insufflation during orogenital sex [3–5]. All of them were pregnant and resulted in death except for four cases. Only one reported that the unborn child survived [6]. Legally, these cases have been considered accidental deaths as the involved parties appeared unaware of any of the consequences from that type of sexual act. However, intentional criminal abortion has also been considered, especially when the woman is in the early stages of pregnancy [3].

19.2 Definition and Epidemiology of Air Embolism

Venous air embolism (VAE) is the entrainment of air from ruptured veins to the central venous system, producing embolism in the right heart or pulmonary artery [6]. VAE has been reported in relation to pregnancy and the postpartum in patients who had orogenital and penile–vaginal intercourse, and is considered a rare but potentially life-threatening event [7,8].

Although there is no definite report of the exact incidence of VAE in pregnancy, Batman et al. [8] reported 18 mortalities as a result of VAE out of 20 million pregnancies. Another more recent review of the literature identified 22 cases of VAE associated with sexual activity; 19 of the 22 incidents occurred during pregnancy or the puerperium, and resulted in the death of 18 of the 22 women involved [7].

19.3 Mechanism of Air Embolism

For VAE to occur, two conditions must be met:

(1) Direct communication between the source of air and vasculature.

(2) A pressure gradient favoring passage of air into the circulation.

During pregnancy and the puerperium, there are direct communication channels between the vagina and the distended uteroplacental vasculature. Air can be introduced into the cervical canal in several ways, such as oral insufflation or the piston-like effect of a penis or finger in the vagina. When air enters the venous circulation and pulmonary vasculature, it can cause serious morbidity as well as cardiac arrest and death [9].

19.4 Pathophysiology

The pathophysiology of VAE from vaginal insufflation can be described as follows. The gravid vagina, being a highly distensible organ, can accommodate more than 1000 mL of air. When air is introduced under pressure, it travels through the dilated cervical canal and dissects beneath the amniotic membranes, where it enters the subplacental sinuses. Once air enters the venous drainage of the uterus, it can rapidly reach the inferior vena cava and from there the right side of the heart [4].

If the volume of introduced air is large (100–300 mL), serious damage can result from the mechanical obstruction of the right ventricular outflow tract as well as from the interaction of the air with blood products. This can produce a surface activity effect in the form of thrombi, increased capillary permeability, and release of biological mediators such as smooth muscle-acting factor [3,10,11].

Systemic arterial occlusion can also result from paradoxical air embolization. Air may reach the arterial circulation through either pulmonary arteriovenous connections or septal cardiac defects [4]. Once air reaches the arterial circulation, it may stay for over 48 hours. This may result in coma secondary to cerebral arterial emboli [12].

On the other hand, the nongravid vagina lacks the distensibility of the gravid one and consequently the invasion of air into the circulation is uncommon. In addition, the uterine venous sinuses are more liable to air entry during pregnancy and the puerperium [10]. Air embolism in the nonpregnant woman can present as pneumoperitoneum. In this condition the patient might complain of lower abdominal, upper quadrant, or shoulder pain but usually completely recovers [11].

19.5 Clinical Picture

Patients with VAE may present with a wide variety of nonspecific symptoms. Compromise of pulmonary or cardiovascular function often dominates the clinical picture. The most serious clinical manifestation of VAE leading to out-of-hospital cardiac arrest should be differentiated from aortic dissection, pericardial tamponade, myocardial infarction, ventricular dysrhythmia, stroke, intracranial bleeding, pulmonary thromboembolism, tension pneumothorax, and acute pulmonary edema. Some are potentially reversible causes for which specific treatment exists and must be considered during any cardiac arrest, particularly if nonshockable rhythms are being monitored [13,14].

The diagnosis of air embolism in fatal cases should be made carefully if there has been a prolonged interval before postmortem. In such cases, it has been shown that gas chromatography can assist in differentiating between genuine cases of air embolism and gas due to decomposition [14–16]. However, if such resources are not available, demonstrating gas within the left side of the heart, ascending aorta, and major branches may indicate that the gas in the right ventricle has been produced during decomposition [17].

19.6 Investigations

Laboratory abnormalities vary according to the severity of the embolism, but they lack specificity. VAE can present with such different ECG patterns as sinus tachycardia, nonspecific ST-segment and T-wave changes, evidence of acute ventricular strain, and different atrial and ventricular dysrhythmias [4].

Chest radiographs are usually normal, but they may later show evidence of pulmonary edema. Arterial blood gases reflect abnormalities in the matching of ventilation and perfusion. Pulmonary artery pressure may remain normal, with an increased central venous pressure, due to the presence of a large air bubble in the outflow tract of the right ventricle. There are three findings which are relatively specific for VAE: X-ray visualization of air in the right heart or pulmonary arteries, air bubbles in the retinal vessels, and the characteristic "mill wheel" murmur. If the air blocking the right ventricle is mechanically separated into smaller bubbles with closed-chest cardiac massage, detection of VAE is very difficult. In cases that lack specific findings, the diagnosis of air embolism is mainly based on the patient's history and the exclusion of other possible causes of out-of-hospital cardiac arrest [4,18].

19.7 Differential Diagnosis

The differential diagnosis for hypotension and coma during pregnancy includes sepsis, eclampsia or seizure, drugs or toxin exposure, acute cerebral event, myocardial infarction, or pulmonary emboli [19]. Amniotic fluid embolism can also be included, as it is accompanied by tachypnea, cyanosis, and pulmonary edema. It usually occurs during labor, cesarean section, or immediately postpartum [20]. Clark et al. [21] reported that the characteristic hemodynamic abnormality after amniotic fluid embolization is left heart failure with marked increases in capillary wedge pressure.

Squamous epithelial cells can be noted in the venous circulation; however, this is also a common finding in healthy gravid women before, during, and after labor [20].

19.8 Management

In spite of the rarity of this entity, pregnant patients should be advised to avoid orogenital sex with air insufflation, as this activity seems to confer an increased risk. Penile–vaginal sex, especially when the level of the uterus is above the level of the heart, may also increase the risk of embolism [22].

In order to minimize the complications of air embolism, accurate diagnosis is mandatory in those pregnant ill women and their unborn children. Management starts with the administration of 100% oxygen, and then turning the patient onto her left side in a head-down position in an attempt to trap the air in the right ventricle [4,23].

In the case of cardiovascular collapse, it is recommended that closed-chest compression is performed and air trapped in the right side of the heart is removed by either catheter or transthoracic puncture. If there is associated cerebral edema, it may be suppressed with corticosteroids [23].

Using hyperbaric oxygen therapy has proved to be specific and effective in treating air embolisms of any etiology; however, its effectiveness is inversely proportional to the delay between the incident and treatment [3,24].

19.9 What Did Dr. Google Say?

19.9.1 Romper.com

This site describes death by sex as a result of air embolism as like an urban legend or a plot for a bad movie. It also mentions how it is commonly believed that oral sex is a safe practice, but that simply blowing air into the vagina could be fatal [25].

Some evidence is mentioned to support the article. According to Healthline, an air or gas embolism can result from an air bubble entering and blocking a blood vessel. In spite of the rare occurrence of such a complication, such a blockage can cause strokes or heart attacks. In addition, the *International Journal of Legal Medicine* states that having oral sex while pregnant could cause an embolism if the partner blows enough air into the vaginal area. The solution to this problem is to simply instruct the partner to avoid it. Finally, deaths have been recorded from air embolism during pregnancy and immediate postpartum periods. The National Center for Biotechnology Information noted that women died from embolisms by having sex shortly after giving birth by spontaneous vaginal delivery (in two cases, the women had sex about a week after giving birth). This can be attributed to the sex, especially with a knee–chest position, which can force air into the vagina and cause air embolism. Again, these are infrequent incidents. In order to be safe, it is advised to follow the doctor's recommendations regarding sexual activity following delivery, which is to postpone sexual activity for at least 6 weeks following delivery.

19.9.2 Fox News

The site describes air embolism as air blown into the vagina that subsequently enters the women's bloodstream and blocks a blood vessel. It also advises pregnant women to prevent their partners from blowing air into their vagina while having oral intercourse during pregnancy [26].

19.9.3 Wikipedia

The site discusses rare causes of embolism during pregnancy, including air embolism caused by air entering the bloodstream from tears in the uterus or genitalia. Also mentioned is that the risk increases during pregnancy. Also reported were cases where attempts were made to induce abortion by syringing, the damage to the placenta allowing air to enter the bloodstream [27].

19.9.4 Metro.co.uk

The article starts by asking whether it is possible to die if someone blows air into the vagina. This is followed by a clear declaration that despite being reported, it is still a rare condition. An embolism is defined as a bubble of air that enters the bloodstream, which can happen in various ways usually related to at-home attempted abortions and, in some cases, during sex.

Evidence was sought from an article published in the *Postgraduate Medical Journal* in 1998 which reported that a UK Department of Health enquiry had found three cases of death by embolism during sexual intercourse and one case of death by embolism during oral sex. Another article published in the *Academic Emergency Medicine Journal* mentioned a similar case of a pregnant woman after her husband had insufflated a large amount of air into her vagina.

Despite the evidence, the article emphasizes the low risk of such an event with a light blow into the vulva or vigorous sex session. The site also contacted a number of UK gynecologists who were not able to speak on the issue since they had had no personal experience of it.

The article ends up by warning females against excess air blown into the vagina, especially those at risk such as pregnant women or those with vaginal injuries. Some alternative therapy products, such as "ozone therapy," pump gas into the vagina using a douche-like mechanism. The companies who manufacture these items assume that the products help with myriad health problems, and that there is no risk in using their products [28].

References

1. O. O. Heid. A strange death trap in pregnancy from air embolism. *Oeff Health Service* 1936;**A2**:720–2.

2. W. D. Ragan. Antepartum air embolism. *J Indiana State Med Assoc* 1981;**1**:30–2.

3. P. Bray, R. A. M. Myers, R. A. Cowley. Orogenital sex as a cause of nonfatal air embolism in pregnancy. *Obstet Gynecol* 1985;**61**: 653–7.

4. F. E. Fyke, F. J. Kazmier, R. W. Harms. Venous air embolism: life threatening complication of orogenital sex during pregnancy. *Am J Med* 1985;**78**:333–6.

5. B. S. Kaufman, S. J. Kaminsky, E. C. Rackow, et al. Adult respiratory distress syndrome following orogenital sex during pregnancy. *Crit Care Med* 1987;**15**:703–4.

6. C. S. Kim, J. Liu, J. Y. Kwon, S. K. Shin, K. J. Kim. Venous air embolism during surgery, especially cesarean delivery. *J Korean Med Sci* 2008;**23**:753–61.

7. A. Truhlar, V. Cerny, P. Dostal, et al. Out-of-hospital cardiac arrest from air embolism during sexual intercourse: case report and review of the literature. *Resuscitation* 2007;**73**:475–84.

8. P. A. Batman, J. Thomlinson, V. C. Moore, et al. Death due to air embolism during sexual intercourse in the puerperium. *Postgrad Med J* 1998;**74**:612–13.

9. C. Jones, C. Chan, D. Farine. Sex in pregnancy. *Can Med Assoc J* 2011;**183**:815–18.

10. P. K. Nelson. Pulmonary gas embolism in pregnancy and the puerperium. *Obstet Gynecol Surv* 1960;**15**:449–81.

11. J. Varon, M. D. Laufer, G. L. Sternbach. Recurrent pneumoperitoneum following vaginal insufflation. *Am J Emerg Med* 1991;**9**:447–8.

12. C. C. Fries, B. Levowitz, S. Adler, et al. Experimental gas embolism. *Ann Surg* 1957;**145**:46–51.

13. M. E. Aronson, P. K. Nelson. Fatal air embolism in pregnancy resulting from an unusual act. *Obstet Gynecol* 1967;**30**:127–30.

14. T. Bajanowski, H. Köhler, A. Du Chesne, et al. Proof of air embolism after exhumation. *Int J Legal Med* 1999;**112**:2–7.

15. I. Pedal, A. Moosmayer, H. J. Mallach, et al. Air embolism or putrefaction? Gas analysis findings and their interpretation. *Z Rechtsmed* 1987;**99**:151–67.

16. G. Pierucci, G. Gherson. Further contribution to the chemical diagnosis of gas embolism. The demonstration of

hydrogen as an expression of "putrefactive component." *Zacchia* 1969;5:595–603.

17. D. I. Rushton, I. M. Dawson. The maternal autopsy. *J Clin Pathol* 1982;**35**:909–21.

18. S. L. Orebaugh, A. Grenvik. Air embolisation. In W. C. Shoemaker, A. Grenvik, eds. *Textbook of Critical Care*, 4th ed. Philadelphia: W. B. Saunders, 2000: 1155–62.

19. A. Fatteh, W. B. Leach, C. A. Wilkinson. Fatal air embolism in pregnancy resulting from orogenital sex play. *Forensic Sci Int* 1973;**2**:247–50.

20. S. L. Clark. New concepts of amniotic fluid embolism: a review. *Obstet Gynecol Surv* 1990;**45**:360–8.

21. S. L. Clark, F. J. Montz, J. P. Phelan. Hemodynamic alterations associated with amniotic fluid embolism: a reappraisal. *Am J Obstet Gynecol* 1985;**151**:617–21.

22. J. P. Nolan, C. D. Deakin, J. Soar, B. W. Böttiger, G. Smith, European Resuscitation Council guidelines for resuscitation 2005. Section 4. Adult advanced life support. *Resuscitation* 2005;**67**(Suppl 1):S39–86.

23. S. B. Alvaran, J. K. Toung, T. E. Graff, et al. Venous air embolism. Comparative merits of external cardiac massage, intracardiac aspiration, and left lateral decubitus position. *Anesth Analg* 1978;**57**:166–70.

24. T. L. Bernhardt, R. W. Goldmann, P. A. Thombs, et al. Hyperbaric oxygen treatment of cerebral air embolism from orogenital sex during pregnancy. *Crit Care Med* 1988;**16**:729–30.

25. L. E. Mack. Here's how vaginal embolisms happen. 2017. www.romper.com/p/how-do-vaginal-embolisms-happen-its-a-rare-but-possible-occurrence-60636 (accessed April 23, 2021).

26. What you need to know about pregnant sex. 2015. www.foxnews.com/health/what-you-need-to-know-about-pregnant-sex (accessed April 23, 2021).

27. Air embolism. Last updated May 10, 2022. https://en.wikipedia.org/wiki/Air_embolism (accessed April 23, 2021).

28. J. Lindsay. Getting freaky: will you really die if someone blows air into your vagina? 2018. https://metro.co.uk/2018/10/25/getting-freaky-will-you-really-die-if-someone-blows-air-into-your-vagina-8050287/ (accessed April 23, 2021).

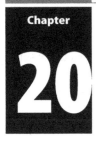

Pelvic and Ovarian Masses during Pregnancy

Elisa Moreno Palacios and Pablo Tobías González

20.1 Introduction

Pelvic masses in pregnant women are rare, although the incidence is increasing with the instauration of routine ultrasound in pregnancy follow-up. Systematic first-trimester ultrasound allows scanning of the uterus, adnexa, pelvis, and abdomen of the patient, looking for possible masses or alterations. Most pelvic masses in pregnant women are incidental findings, but occasionally raising the doubt of malignancy. The differential diagnosis of pelvic masses in pregnant women should include gynecological and inflammatory/infectious processes, as well as nongynecological pathology such as appendicitis, diverticulitis, and others that can confusingly present as adnexal masses. The most common pelvic masses in pregnant women are uterine fibroids and adnexa cyst.

20.2 Myomas

Myomas, commonly known as fibroids, are the most frequent solid benign tumor of the uterus that affect women in reproductive age. The prevalence is variable among different studies and countries, but has been reported as high as 80% in women who have reached the age of 50 [1]. Myomas are reported in about 3–12% of pregnant women, varying with ethnicity (18% in African-American women, 8% in Hispanic women, and 10% in White women) and age, with prevalence as high as 25% in older women undergoing ovum donor recipient in vitro fertilization (IVF) [2].

Most pregnant women with myomas are asymptomatic, with only 10–30% developing complications during gestation, delivery, or puerperium. The most commonly reported symptom is pain; approximately 5–21% of women with myomas will require hospitalization for pain control during pregnancy.

Myomas tend to grow through pregnancy, with a mean increase in volume of 12%, but as high as 25% in a low percentage of myomas; it has been observed that larger myomas (>5 cm) are more likely to grow. It was widely thought that myomas grow rapidly during pregnancy under the influence of hormone stimulation and increased blood flow. Current evidence from in vitro studies has related the exponential increase in human chorionic gonadotropin (hCG) and the kinetics of its receptor to the enlargement of fibroids. Myomas suffer the same process of hyperplasia and hypertrophy as uterine muscle [2].

Pain has been associated with the rapid growth of myomas, especially during the first half of pregnancy. The rapid enlargement of the myoma leads to edema and central necrosis, with consequent prostaglandin release causing the pain [3]. Central necrosis, also called red degeneration, is characterized by acute focal abdominal pain, mild fever, nausea and vomiting, tenderness over the myoma, and leukocytosis. Pain can also result from torsion of a pedunculated fibroid, caused by obstruction of the blood supply. Torsion is more likely to occur in the first trimester or after delivery, as there is more space in the abdominal cavity, although it is rare.

Uterine myomas have been associated with an increased risk of obstetric complications, such as miscarriage, preterm birth, fetal malpresentation, cesarean section, placenta previa, and peripartum hemorrhage. The most important risk factors for obstetric morbidity are related to the number, localization, and size of myomas [4].

With regard to the number of fibroids, Ciavattini et al. [5] showed that women with two or more fibroids display a higher risk of preterm labor and cesarean section. With regard to the size of myomas, larger fibroids (mostly defined as >5 cm) are associated with delivery at earlier gestational age, higher rates of hemorrhage, increased estimated blood loss during delivery, and higher rates of admission for pain-related symptoms. Furthermore, the risk of cesarean section has been reported to be greater in women with larger myomas and higher total fibroid volume [2].

Regarding the localization of myomas, submucosal and intramural myomas are associated with more complications compared with subserosal myomas, which have not shown any association with pregnancy complications. However, this assertion is not completely reassuring, as there seems to be an increased risk of miscarriage of 1.7 in women with fibroids, independent of location.

With respect to pain during sexual intercourse, there are no published data on pregnant women with myomas. In 2015, David et al. [6] published a retrospective study that included 1548 patients with myomas, observing a moderate correlation between dyspareunia and the presence of myomas in nonpregnant women, the intensity of the pain being uninfluenced by the number, size, or location of the myomas. However, this study has important limitations: It is a retrospective study that only included patients with myomas seeking medical treatment, and it is well known that only 10–20% of women with myomas are symptomatic.

Management of myomas during pregnancy is merely conservative. Myomectomy is contraindicated during pregnancy due to the possibility of significant complications such as pregnancy interruption and severe bleeding. If complications such as specific pain appear during pregnancy, treatment should be symptomatic, with analgesia and hospitalization if required. Surgery should be limited to symptomatic torsion of peduncular myomas or in selected cases during cesarean section because of the significant risk of hemorrhage.

In conclusion, pregnant women with myomas should be considered at high risk because of the associated adverse obstetric outcomes. Surgical treatment is not indicated during pregnancy. Myomectomy should generally be deferred until after birth, although myomas should be reevaluated in the postpartum as they tend to partially regress after delivery.

20.3 Adnexal Masses

Adnexal masses detected during pregnancy represent both a diagnostic and management challenge. During the last few years, there has been an increasing trend in the incidence of adnexal masses diagnosed during pregnancy due to the use of routine ultrasound in pregnancy follow-up. The reported incidence of adnexal masses detected during pregnancy varies from 0.15 to 5.7% [7].

In general, most adnexal masses are diagnosed in the first and second trimester. Symptoms are rare, with 65–80% of patients being asymptomatic. Functional ovarian cysts tend to regress spontaneously. Nevertheless, when the adnexa mass persists beyond 16–19 weeks of pregnancy, pathology should be suspected.

When an adnexal mass is diagnosed in a pregnant woman, the main concern is to exclude malignancy. The incidence of malignant masses during pregnancy range from 0.8 to 13%. The reported incidence of ovarian cancer in pregnant women varies from 1 in 15 000 to 1 in 32 000 [7]. Pelvic ultrasound is the technique of choice for evaluating adnexa masses. There are a series of ultrasonographic features that should raise suspicion of malignancy, such as the presence of solid components, multiloculated large tumors with increased wall thickness and maximum diameter over 6 cm, gross internal septa (>2-3 mm), papillary projections, decreased resistance in blood flow during Doppler examination, or pelvic free fluid. Based on ultrasonographic features, adnexal masses are categorized as low, intermediate, or high risk of malignancy. Low-risk ovarian cysts are typically anechoic and unilocular with thin walls. Intermediate-risk masses are not completely anechoic and/or unilocular, but do not have clear malignant characteristic. High-risk masses are generally solid, multilocular, large (>6 cm) with thick walls. If the adnexal mass is not properly visualized and characterized with ultrasound, magnetic resonance imaging can provide more information and is safe during pregnancy [8].

Complementary tests such as tumor markers are of low utility in pregnant women because of the physiological elevation of cancer antigen (CA)-125 and hCG during the first trimester. Tumor markers cannot be used to exclude malignancy in pregnant women.

Pregnant women with adnexal masses are at risk of ovarian torsion. It has been reported that there is a higher risk of torsion in patients with ovarian cysts of specifically 6–8 cm and which occur between weeks 10 and 17 of pregnancy. Ovarian torsion should be suspected in pregnant women with an ovarian cyst that presents with acute abdominal pain [9]. Ovarian hyperstimulation is also a risk factor for ovarian torsion: If a patient who is pregnant via an assisted reproductive technique presents with intense unilateral pelvic pain, ovarian torsion should be suspected as the first diagnosis [10].

Management of adnexal masses during pregnancy is controversial, as surgery is associated with risks for the mother and the fetus, and conservative management can lead to ovarian torsion or abdominal spread of a tumor if it is a carcinoma. If the patient is asymptomatic and ultrasound reveals a low-risk ovarian cyst, observation and follow-up is reasonable. Surgery is indicated in the pregnant patient with an enlarging cyst, rupture, torsion, hemorrhage, or high suspicion of malignancy. Recommended timing of surgery is during the second trimester (16–20 weeks) in order to avoid the risk of miscarriage if performed during the first trimester and the risk of preterm delivery if carried out later when the enlarged gravid uterus limits surgery. Symptomatic patients are an exception, as surgery should be performed at the time of presentation to avoid further risks. Intermediate- or low-risk adnexal masses are usually monitored closely, with frequent ultrasound. On the other hand, in high-risk ovarian cysts or adnexal masses associated with ascites prompt surgery is indicated.

Laparoscopic resection is preferred over laparotomy in pregnant women, as in non-pregnant patients. The advantages of laparoscopy over laparotomy include shorter hospital stay, less postoperative pain, minor uterine manipulation, and prompt postoperative ambulation reducing the risk of thrombosis, which is increased during pregnancy.

No specific published data has been found relating intercourse with complications of adnexal masses during pregnancy. In theory, sexual intercourse in patients with adnexal masses can cause torsion, rupture, and/or hemorrhage of an ovarian cyst. Therefore, there is no strong evidence to recommend avoiding sexual intercourse in patients with ovarian hyperstimulation or ovarian cyst, although it may seem a reasonable recommendation where there are larger ovaries as these have a higher propensity to torsion.

In summary, most adnexal masses diagnosed during pregnancy are incidental benign findings. Adnexal masses in pregnant women should be evaluated with ultrasound as for nonpregnant premenopausal women. Surgery should be limited to cases with high suspicion of malignancy or severe acute complications. Asymptomatic low/intermediate-risk adnexal masses should be managed with frequent ultrasound follow-up.

20.4 What Did Dr. Google Say?

As with published studies, very limited data about pregnancy with pelvic masses and sex was found during the revision for this chapter. After introducing the terms "sex OR intercourse," "pregnancy," and "fibroid OR myoma OR pelvic mass OR ovarian cyst OR ovarian tumor" in a search engine, almost all the results address the issue of sex with fibroids or pelvic masses outside of pregnancy.

Many sites comment on the implications of fibroid or adnexal masses during pregnancy: possible growth, symptoms, treatment, labor complications, and their impact on fertility. Unfortunately, there is no mention about sexual intercourse during pregnancy. Pain during sex is frequently mentioned outside of pregnancy.

As examples of the limited results found, at www.thebump.com the corpus luteum is mentioned as the possible origin of pain during intercourse during the first trimester [11]. Other sites mention pelvic masses as a cause of pain during sex in pregnancy [12,13]. Most sites recommend consulting a healthcare provider in cases of severe or persistent pain or if it is associated with bleeding.

References

1. G. A. Vilos, C. Allaire, P. Y. Laberge, N. Leyland. The management of uterine leiomyomas. *J Obstet Gynaecol Can* 2015;**37**:157–78.

2. G. N. Milazzo, A. Catalano, V. Badia, M. Mallozzi, D. Caserta. Myoma and myomectomy: poor evidence concern in pregnancy. *J Obstet Gynaecol Res* 2017;**43**:1789–804.

3. P. C. Klatsky, N. D. Tran, A. B. Caughey, V. Y. Fujimoto. Fibroids and reproductive outcomes: a systematic literature review from conception to delivery. *Am J Obstet Gynecol* 2008;**198**:357–66.

4. F. Parazzini, L. Tozzi, S. Bianchi. Pregnancy outcome and uterine fibroids. *Best Pract Res Clin Obstet Gynaecol* 2016;**34**:74–84

5. A. Ciavattini, N. Clemente, G. Delli Carpini, et al. Number and size of uterine fibroids and obstetric outcomes. *J Matern Fetal Neonatal Med* 2015;**28**:484–8.

6. M. David, C. M. Pitz, A. Mihaylova, F. Siedentopf. Myoma-associated pain frequency and intensity: a retrospective evaluation of 1548 myoma patients. *Eur J Obstet Gynecol Reprod Biol* 2016;**199**:137–40.

7. A. Mukhopadhyay, A. Shinde, R. Naik. Ovarian cysts and cancer in pregnancy.

Best Pract Res Clin Obstet Gynaecol 2016;**33**:58–72.

8. A. M. Hakoun, I. AbouAl-Shaar, K. J. Zaza, H. Abou-Al-Shaar, M. N. A. Salloum. Adnexal masses in pregnancy: an updated review. *Avicenna J Med* 2017;**7**:153–7.

9. V. Asfour, R. Varma, P. Menon. Clinical risk factors for ovarian torsion. *J Obstet Gynaecol* 2015;**35**:721–5.

10. S. M. Hilbert, S. Gunderson. Complications of assisted reproductive technology. *Emerg Med Clin North Am* 2019;**37**:239–49.

11. K. Miller. Why you might be experiencing painful sex during pregnancy. 2020. www .thebump.com/a/pain-during-sex (accessed September 20, 2021).

12. *5 Reasons you may be experiencing painful sex during pregnancy. www.parents.com/ pregnancy/my-life/sex-relationship/ painful-sex-during-pregnancy/ (accessed September 20, 2021).*

13. Kidadl Team. Painful sex during pregnancy: tips to help. 2021. https:// kidadl.com/articles/painful-sex-during-pregnancy-tips-to-help (accessed September 20, 2021).

Chapter

21

Sexually Transmitted Infections and Pregnancy

María Serrano Velasco and Cristina González Benítez

21.1 Introduction

Sexually transmitted infections (STIs) are a major global public health problem. The World Health Organization (WHO) recently published a document that imparts keys messages and summarizes the magnitude of the problem [1]:

- More than 1 million STIs occur every day.
- An estimated 376 million infections of chlamydia, gonorrhea, syphilis, and trichomoniasis occur every year.
- More than 500 million people have a herpes simplex virus (HSV1 or HSV2) genital infection.
- Approximately 300 million women have a human papillomavirus (HPV) infection and this number is likely similar in men.
- The majority of STIs occur without symptoms.
- Some STIs can increase the risk of human immunodeficiency virus (HIV) acquisition threefold or more.

This chapter documents the main STIs that are relevant in pregnancy. Some STIs can cause infertility, some may affect the normal course of pregnancy or the development of the fetus, and others can be transmitted to the newborn and cause chronic illness.

Some STIs have a cure or a vaccine, but only through major efforts aimed at primary prevention (vaccination, sex education), early detection (screening at the beginning of pregnancy and, in people at risk, accessible diagnostic tests with the first symptoms), and effective treatment will we be able to fight efficiently against them.

21.1.1 Screening of STIs in Pregnancy

All pregnant women should be tested for hepatitis B virus (HBV), syphilis, and HIV in the first trimester of pregnancy. In addition, the Centers for Disease Control and Prevention (CDC) recommends that women under 25 years of age or with risk factors for STIs be screened for *Chlamydia trachomatis* and *Neisseria gonorrhoeae* infection [2]. Risk factors for acquiring an STI include new or multiple sex partners, a sex partner with concurrent partners, or a sex partner with an existing STI; inconsistent condom use among persons who are not in mutually monogamous relationships; previous or concurrent STI; and exchanging sex for money or drugs.

The determination of antibodies against hepatitis C virus (HCV) is recommended for all pregnant women unless they live in an environment where the prevalence is less than 0.1%, and regardless of the local prevalence if the patient is at risk of acquiring it (sexual partner being a virus carrier, parenteral drug user, recipient of potentially contaminated blood products, or patient on hemodialysis) [3].

If the patient is HIV positive, the tests described should be performed at the preconception visit (syphilis, HBV, *Chlamydia trachomatis*, and *Neisseria gonorrhoeae*), adding *Trichomonas vaginalis* and HCV. There are high rates of STIs in the HIV-positive population and existing STIs can also increase the risk of HIV transmission [4].

If the pregnant patient is at high risk for acquisition of STIs, the tests should be repeated in the third trimester.

21.1.2 Cervical Cancer Screening in Pregnancy

When a patient attends the first pregnancy visit, it is important to ascertain whether she has undergone correct cervical cancer screening. The European guidelines recommend that invitation to cervical cancer screening should begin between 20 and 30 years of age [5]. The only primary screening test currently recommended by the European Union for cervical cancer in women under 35 years of age is cervical cytology. The most appropriate interval between cytologies is 3 years [6].

Routine primary screening for HPV should therefore not begin before 30 years of age [7]. The screening interval for women with negative HPV primary screening results should be at least 5 years. Screening with cytology every 3 years from the age of 30 is also acceptable.

Immunosuppressed patients should start screening earlier and undergo more frequent controls, since cytopathological and histopathological lesions of the cervix are five to six times more common in HIV-positive than HIV-negative women.

21.2 Main STIs in Pregnancy

21.2.1 Syphilis

Epidemiology

At present there are 18 million estimated prevalent cases of syphilis worldwide [8].

Etiological Agent

Treponema pallidum (spirochete bacterium).

Transmission

Sexual contact through intact or eroded skin or mucosa. There is also blood transmission since the bacterium spreads through the lymphatic and blood vessels and transplacentally.

Clinical Presentation

We can differentiate early syphilis (primary, secondary, and early latent) and late syphilis (tertiary and late latent).

- **Primary syphilis**: The syphilitic chancre appears 9–90 days after contact. It is indurated, without exudation, not very painful, and usually on the external genitalia, and is accompanied generally by bilateral adenopathy. It disappears in 3–6 weeks.

- **Secondary syphilis**: Due to the spread of the bacterium 2–8 weeks after the appearance of the chancre, general flu-like symptoms and symptoms in various organs are produced. The most characteristic symptom is the maculopapular rash on palms and soles that erodes in areas of friction and produces flat condylomata. Other symptoms include meningism, headache, glomerulonephritis, osteitis, synovitis, digestive disorders, hepatitis, and pharyngitis. This phase lasts 2–6 weeks.
- **Latent syphilis**: Characterized by the absence of symptoms, and only detectable by serology. It can be early latent (<12 months from infection) or late latent (>12 months, or time since infection unknown). An infected person can stay in this phase for their entire life without moving on to the next stage.
- **Tertiary syphilis**: After one or several decades of latency. Possible manifestations include neurosyphilis (tabes dorsalis, general paralysis), cardiovascular syphilis with destruction of the great vessels (aortic arch), iritis and chorioretinitis, and tuberous syphiloderma on skin, gums (asymptomatic nodules that later become necrotic and drain necrotic material), bones, liver, oral mucosa, or upper respiratory tract.

Gynecologic/Obstetric Implications

The effects on the fetus are devastating if syphilis is not detected and treated early, including stillbirth, neonatal death, preterm delivery, low-birthweight babies, and infected infants [9]. Most of the untreated primary and secondary infections that occur during pregnancy and half that occur in the latent phase have adverse effects on pregnancy. Most of the transmission to the fetus occurs in late pregnancy (after 28 weeks) and treatment before this period will usually prevent congenital features [10].

Diagnosis

- **Direct diagnosis**: Fresh examination with dark-field microscopy, direct immunofluorescence (DFA-TP), and nucleic acid amplification techniques (NAAT). Culture is only used in research.
- **Indirect diagnosis**: Valid for screening and diagnosis. There are two types of serological tests: nontreponemal and treponemal. For an accurate diagnosis both tests must be positive.
  - Reaginic or nontreponemic tests (NTT): These are good markers of activity and response to treatment. They are not very specific and can give false-positive results in pregnancy and other cases. The most widely available nontreponemal tests are the microscopic Venereal Diseases Research Laboratory (VDRL) and the macroscopic rapid plasma reagin (RPR) tests. The RPR test has become the standard screening test while the VDRL is used for the diagnosis of neurosyphilis. The enzyme-linked immunosorbent assay (ELISA) technique is used for population screening [10].
  - Nonreaginic or treponemic tests (TT): These confirm a positive result of nontreponemal tests but can remain positive for life, so they can indicate a current or past infection. Treponemal tests include the *Treponema pallidum* hemagglutination assay (TPHA), the *Treponema pallidum* particle agglutination assay (TPPA), and the fluorescent treponemal antibody absorption (FTAABS) tests.
  - Rapid syphilis tests (RST): These provide treponemal antibody results in 10–15 minutes and can be performed on-site in any setting since they do not require refrigerated storage or laboratory equipment [8].

Treatment

The first- and second-line treatment of early syphilis is the same as that in the non-pregnant population.

- Preferred therapy: Single dose of benzathine penicillin G (BPG) 2.4 million units intramuscularly (IM). One injection of 2.4 million units or 1.2 million units in each buttock.
- Alternative therapy: Procaine penicillin 600 000 units IM daily for 10–14 days, i.e. if BPG is not available.

In the case of penicillin allergy in pregnant women, doxycycline cannot be used, so it would be necessary to attempt penicillin desensitization [11]. If this option is impossible, WHO STI guidelines suggest using erythromycin 500 mg orally four times daily for 14 days or ceftriaxone 1 g IM daily for 10–14 days [12], but erythromycin and azithromycin do not cross the placental barrier completely, so it is necessary to treat the newborn infant soon after delivery.

The treatment of late syphilis or unknown state in pregnant women is as follows:

- Preferred therapy: The WHO STI guidelines recommend BPG 2.4 million units IM once weekly for three consecutive weeks.
- Alternative therapy: Procaine penicillin 1.2 million units IM once daily for 20 days. In case of allergy or if the previous medications are unavailable, erythromycin 500 mg orally four times daily for 30 days can be used.

Treatment of Contacts

A person who has sexual contact with a patient with primary syphilis in less than 90 days should be treated. The rest should have serological tests if available.

Follow-Up

Globally, many studies have confirmed that follow-up is suboptimal. For early syphilis, minimum clinical and serological (VDRL/RPR) follow-up should be at 1, 3, 6, and 12 months [11]. After treatment of early syphilis, the titer of an NTT taken at day 0 (e.g. VDRL and/or RPR) should decline by two or more dilution steps (fourfold or greater decrease in antibody titer) within 6 months.

21.2.2 Hepatitis B

Epidemiology

Despite the existence of a vaccine, HBV infection is endemic. An estimated 240 million people are affected, with South and East Asia being the most prevalent areas worldwide [13]. In areas of medium and high endemicity, mother–child transmission is responsible for the majority of chronic hepatitis. Screening in pregnancy, treatment of pregnant women with high levels of HBV DNA, and vaccination in infancy have been crucial in reducing infection rates significantly.

Etiological Agent

Hepatitis B virus (DNA virus), family *Hepadnaviridae*.

Transmission

HBV transmission occurs through infected body fluids, including blood, semen, vaginal secretions, breast milk, and saliva.

Clinical Presentation

The symptoms of acute infection can occur between 30 and 180 days after exposure and initially symptoms of gastroenteritis may appear before the typical symptoms of hepatitis (nausea, pain in the right upper quadrant, jaundice). Infrequently, encephalopathy can occur. Fulminant hepatitis in the general population is rare (<0.5–1%) [14].

Pregnancy is normally well tolerated in patients with chronic HBV infection unless there is advanced liver dysfunction [15]. Physiological changes in pregnancy can mask decompensation.

Gynecologic/Obstetric Implications

There are usually no serious effects on the fetus except in the case of liver cirrhosis due to previous chronic hepatitis. In these cases, intrauterine growth restriction, intrauterine infection, preterm delivery, and intrauterine fetal demise may appear.

The mother–child transmission rate increases as pregnancy progresses and has been reported to be as high as 90% without the use of active and passive immunization.

Diagnosis

At the first prenatal visit, the determination of HB antigen (HBsAg) is recommended and, if positive, other HBV markers should be tested. If acute hepatitis is suspected at any time during pregnancy, the tests should be repeated. In addition, a differential diagnosis should be made with other possible causes of liver disease in pregnancy.

Treatment

The treatment of acute hepatitis in pregnant women is supportive except in severe cases. In the third trimester, in cases of high viral load treatment is recommended in order to avoid vertical transmission as much as possible.

The management of the pregnant woman with chronic HBV infection should be carried out in consultation with a hepatologist. If the patient was already receiving treatment before the pregnancy and it cannot be terminated, she should be switched to tenofovir disoproxil fumarate (TDF).

In general, for pregnant women with a viral load in excess of 2×10^5 IU/mL ($>10^6$ copies/mL), antiviral therapy is recommended. This begins at 28–30 weeks of gestation. The two preferred treatments are TDF (300 mg daily) or lamivudine (100 mg daily).

Follow-Up

For acute HBV infection, follow-up is needed to ensure that HBsAg is cleared. Notification and consideration of possible contagion to the cohabiting partner is important.

In pregnant women with chronic HBV infection without severe liver dysfunction, biochemical monitoring is performed quarterly and for up to 6 months after delivery. HBV DNA should be quantified if there is an increase in alanine aminotransferase (ALT) and also at weeks 26–28 of gestation to determine the need for treatment in the third trimester in order to reduce vertical transmission. Children can be breastfed after receiving HBV immune globulin (HBIG) and the first dose of vaccine.

21.2.3 Hepatitis C

Epidemiology

HCV is a worldwide endemic infection with an average prevalence of 1.6%. However, it reaches 4% in sub-Saharan Africa and Central Asia [16]. Only 15–45% of infected patients clear the virus spontaneously. There is no effective vaccine against HCV and serious complications such as liver cirrhosis and hepatocarcinoma are not uncommon.

Etiological Agent

Hepatitis C virus (RNA virus), family *Flaviviridae*.

Transmission

Heterosexual transmission is rare. Transmission through blood is much more efficient than through other fluids. Reinfection and superinfection are possible.

Clinical Presentation

Acute infection has the same nonspecific symptoms as in nonpregnant patients and in other types of hepatitis (general discomfort, fatigue, or nausea). On rare occasions jaundice develops, with choluria and acholia.

Gynecologic/Obstetric Implications

The majority of neonates are infected perinatally. The most important factors for transmission are maternal viremia in pregnancy and delivery and HIV coinfection. Other risk factors include invasive prenatal testing, prolonged rupture of membranes, and invasive obstetric procedures. However, the genotype of the virus, the mode of delivery, and even breastfeeding do not seem to be associated with an increased risk of transmission. Transmission is approximately 5%, but up to 10% in HIV-positive patients.

Virus infection does not appear to have prenatal implications. Newborns are usually asymptomatic, but progression to chronicity is usually 80% [17].

Diagnosis

The indications for screening with HCV serology have been discussed at the beginning of the chapter.

If recent infection is suspected (<3 months), testing for HCVAg or HCV RNA should be performed (mean seroconversion after infection is 65 days) [14]; 71% of patients rapidly normalize ALT levels in blood.

Specific antibody/antigen testing for verifying the diagnosis is available, but might not differentiate between acute and chronic forms of HCV infection.

Treatment

Direct-acting antiviral agents are highly effective and fairly well tolerated, but in many countries treatment is only financed for chronic hepatitis (>6 months duration). Treatment of women prior to becoming pregnant is essential to reduce vertical transmission.

Women who were treated with a ribavirin-containing regimen should avoid pregnancy for at least 6 months afterwards.

Follow-Up

Patients with acute HCV infection should be followed with 4-weekly HCV RNA quantitation to detect spontaneous clearing of the disease. It is important the patient is followed up by a hepatologist in case of chronic hepatitis.

21.2.4 Genital Herpes

Epidemiology

It is estimated that 67% of the world population is infected by one of the two types of herpes simplex (HSV1 and HSV2) [18].

Etiological Agent

Herpes simplex virus 1 and 2 (DNA virus), family *Herpesviridae*.

Transmission

Normally occurs through the skin due to typical viral lesions, although there may be genital viral excretion when the lesions have not yet appeared. Vertical transmission is possible, with a very low intrauterine incidence (5%), mostly perinatal (85%) and postnatal (10%) [19].

Gynecologic/Obstetric Implications

Although infrequent, if intrauterine infection occurs there are alterations of the central nervous system (CNS) in two-thirds of neonates (microcephaly, ventriculomegaly, porencephaly, calcifications, and hemorrhagic infarcts). They can also have ocular, liver, and bone involvement. Mortality is 45% and psychomotor retardation is frequent. Perinatal infection manifests at 10–12 days of life with skin (80%), oral, and/or ocular involvement. Postnatal disease can be localized in the CNS (30–35%) or disseminated (25%).

Clinical Presentation

Symptoms in pregnant women are the same as those in nonpregnant women. Primary infection can be asymptomatic in up to two-thirds of cases. Patients may have prodromes with general malaise, inguinal lymphadenopathy, and dysuria. Later, papules appear, become vesicles and break early, causing painful erosions. In recurrent cases, the prodromes are usually milder.

Diagnosis

Although the virus can be cultured, the preferred method is polymerase chain reaction (PCR) determination of viral DNA in the lesions. Seroconversion usually occurs at 90 days [20].

Treatment

Treatment in pregnancy is only indicated if the woman is very symptomatic or the lesions appear near delivery. Oral acyclovir 400 mg three times daily or oral valacyclovir

500 mg twice daily can be used. In primary infection, the duration of treatment will be 7–10 days and in recurrences 3–5 days.

In women with recurrent herpes (six or more episodes per year), suppressive treatment should be undertaken from week 36 until delivery or earlier if there is a risk of premature delivery. In concomitant HIV and herpetic infection, treatment should begin at week 32 due to a higher risk of prematurity. Suppressive treatment is carried out with the same drugs and doses. If there is an outbreak in the 6 weeks prior to delivery, cesarean section is mandatory to prevent neonatal infection.

21.2.5 Human Immunodeficiency Virus

It is estimated that 1.3 million HIV-infected women become pregnant each year. The vertical transmission of HIV constitutes 9% of new infections globally, with infected children doomed to an early death [21].

Of pregnant women with HIV, 86% are in sub-Saharan Africa. Efforts aimed at prevention, early detection, and adherence to treatment are key to reducing transmission rates.

Etiological Agent

Human immunodeficiency virus 1 and 2 (RNA retrovirus), family *Retroviridae*.

Transmission

HIV transmission requires contact with body fluids, specifically blood, semen, vaginal secretions, breast milk, or exudates from wounds or lesions on the skin or mucosa, which contain HIV free virions or infected cells. Contagion from saliva or cough/sneeze drops is highly unlikely.

Gynecologic/Obstetric Implications

Vertical transmission can occur in utero (especially in the third trimester) due to alteration in the integrity of the placenta and passage of maternal blood, intrapartum due to contamination of the fetal mucosa with maternal secretions and blood (depending on the time of rupture of membranes and duration of labor), and during breastfeeding.

In developed countries, combined antiretroviral therapy (ART) has managed to reduce vertical transmission from 20–30% to less than 1%.

Clinical Presentation

At the time of infection, approximately 10–60% of people are asymptomatic. Sometimes within 2–4 weeks nonspecific symptoms may appear (fever, headache, lymphadenopathy, sore throat, rash, myalgia/arthralgia, diarrhea, and weight loss). Sometimes opportunistic infections, as well as different cancers resulting from the immunosuppression produced by the virus, provide alarm signals.

HIV-infected women have a higher frequency of gynecological complications, such as candidal vulvovaginitis, other STIs, vaginitis or pelvic inflammatory disease (PID), menstrual abnormalities, and premalignant and malignant lesions of the cervix and the rest of the lower genital tract.

Diagnosis and Control

In addition to serological screening at the beginning of pregnancy in all women, repeat screening is recommended in the third trimester.

In the case of a diagnosis of HIV infection, it is advisable to perform hepatitis A virus (HAV), HBV and HCV serologies, since coinfection is common, as well as screening for other STIs [22].

Viral RNA will be determined frequently during pregnancy to monitor response to treatment and keep viral load low. At 16–24 weeks after the start of treatment, complete viral suppression should be achieved.

The CD4 lymphocyte count should be performed at least every 3 months in the case of recent diagnosis.

Management of the Pregnant Woman with HIV

Education about the importance of avoiding risky habits (drug use, unprotected sexual practices, etc.) and carrying out a complete physical examination to detect concomitant pathologies is essential, since this is crucial for reducing vertical transmission. It is also important to date the pregnancy correctly, since if the viral load is more than 1000 copies/mL, a cesarean section should be scheduled at 38 weeks of gestation to reduce mother–child transmission.

Use of HAV and HBV vaccines, the inactivated influenza vaccine, pneumococcal vaccine, and reduced tetanus and diphtheria toxoids is recommended.

The recommendation to breastfeed depends, among other things, on the resources of the country concerned, since in those without resources the benefits probably outweigh the risks.

Treatment

As soon as the diagnosis is known, treatment of the pregnant woman should be started and continued for life. The general regimen recommended by the WHO in 2019 includes tenofovir, lamivudine (or emtricitabine), and dolutegravir [23].

Pregnancy affects ART selection, so ideally it should be planned, something that can often only be done in resource-rich countries. If the woman is starting treatment and wants a short-term pregnancy, raltegravir plus tenofovir disoproxil fumarate/emtricitabine (TDF-FTC) is usually used [24]. If the woman was already under treatment when she decided to plan a pregnancy, the risks and benefits of continuing with the same treatment should be discussed. In general, it is recommended to change cobicistat because during pregnancy the levels of the drug decrease, increasing the risk of losing virological suppression. Dolutegravir slightly increases the risk of a neural tube defect.

21.2.6 Chlamydia

Epidemiology

The approximate prevalence in sexually active people between 18 and 26 years of age in Europe and countries with high resources is approximately 2.5–7% [25].

Etiological Agent

Chlamydia trachomatis (obligate intracellular bacterium).

Transmission

Through contact of the different mucous membranes during the sexual act. Using estimation models, transmissibility seems to be 10% for a single act and spontaneous clearance seems to be 54, 82, and 94% in the first, second, and third years, respectively. There is also mucosal infection of the newborn through the birth canal.

Gynecologic/Obstetric Implications

Chlamydia trachomatis can cause infertility by altering the anatomy and function of the tubes and endometritis. It can facilitate extrauterine gestation. It can also create infertility in men.

The risk of vertical transmission to the neonate is 50–75%, who may develop ophthalmitis and pneumonia.

Clinical Presentation

Asymptomatic infection is the norm (70–95%). In women, voiding and vaginocervicitis symptoms may occur (leukorrhea, localized pain, bleeding during sex, friable tissues). If the infection does not resolve, it may rise from the lower genital tract and produce the typical symptoms of PID (pain on cervical mobilization, abdominal pain, fever, dyspareunia), with abscess formation and pelvic and perihepatic adhesions (Fitz-Hugh–Curtis syndrome).

Anorectal, pharyngeal, and ophthalmic clinical manifestations in women are rare, as is lymphogranuloma venereum.

In pregnancy, therefore, symptoms (if present) are usually limited to urethritis and cervicovaginitis, which can be confused with the physiological condition of the woman at that time.

Diagnosis

NAATs are recommended for diagnosis. Results can be positive only 1–3 days after exposure. In women, the sample must be cervical. If the appropriate kits are not available, a urine sample can be taken.

The diagnosis with serology is not recommended since only invasive infections will generate detectable antibodies.

Treatment

The preferred treatment for pregnant women is azithromycin 1 g orally as a single dose. Possible alternatives include amoxicillin 500 mg three times daily for 7 days or erythromycin 500 mg four times daily for 7 days. Doxycycline is contraindicated in pregnancy.

The WHO STI guidelines recommend ocular prophylaxis for all newborns with tetracycline hydrochloride 1% eye ointment. Another option is erythromycin 0.5% eye ointment. This prophylaxis will also protect them from a possible gonococcal infection.

21.2.7 Gonorrhea

Epidemiology

In 2012, the WHO estimated that there were 78 million cases of gonorrhea in the world [26]. In the European Union, it is the second most common bacterial STI after chlamydia [27].

Etiological Agent

Neisseria gonorrhoeae (Gram-negative bacterium).

Transmission

Very similar to that of chlamydia, as well as the risk of vertical transmission at birth.

Gynecologic/Obstetric Implications

The organism can cause infertility in both genders, ectopic pregnancy, and conjunctivitis in the newborn that can lead to blindness if not properly treated.

Clinical Presentation

The clinical manifestations are also similar to those of chlamydia. The woman is often asymptomatic, while at other times she may present with dysuria, leukorrhea, and a hyperemic and friable cervix or the typical signs of PID if the disease progresses. It can rarely produce bacteremia with skin lesions, arthralgia, fever, or symptoms of disseminated gonorrhea (arthritis and tenosynovitis).

Diagnosis

The Gram-negative intracellular diplococcus can be directly visualized in a urethral or cervical discharge sample, can be detected with high sensitivity with NAATs, or can be cultured. In fact, it is recommended that a culture with an antibiogram is always performed in all diagnoses of gonorrhea.

If the pregnant woman is under 25 years old, has risk factors for STIs, or is HIV positive, she should be screened at the beginning of pregnancy or if she has suspicious symptoms at any time during the pregnancy.

Treatment

One of the main problems in the treatment of gonorrhea is the increase in antibiotic resistance, because of which the WHO STI guidelines recommend that local resistance data should guide therapy. In general, in pregnant and nonpregnant women, dual therapy with ceftriaxone 250 mg IM as a single dose (or cefixime 400 mg orally as a single dose) plus azithromycin 1 g orally as a single dose is indicated as the treatment of choice. European guidelines use increased doses.

If there is treatment failure, it is suggested that the same regimen be maintained but doubling the dose or substituting the cephalosporins with gentamicin 240 mg IM as a single dose or spectinomycin 2 g IM as a single dose *plus* azithromycin 2 g orally as a single dose.

Neonate prophylaxis is the same as for chlamydia.

21.2.8 Trichomoniasis

Epidemiology

Although its prevalence is difficult to estimate, it is the most common nonviral STI. It affects between 1 and 8% of symptomatic women of reproductive age [14].

Etiological Agent

Trichomonas vaginalis (anaerobic microaerophilic protozoan).

Transmission

By infected genital secretions during sexual contact via mucous membranes.

Gynecologic/Obstetric Implications

Trichomonas vaginalis can cause premature rupture of membranes, preterm delivery, or low birthweight. It can also cause infection of the newborn during delivery.

Clinical Presentation

It is estimated that 80% of all infections are asymptomatic. If there are symptoms, they usually include vulvovaginitis and urethritis. Itching and foul-smelling leukorrhea are the most common. Strawberry cervix (caused by vascular dilation and pinpoint hemorrhages) and foamy leukorrhea, when they appear, are characteristic of this infection.

Diagnosis

The fresh visualization of the mobile parasite is fast and cheap, although the sensitivity is low (51–65% in vaginal samples). Microscopic evaluation can also be done using various dry stains, or combined with culture (almost 100% sensitivity). NAAT is useful if the microscopic test is negative or in the absence of diagnosis; it has high sensitivity and specificity.

In HIV-positive pregnant women, the test is indicated as a screening at the beginning of pregnancy, since it is a risk factor for vertical transmission of HIV.

Treatment

The main and almost only treatment against *Trichomonas vaginalis* is the nitroimidazoles (metronidazole and tinidazole), but the first should be avoided in the first trimester of pregnancy and the second throughout it.

The usual treatment is 2 g orally in a single dose; in cases of failure the dose is 500 mg twice daily for 7 days.

Follow-Up

It is advisable to repeat the detection tests 3 months after treatment, given the high rate of reinfection and the increasing existence of resistance to treatment.

21.2.9 Human Papillomavirus

Epidemiology

HPV is considered the cause of nearly all cervical cancers. There were an estimated 570 000 new cases in 2018 and almost 90% of deaths from this cause occurred in low- and middle-income countries [28].

Some types of HPV cause condylomata acuminata. It is difficult to establish the incidence and prevalence worldwide since there are no registries in many countries. Each year in the USA, between 500 000 and 1 million new cases of condylomas are diagnosed [29].

Etiological Agent

Human papillomavirus (DNA virus), family *Papillomaviridae*. There are more than 100 types. Of the ones that have tropism for the genital tract, there is most interest in the following:

- High risk: 16, 18, 31, 33, 35, 39, 45, 51, 52, 56, 58, 59, 66, and 68, with oncogenic capacity.
- Low risk: 6 and 11, which cause condylomata acuminata in 90% of cases.

Transmission

Occurs through contact with the skin or infected mucous membranes during sexual intercourse. Vertical transmission is possible and can be intrauterine, via the birth canal, or postnatal.

Gynecologic/Obstetric Implications

There is no evidence of any type of harm to the fetus or the neonate due to the transmission of high-risk HPV.

The low-risk HPV that cause condylomata acuminata can lead to recurrent laryngeal or respiratory papillomatosis, a rare entity in which condylomas are found in the larynx or along the respiratory tract. The greatest risk of transmission for the newborn is the maternal history of genital condylomatosis during pregnancy and not its transmission via the birth canal [30].

Clinical Presentation

There are two types of clinical presentation depending on whether it is high- or low-risk HPV.

- **High-risk HPV**: Occurs asymptomatically while producing premalignant lesions of the cervix (cervical intraepithelial neoplasia or CIN) that can only detected by cytology. In case of viral persistence over the years, it can progress to cervical cancer and the symptoms will mainly be bleeding with or without sexual intercourse and, in more advanced cases, locoregional invasion, pain, or involvement of adjacent structures (ureters, rectum). Especially in immunosuppressed patients, high-risk HPV can also produce lesions in other locations of the lower genital tract, such as the vagina, vulva, or anus.
- **Low-risk HPV**: Causes condylomata acuminata. As pregnancy is a state of relative immune tolerance, condylomas tend to proliferate more than in nonpregnant women.

Diagnosis

The gold standard for the diagnosis of premalignant or malignant cervical lesions is colposcopy and biopsy once abnormalities have been detected on the screening cytology or a positive endocervical high-risk HPV test has been detected.

Visualization with colposcopy in premalignant lesions will reveal an acetowhite epithelium possibly accompanied by mosaic or dotted vascular patterns that may be friable in cases of high-grade premalignant lesions (high-grade squamous intraepithelial lesion or HSIL).

In the case of cancer, an excretory or bleeding mass can be seen, with aberrant vascularization.

Pregnant patients exhibit a phenomenon called deciduosis, which involves decidualization of the cervical stroma that sometimes falsely reproduces the appearance of a cervical lesion, so especially in this case, colposcopy must be performed by expert professionals.

Treatment

There is no proven effective medical treatment for premalignant cervical lesions. Surgical treatment (cervical conization) is not indicated in pregnancy unless there is a suspicion of cancer. Therefore, during this period, if HSIL is diagnosed, quarterly cytology and colposcopy monitoring will have to be performed until the end of pregnancy, with subsequent reassessment 6–8 weeks after delivery. Vaginal delivery is not contraindicated.

In the case of genital warts, medical treatment with immunomodulators or cytotoxic agents should be avoided, and trichloroacetic acid, cryotherapy, or surgery can be applied. Cesarean delivery will only be indicated if the condylomas cause significant obstruction to the birth canal.

21.3 What Did Dr. Google Say?

An Internet search for patient-available information was carried out for STIs in pregnancy and for each of the above-mentioned conditions specifically in pregnancy.

When using the terms "sexual transmitted infection OR sexual transmitted disease" and "during pregnancy OR pregnancy," most of the results indicated sites that comment on the implications of PID in fertility and chronic pelvic pain. Some of the results are from clinics that offer testing and/or treatment and follow-up of STIs. The risk of premature delivery in patients with bacterial vaginosis and the increased probability of an ectopic pregnancy after PID are discussed on some sites [31]. The possibility of vertical transmission is also sometimes noted [32,33]. The recommendations of different societies regarding STI screening during pregnancy are easily located.

Searching for the specific conditions provides more fruitful results. The CDC site is frequently one of the top ten results, with information on the symptoms of the diseases, their prevention, and treatment. Examples of some of the conditions are briefly described.

- **Syphilis**: The symptoms of congenital syphilis are detailed on some sites (e.g. bone and tooth deformities, kidney damage) [34,35]. Treatment with penicillin is also mentioned, as well as the need for early treatment [35].
- **Hepatitis B**: On the Hepatitis B Foundation website, the high rate of vertical transmission is described, as well as the possibility of treatment during pregnancy but, most prominently, treatment of the newborn to prevent vertical transmission [36].
- **Hepatitis C**: The long-term effects of HCV, the indications for testing during pregnancy, the chances of vertical transmission, and the possibility of breastfeeding in HCV-positive mothers among other issues is covered in an article at Caring for Kids [37].
- **Genital herpes**: Possible fetal malformations in the case of vertical transmission are noted at www.pressreader.com [34]. The National Health Service (NHS) is one of the top results, briefly mentioning the neonatal repercussions and the need to consult a general provider or midwife if suffering from genital herpes [38].
- **HIV**: Using three different search engines, the sites of the CDC and American College of Obstetricians and Gynecologists (ACOG) are the two top results. Transmission, prevention, treatment, screening indications, and obstetric implications are reviewed.

In conclusion, accurate information can easily be found on the Internet, provided it is adequately selected. Sites from medical societies or associations are recommended.

References

1. World Health Organization. *Sexually transmitted infections: evidence brief.* WHO/RHR/19.22. Geneva: World Health Organization, 2019.

2. K. A. Workowski, G. A. Bolan, Centers for Disease Control and Prevention. Sexually transmitted diseases treatment guidelines, 2015. *MMWR Recomm Rep* 2015;**64**(RR-03):1–137.

3. S. Schillie, C. Wester, M. Osborne, L. Wesolowski, A. B. Ryerson. CDC recommendations for hepatitis C screening among adults: United States, 2020. *MMWR Recomm Rep* 2020;**69**:1–17.

4. Centers for Disease Control and Prevention. *Sexually Transmitted Disease Surveillance 2018.* Atlanta, GA: Department of Health and Human Services, 2019. www.cdc.gov/std/stats18/STDSurveillance2018-full-report.pdf (accessed March 14, 2021).

5. L. von Karsa, J. Dillner, E. Suonio, et al. *European Guidelines for Quality Assurance in Cervical Cancer Screening,* 2nd ed. Luxembourg: Publications Office of the European Union, 2015.

6. D. Saslow, D. Solomon, H. W. Lawson, et al. American Cancer Society, American Society for Colposcopy and Cervical Pathology, and American Society for Clinical Pathology screening guidelines for the prevention and early detection of cervical cancer. *Am J Clin Pathol* 2012;**137**:516–42.

7. G. Ronco, J. Dillner, K. M. Elfström, et al. Efficacy of HPV-based screening for prevention of invasive cervical cancer: follow-up of four European randomised controlled trials. *Lancet* 2014;**383**:524–32.

8. World Health Organization. *WHO Guideline on Syphilis Screening and Treatment for Pregnant Women.* Geneva: World Health Organization, 2017. Licence: CC BY-NC-SA 3.0 IGO.

9. M. Alsina, O. Arencibia, C. Centeno, et al. *AEPCC-Guía: Infecciones del Tracto Genital Inferior.* Publicaciones AEPCC, 2016.

10. J. M. Boot, A. P. Oranje, R. de Groot, G. Tan, E. Stolz. Congenital syphilis. *Int J STD AIDS* 1992;**3**:161–7.

11. M. Janier, M. Unemo, N. Dupin, et al. 2020 European guideline on the management of syphilis. *J Eur Acad Dermatol Venereol* 2021;**35**:574–88.

12. World Health Organization. WHO Guidelines for the Treatment of *Treponema pallidum* (Syphilis). Geneva: World Health Organization, 2016.

13. World Health Organization. *Guidelines for the Prevention, Care and Treatment of Persons with Chronic Hepatitis B Infection.* Geneva: World Health Organization, 2015. www.who.int/publications/i/item/9789241549059 (accessed March 14, 2021).

14. G. Brook, N. Brockmeyer, T. van de Laar, S. Schellberg, A. J. Winter. European guideline for the screening, prevention and initial management of hepatitis B and C infections in sexual health settings. *Int J STD AIDS* 2018;**29**:949–67.

15. H. Lee, A. S. F. Lok. Hepatitis B and pregnancy. UpToDate, 2021. www.uptodate.com/contents/hepatitis-b-and-pregnancy

16. E. Gower, C. Estes, S. Blach, K. Razavi-Shearer, H. Razavi. Global epidemiology and genotype distribution of the hepatitis C virus infection. *J Hepatol* 2014;**61**(1 Suppl): S45–57.

17. E. Goldberg, D. J. O'Donovan. Vertical transmission of hepatitis C virus. UpToDate, 2022. www.uptodate.com/contents/vertical-transmission-of-hepatitis-c-virus

18. K. J. Looker, A. S. Magaret, K. M. E. Turner, et al. Global estimates of prevalent and incident herpes simplex type 2 infections in 2012. *PLoS ONE* 2015;**10**:e114989.

19. F. Baquero Artigao, L. M. Prieto Tato, J. T. Ramos Amador, et al. The Spanish Society of Pediatric Infectious Diseases guidelines on the prevention, diagnosis and treatment of neonatal herpes simplex infections. [In Spanish] *Ann Pediatr (Barc)* 2018;**89**:64.e1–10.

20. R. Patel, O. J. Kennedy, E. Clarke, et al. 2017 European guidelines for the management of genital herpes. *Int J STD AIDS* 2017;**28**:1366–79.

21. World Health Organization. *Global Guidance on Criteria and Processes for Validation: Elimination of Mother-to-Child Transmission of HIV and Syphilis*, 2nd ed. Geneva: World Health Organization, 2017.

22. B. Hughes, S. Cu-Uvin. Prenatal evaluation of women with HIV in resource-rich settings. UpToDate, 2022. www.uptodate.com/contents/prenatal-evaluation-of-women-with-hiv-in-resource-rich-settings

23. World Health Organization. *Policy Brief: Update of Recommendations on First- and Second-line Antiretroviral Regimens.* Geneva: World Health Organization, 2019. https://apps.who.int/iris/handle/10665/325892 (accessed March 14, 2021).

24. Panel on Antiretroviral Guidelines for Adults and Adolescents. *Guidelines for the Use of Antiretroviral Agents in Adults and Adolescents with HIV.* Washington, DC: Department of Health and Human Services, 2021. https://clinicalinfo.hiv.gov/sites/default/files/guidelines/archive/AdultandAdolescentGL_2021_08_16.pdf (accessed March 14, 2021).

25. E. Lanjouw, S. Ouburg, H. J. de Vries, et al. 2015 European guideline on the management of *Chlamydia trachomatis* infections. *Int J STD AIDS* 2016;**27**:333–48.

26. World Health Organization. *WHO Guidelines for the Treatment of Neisseria gonorrhoeae.* Geneva: World Health Organization, 2016.

27. M. Unemo, J. D. C. Ross, A. B. Serwin, et al. 2020 European guideline for the diagnosis and treatment of gonorrhoea in adults. *Int J STD AIDS* 2020; DOI: https://doi.org/10.1177/0956462420949126.

28. J. Ferlay, M. Ervik, F. Lam, et al. *Global Cancer Observatory: Cancer Today.* Lyon, France: International Agency for Research on Cancer, 2018.

29. N. Muñoz, S. K. Kjaer, K. Sigurdsson, et al. Impact of human papillomavirus (HPV)-6/11/16/18 vaccine on all HPV-associated genital diseases in young women. *J Natl Cancer Inst* 2010;**102**:325–39.

30. M. J. Silverberg, P. Thorsen, H. Lindeberg, L. A. Grant, K. V. Shah. Condyloma in pregnancy is strongly predictive of juvenile-onset recurrent respiratory. *Obstet Gynecol* 2003;**101**:645–52.

31. Blue Water Medical. Sexually transmitted infection. www.bluewatermedical.com.au/sti/ (accessed September 19, 2021).

32. NewDay Women's Clinic. Free STI testing and treatment: learning about your sexual health. https://ndwomensclinic.com/services/sti/ (accessed September 19, 2021).

33. W. Owoo. Sexual transmitted infections. 2013. http://academic.macewan.ca/preconceptionhealth/2013/03/04/sexual-transmitted-infections/ (accessed September 19, 2021).

34. G. Vaidah Mashangwa. Sexually transmitted diseases: a major health concern. www.pressreader.com/zimbabwe/chronicle-zimbabwe/20151121/281616714273006 (accessed September 19, 2021).

35. March of Dimes. Syphilis in pregnancy. 2017. www.marchofdimes.org/complications/syphilis-in-pregnancy.aspx (accessed September 19, 2021).

36. Pregnancy and hepatitis B. 2020. www.hepb.org/treatment-and-management/pregnancy-and-hbv/ (accessed September 19, 2021).

37. Caring for Kids. Hepatitis C in pregnancy. 2021. www.caringforkids.cps.ca/handouts/pregnancy-and-babies/hepatitis_c_in_pregnancy (accessed September 19, 2021).

38. National Health Service. Genital herpes. 2020. www.nhs.uk/conditions/genital-herpes/ (accessed September 19, 2021).

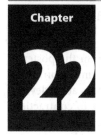

Sex for Induction of Labor

Jazleen Dada and Stefania Ronzoni

22.1 History of Sex and Induction of Labor

35wTherelationshipbetweensexualintercourseanditsroleinonsetofspontaneouslaborhasbeen questionedfordecades.Inthe1950s,academicobstetricianscautionedagainstintercourseinlate pregnancyforfearofpretermbirthandintroductionofintra-amnioticinfection,despiteminimal high-qualityevidencetosupporttheseoutcomes[1].

In the 1970s and 1980s, the debate continued and the notion that coitus could be linked to preterm birth, amnionitis, lower APGAR scores, and meconium-stained amniotic fluid persisted. These studies argued that coitus could cause potential direct harm to the fetus. However, most of these studies were observational and limited by small sample sizes, selection of questionable control groups, retrospective data, or multiple comparators [2–7].

Ultimately, more robust studies have since emerged revealing that in the majority of low-risk pregnancies at term there is no confirmed association between coitus in pregnancy and the aforementioned adverse outcomes of pregnancy [8]. Indeed, among the general population today, the use of intercourse for the induction of labor is regarded by many as a recommended and "natural" method for initiating labor [9].

For many physicians, midwives, and other healthcare providers the question at times remains unclear. Does increasing the frequency of sexual intercourse hasten the onset of spontaneous labor at term in pregnancy and what does the evidence say?

22.2 Physiological Explanations

Three theories have been proposed in the literature to offer physiological explanations for why this induction of labor may occur or be more likely following sex.

22.2.1 Sperm Is a Natural Source of Prostaglandins

As discussed in previous chapters, human semen is known to be a rich source of prostaglandins E and F2α [10]. Both of these prostaglandins are utilized in synthetic formulations at higher doses to induce labor artificially. To further demonstrate this, studies have been carried out in which researchers have collected samples of cervical mucus 2–4 hours following coitus. These samples have been found to exhibit prostaglandin concentrations 10–50 times higher than the levels in the cervical mucus at baseline [11].

22.2.2 Breast Stimulation Leads to Increased Production and Release of Endogenous Oxytocin

Stimulation of the breast and nipples causes the release of oxytocin from the posterior pituitary in the brain (see Chapter 23 for more details on nipple stimulation). This endogenous oxytocin then binds to and acts on uterine oxytocin receptors at the level of the gravid uterus. Theoretically, this leads to initiation and maintenance of contractions in labor. This technique has been described for induction and augmentation of labor through history in many different cultures and by the medical literature in the eighteenth and nineteenth centuries for management of prolonged labor [12]. An observational study in the 1980s reproduced this phenomenon whereby bilateral breast stimulation was used to successfully evoke uterine contraction stress testing in direct comparison with oxytocin administration [13]. More recently in 2018, a small Japanese study by Takahata et al. [14] reported confirmation of higher median oxytocin levels 30 minutes after breast stimulation, with the highest levels following 3 days of stimulation. The exact mechanism remains unclear. A direct relationship between oxytocin levels and intrapartum uterine response to breast stimulation has not been clearly established.

A Cochrane review in 2005 by Kavanagh et al. [15] specifically considered evidence for breast stimulation for cervical ripening and induction of labor. A total of six trials were included internationally with a total of 719 participants. The participants performed either hand massage or pump stimulation of the breasts one side at a time for between 1 and 3 hours per day. Ultimately, there was evidence to suggest a significant reduction in the number of women not in labor at 72 hours when compared with no intervention. However, this result was only significant in the presence of an already ripened cervix or favorable Bishop score. This intervention has not been found to make a significant difference in those with an unfavorable cervix. Interestingly, the rate of postpartum hemorrhage was also reduced in the breast stimulation group in comparison to no intervention. There was no difference in the cesarean section rate, no meconium, and no cases of uterine hyperstimulation between groups.

22.2.3 Female Orgasm and Mechanical Effect of Sex Can Encourage Uterine Contraction

Early research conducted into orgasm in pregnant women demonstrated that uterine contraction patterns could be produced secondary to orgasm [16] (see Chapter 4 for more details on orgasm). This may be mediated through release of endogenous oxytocin or a mechanical effect from physical stimulation of the lower uterine segment [17]. Equally, these recorded uterine contractions during orgasm have been associated with transient and immediate fetal heart rate changes following orgasm [18]. As such, there was initial concern that women with orgasm had an increased risk of preterm labor. More recently, orgasm has not been reported to be associated with labor onset or adverse pregnancy outcomes [8].

22.3 What Does the Current Medical Literature and Most Recent Evidence Say?

Overall, studies exploring sex as a method for induction of labor are limited in quantity and quality. Available reviews conducted with the highest level of evidence in this area include a Cochrane Review from 2001 and, more recently, a meta-analysis from Carbone et al. in 2019.

The only available Cochrane review on sexual intercourse for cervical ripening and induction of labor offers limited insight. A single trial is included and analyzed in this review, which included a sample size of just 28 women. This solitary trial offered limited data and was insufficiently powered to draw any relevant conclusions. The main conclusion was that the role of sex as a method for induction of labor remained uncertain and the need for further study and well-designed randomized control trials in this area is warranted [19].

The recent 2019 meta-analysis from Carbone et al. [20] included three high-quality randomized controlled trials with a total of 1483 pregnant women. The intervention groups were advised either to have sexual intercourse as frequently as possible to avoid medical induction or coitus at least twice a week until delivery. The control groups were neither encouraged nor discouraged from sexual intercourse or remained abstinent. Both groups consisted of low-risk pregnant women with singleton fetuses in cephalic presentation at term. Ultimately, the meta-analysis revealed that those randomly assigned to the intervention or coitus group achieved spontaneous labor at the same rate as those in the control group. There was also no detectable difference in pregnancy duration, premature rupture of membranes, induction of labor for post-term pregnancy, epidural use, oxytocin augmentation, cesarean section rate, postpartum hemorrhage, newborn birthweight, or neonatal intensive care unit admissions. The only other significant outcome of this analysis was a lower incidence of emergency cesarean sections due to abnormal fetal heart rate patterns in women advised to have coitus compared with control subjects, for which there was no proposed physiological explanation. None of the trials demonstrated evidence of harm or adverse maternal or pregnancy outcomes.

22.4 What Are the Limitations of the Literature?

Despite meta-analysis having the highest quality of evidence, there are limitations to our current available evidence. These studies demand accurate reporting of coitus, which is often completed through patient self-reporting and patient diaries. This method of data collection is not always reliable. There is also no distinction between condom use, volume of ejaculate, sperm prostaglandin concentration, timing of breast/nipple stimulation, duration of intercourse, role of masturbation, and frequency of orgasm reported. These factors have the potential to influence outcome, in accordance with the physiological hypothesis of methods of induction. The control arm in each study should ideally practice abstinence. Exposure to sexual intercourse is also difficult to measure over time and at different gestational ages. In order to reach significance with these variables, larger patient populations and further meticulously planned randomized controlled trials are required.

22.5 Does Sex in Pregnancy Affect Induction and Spontaneous Onset of Labor?

To summarize, according to the most recent and up-to-date literature, there is no current strong evidence to suggest sex is an effective means of induction of labor. The results of previous observational and historical studies have been mixed and are likely subject to a high risk of bias.

None of the high-quality studies showed evidence of harm to pregnancy outcomes such as preterm birth in a low-risk patient population. Sex is considered safe for most pregnancies and should not be restricted. This is reflected in most national guidelines and by the National Collaborating Centre for Women's and Children's Health in the UK with regard to antenatal care in pregnancy. Psychological benefits are potentially gained from sexual intercourse in pregnancy as it leads to increased bonding in the parent dyad. In a high-risk pregnancy or pregnancy complicated by premature rupture of membranes with a low-lying bleeding placenta or by short cervix, sexual intercourse may be contraindicated, as discussed in other chapters.

Further research and superior-quality evidence is required in this area, especially in order to better define the effects of seminal prostaglandins, breast/nipple stimulation, and orgasm during intercourse and their relation to cervical ripening. This may help better determine whether sex is an effective means of induction of labor.

22.6 What Did Dr. Google Say?

According to survey data collected in the USA from the Listening to Mothers III survey 2013, approximately 22% of mothers attempted to induce their own labor. The most common methods for self-induction included walking/physical activity, engaging in sexual intercourse, nipple stimulation, and ingestion of dietary items that trigger labor. Patients who carry out a quick internet search will be faced with many of these "natural" methods of induction, including sexual intercourse. Clearly, some women are motivated to undergo and prefer nonhormonal induction before medical methods. Reported concerns include over-medicalization and fear of adverse outcomes secondary to hormonal methods of induction. Expectant patients may encounter resources that criticize these medical approaches as inconsistent with "natural" or "normal" labor. Therefore, patient must be cautious of medical misinformation and myths they may encounter online and through social media.

Much of the information pertaining to "natural" or "nonhormonal" methods are featured on blogs, women's magazine articles, YouTube videos, Instagram posts, and podcasts. Most are described in comparison to medical methods of induction like amniotomy, oxytocin administration, balloon catheter, or vaginal prostaglandins for induction of labor.

22.6.1 Exercise/Physical Activity

The most-suggested option for nonhormonal induction is that of physical activity and exercise beyond term pregnancy to try to promote induction and spontaneous onset of labor. The online consensus supports this option and encourages it, stating there is minimal to no harm. Particular yoga poses, hip/pelvic-focused and inflatable exercise ball-related activities, and just walking in general are described, with guidance to avoid overexertion or extreme sports.

To date only one randomized controlled trial has been completed [21], reporting that walking for 30 minutes three times per week at 4 km/h from 38 weeks onward is safe and may contribute to spontaneous onset of labor and increased vaginal delivery rates. All other studies have been observational. This amount of activity also falls safely within the 2019 guidance from the American College of Physicians on exercise during pregnancy.

22.6.2 Sexual Intercourse

Sex is almost unanimously supported by online sources as a method of induction. Most report that coitus has been evidenced by science to be a reliable source of nonhormonal induction. There are even obstetrician and gynecologist online influencers who reiterate this claim. Some sources do not go as far as to claim this association to be fact but recommend it regardless as there is no harm in most uncomplicated pregnancies, which is in line with actual practice. Seminal prostaglandins, breast/nipple stimulation, and orgasm are all mentioned as potential physiological mechanisms. The psychological and emotional benefits of sex are also mentioned. There is minimal advice on frequency, optimal sexual positioning, and role of masturbation, which patients continue to question online.

22.6.3 Acupuncture

Acupuncture techniques have been documented and utilized in medicine for greater than 2000 years in Asia. It is also a popular therapy that is listed online as an option for cervical ripening. The underlying mechanism is not clearly understood and hypotheses suggest that stimulation of the uterus and cervix via pressure points upregulate blood and hormonal flow to the uterus and may decrease overall stress. Many local advertisements immediately arise when this topic is inserted into a search engine. These private clinics/businesses make claims regarding successful increase in induction of labor yet share hyperlinks to nonreputable sources. Notably, not all acupuncturists are formally trained and licensed and no uniform stimulation regimen for induction of labor has been identified. Most online sources support its use in induction of labor and do not report any harmful maternal or fetal side effects.

A 2017 Cochrane review on acupuncture for induction of labor analyzed 22 trials including 3456 pregnant women with a moderate risk of bias. Based on the results, acupuncture does not reduce the need for cesarean section but may improve the cervical readiness for labor. There was no evidence of benefit from acupressure in nonlaboring women. Overall, the technique was found to be safe in pregnancy. There is a low incidence of adverse effects, which are typically not directly related to pregnancy, such as fainting, reductions in blood pressure, drowsiness, discomfort, and localized bleeding or bruising. Furthermore, appropriately powered randomized trials are necessary to examine the effectiveness of acupuncture on the clinical outcomes, especially with regard to measurements of cervical change (i.e. Bishop score) [22].

22.6.4 Castor Oil

Castor oil is a recognized source of ricinoleic acid and is known to act as a powerful laxative. There are anecdotal reports of its use as far back as ancient Egypt for its role in stimulating labor onset. The mechanism of action is believed to be via direct irritation of the gastrointestinal tract, which in turn causes irritation and stimulation of the uterus, causing contractions. The majority of articles do not specify a standard dosage, frequency, and timing of castor oil ingestion. Some do advise that consumption may result in diarrhea and dehydration. There is also mention of the potential for castor oil to penetrate the placenta and influence timing of meconium. Online sources tend to offer castor oil as an option for induction of labor following exercise, sexual intercourse, and acupuncture but do warn of potential gastrointestinal side effects.

A 2013 Cochrane review on castor oil for cervical priming and induction of labor included three randomized controlled trials involving 233 women with Bishop score less than six. All patients in the intervention groups received a single 60-mL dose of castor oil. The authors found no differences in rates of cesarean section, use of forceps, episiotomy, hemorrhage, meconium-stained amniotic fluid, neonatal intensive care unit (NICU) admissions, maternal death, stillbirth, or uterine rupture between the two groups. Once all results were combined it was found that there was insufficient evidence to show the effects of castor oil on ripening the cervix or inducing labor or compare it with other methods of induction. The review found that most women who took castor oil by mouth felt nauseous. More research is needed into the effects of castor oil for induction of labor [23].

22.6.5 Herbal Therapies (Red Raspberry Leaf and Pineapple)

Red raspberry leaf can be consumed in either tea or tablet formulations. Traditionally, this plant has been used in the treatment of conditions related to the gastrointestinal tract and in menstruation and pregnancy/childbirth. Online sources describe its hypothesized ability to act on and strengthen the uterine muscle fibers and promote a faster healthier labor as well as prevent excessive bleeding postpartum. Highlighted risks according to internet sources caution against potential risks of diuretic effect, gastrointestinal upset, and possibility of miscarriage in the first trimester. The majority of articles do not specify a standard dosage, frequency, and timing of ingestion. In addition to red raspberry leaf, recently pineapple has also been suggested as a herbal or ingestible therapy on social media.

There is limited evidence in the medical literature with regard to red raspberry leaf and further high-quality studies need to be conducted. A single, double-blind, randomized controlled trial published by Simpson et al. in 2001 included 192 low-risk pregnant patients. Recruited patients were randomly assigned to raspberry leaf tablets or placebo tablets starting at 32 weeks of gestation until the beginning of labor. In terms of outcomes, they found that raspberry leaf was not significantly different from placebo with regard to any outcome measured. The outcomes measured were maternal blood loss, maternal blood pressure, meconium-stained fluid, Apgar scores of the baby, birthweight, NICU admission, length of pregnancy, need for medical induction of labor with oxytocin, artificial rupture of membranes, request for an epidural, length of any stages of labor, or type of birth (vaginal or cesarean section). There were also no significant differences between groups with regard to side effects [24].

Regrettably, there are no clinical research or evidence-based human studies on pineapple for nonhormonal induction of labor. However, this method is also not likely to be harmful but may result in gastrointestinal upset or reflux.

22.6.6 Hypnosis

Hypnosis or hypnobirthing techniques have been used in pregnancy to bring the patient into a state of deep relaxation and prohibit external distractions so that they may focus instead on specific thoughts and feelings. This can be helpful in cases of extreme maternal anxiety. This technique is performed through a number of meditations, visualizations, and breathing exercises. Advantages are stated to be possible avoidance of medical induction methods and less reliance on pain relief while in labor. This form of hypnosis denies claims of brainwashing, loss of awareness, or loss of free will. There are no clear associated risks.

A 2014 Cochrane review on hypnosis for induction of labor unfortunately found no randomized controlled trials during the search strategy and was therefore unable to assess the hypothesis [25].

22.7 Conclusion

In low-risk pregnancies at term, sexual intercourse, breast/nipple stimulation, and orgasm offer plausible explanations for the release of prostaglandins via semen and endogenous oxytocin to ultimately promote cervical ripening. The current medical literature on this topic is limited but there is no evidence to suggest that sex at term has an effect on spontaneous onset of labor, cesarean delivery rates, or neonatal outcomes. Simultaneously, there are no known harmful consequences in engaging in sexual activity for those patients with low-risk pregnancies. None of the popularized "nonhormonal" methods of induction reviewed in this chapter have been found to modify or have an effect on the spontaneous onset of labor.

References

1. W. E. Pugh, F. L. Fernandez. Coitus in late pregnancy: a follow-up study of the effects of coitus on late pregnancy, delivery, and the puerperium. *Obstet Gynecol* 1953;2:636–42.

2. R. C. Goodlin, D. W. Keller, M. Raffin. Orgasm during late pregnancy: possible deleterious effects. *Obstet Gynecol* 1971;38:916–20.

3. N. N. Wagner, J. C. Butler, J. P. Sanders. Prematurity and orgasmic coitus during pregnancy: data on a small sample. *Fertil Steril* 1976;27:911–15.

4. J. G. Grudzinskas, C. Watson, T. Chard. Does sexual intercourse cause fetal distress? *Lancet* 1979;314:692–3.

5. R. L. Naeye. Coitus and associated amniotic-fluid infections. *N Engl J Med* 1979;301:1198–200.

6. J. L. Mills, S. Harlap, E. E. Harley. Should coitus late in pregnancy be discouraged? *Lancet* 1981;318:136–8.

7. M. A. Klebanoff, R. P. Nugent, G. G. Rhoads. Coitus during pregnancy: is it safe? *Lancet* 1984;324:914–17.

8. P. C. Tan, C. M. Yow, S. Z. Omar. Coitus and orgasm at term: effect on spontaneous labor and pregnancy outcome. *Singapore Med J* 2009;50:1062–7.

9. J. Schaffir. Survey of folk beliefs about induction of labor. *Birth* 2002;29:47–51.

10. R. J. Cenedella. Prostaglandins and male reproductive physiology. *Adv Sex Horm Res* 1975;1:325–58.

11. M. Toth, J. Rehnstrom, A. R. Fuchs. Prostaglandins E and F in cervical mucus of pregnant women. *Am J Perinatol* 1989;6:142–4.

12. P. Curtis. Breast stimulation to augment labor: history, mystery, and culture. *Birth* 1999;26:123–6.

13. E. L. Capeless, L. I. Mann. Use of breast stimulation for antepartum stress testing. *Obstet Gynecol* 1984;64:641–5.

14. K. Takahata, S. Horiuchi, Y. Tadokoro, et al. Effects of breast stimulation for spontaneous onset of labor on salivary oxytocin levels in low-risk pregnant women: a feasibility study. *PLoS ONE* 2018;13:e0192757.

15. J. Kavanagh, A. J. Kelly, J. Thomas. Breast stimulation for cervical ripening and induction of labour. *Cochrane Database Syst Rev* 2005;(3):CD003392.

16. W. H. Masters, V. E. Johnson. *Human Sexual Response*. Boston: Little, Brown, 1966.

17. R. C. Goodlin, W. Schmidt, D. C. Creevy. Uterine tension and fetal heart rate during maternal orgasm. *Obstet Gynecol* 1972;**39**:125–7.

18. B. Chayen, N. Tejani, U. L. Verma, et al. Fetal heart rate changes and uterine activity during coitus. *Acta Obstet Gynecol Scand* 1986;**65**:853–5.

19. J. Kavanagh, A. J. Kelly, J. Thomas. Sexual intercourse for cervical ripening and induction of labour. *Cochrane Database Syst Rev* 2001;(2): CD003093.

20. L. Carbone, V. De Vivo, G. Saccone, et al. Sexual intercourse for induction of spontaneous onset of labor: a systematic review and meta-analysis of randomized controlled trials. *J Sex Med* 2019;**16**:1787–95.

21. I. B. Pereira, R. Silva, D. Ayres-de-Campos, N. Clode. Physical exercise at term for enhancing the spontaneous onset of labor: a randomized clinical trial. *J Matern Fetal Neonatal Med* 2020;**29**:1–5.

22. C. A. Smith, M. Armour, H. G. Dahlen. Acupuncture or acupressure for induction of labour. *Cochrane Database Syst Rev* 2017;(10):CD002962.

23. A. J. Kelly, J. Kavanagh, J. Thomas. Castor oil, bath and/or enema for cervical priming and induction of labour. *Cochrane Database Syst Rev* 2013;(7): CD003099.

24. M. Simpson, M. Parsons, J. Greenwood, K. Wade. Raspberry leaf in pregnancy: its safety and efficacy in labor. *J Midwifery Womens Health* 2001;**46**:51–9.

25. D. Nishi, M. N. Shirakawa, E. Ota, N. Hanada, R. Mori. Hypnosis for induction of labour. *Cochrane Database Syst Rev* 2014;(8):CD010852.

Chapter 23

Nipple Stimulation during Pregnancy

Doron Kabiri, Gali Gordon, and Yossef Ezra

23.1 Introduction

Stimulation of the nipple is known to release oxytocin from the pituitary gland, which in turn causes uterine contraction during pregnancy and in the postpartum period, which is elaborated in this chapter. Consequently, it has been ideated to serve as a method of induction of labor (IOL) and as one of the available measures to deal with postpartum hemorrhage (PPH).

23.2 Nipple Stimulation and Induction of Labor

The exact method of performance of nipple stimulation, length of time, or frequency needed to produce adequate amounts of oxytocin for the onset of labor, yet not excessive so as to avoid uterine hypercontractility and subsequent fetal distress, is unknown. Furthermore, it is of importance to note that this maneuver may cause discomfort despite popular belief.

The efficacy and safety of nipple stimulation in IOL is controversial. A Cochrane systematic review regarding breast stimulation for IOL originally published in 2005 and revisited in 2009, with no further findings, included six randomized controlled trials comprising 719 pregnant women at term [1]. The effects of breast stimulation, using various predetermined methods, were compared to either placebo or administration of oxytocin. Results revealed a significant reduction in women not in labor after 72 hours in the breast stimulation group compared with the no intervention group but not the oxytocin group. In addition, the difference in cesarean section rate did not reach statistical significance across all comparisons. However, there was a significant reduction in PPH.

In support of these findings, a more recent study conducted in India and published in 2014 [2] compared two groups (breast stimulation vs. no intervention) of 100 participants. In this study, the authors found more favorable Bishop score and shorter period of gestation, and an increase in favor of vaginal delivery and a decrease in the rate of cesarean section for failed induction when breast stimulation was performed. Moreover, no significant difference was observed in adverse fetal or obstetric outcomes.

A randomized controlled trial conducted in Turkey and published in 2015 compared nipple stimulation to manual uterine stimulation or no intervention in 390 participants before labor [3]. Similarly, results showed a significant increase in Bishop scores, reduction in duration of the first, second, and third stages of labor, and a reduction in the rate of cesarean deliveries in the nipple stimulation group compared with the nonintervention control group but not the uterine stimulation group.

Most recently, a small study conducted in Japan and published in 2018 that included 42 low-risk primiparous women, who were divided into breast stimulation group and nonintervention control group, found a significant increase in oxytocin levels in saliva in the intervention group [4]. Contrary to previously mentioned studies, there was no significant difference in the rate of spontaneous onset of labor, nor in other delivery outcomes, between the groups.

Adverse events associated with antepartum nipple stimulation have been reported in several studies [4–8]. In these reports, nipple stimulation resulted in uterine hyperstimulation and consequently profound fetal bradycardia and even placental abruption. In general, fetal distress was reported to be temporary in most cases and without repercussions; however, one of the trials, which was conducted on a high-risk population, was halted due to four instances of perinatal deaths, three of which occurred in the breast stimulation arm. There was also one reported case of fatal placental abruption at 28 weeks of gestation following 5 minutes of breastfeeding. Despite the encouraging results of nipple stimulation on the success rate of cervical maturation, it is important to note that it may lead to increased interventions and sometimes to severe outcomes.

23.3 Nipple Stimulation and Postpartum Hemorrhage

Postpartum hemorrhage is one of the main obstetric causes of morbidity and mortality of women worldwide [9]. One of the main reasons for PPH is uterine atony. The known risk factors for uterine atony are high-order parity, nonemptying urinary bladder, and hyperextended uterus before labor and delivery as in multifetal pregnancy, polyhydramnios, and fetal macrosomia. After delivery of the placenta, the spiral arteries are issuing blood and coagulation factors into the uterine cavity and mechanical obstruction caused by an efficient uterine contraction are needed to allow the formation of the primary blood clot to prevent PPH. When uterine atony occurs due to inefficient uterine contraction, it may prevent this process. Prompt treatment of the factors causing uterine atony would prevent excessive blood loss; these interventions include emptying the urinary bladder, ensuring complete expulsion of the placenta, manual uterine massage, and administration of uterine stimulating agents such as oxytocin and prostaglandins. Active management of the third stage of labor is now an evolving issue and is recommended to prevent the complications of PPH [10]. Breast stimulation, by stimulating endogenous oxytocin secretion, may have an additional positive effect on uterine contraction after labor and delivery in preventing PPH.

Very few studies have been performed to assess the effect of nipple stimulation or breastfeeding on the incidence and severity of PPH. Irons et al. [11] compared, in their randomized controlled trial of 14 cases, the effect of nipple stimulation and Syntometrine on uterine activity and found similar effects on the third stage of labor and blood loss. Bullough et al. [12] compared 2104 and 2123 early breastfeeding and nonbreastfeeding women, respectively. All women were evaluated for bleeding immediately after birth. In this large trial the authors found no difference in the incidence of PPH between the groups. Kim et al. [13] evaluated the third stage of labor in 87 women randomized for nipple stimulation or intravenous oxytocin; the results were comparable.

A recent review of the Cochrane database that was published in 2015 included 4608 women in four studies that assessed blood loss in the third stage of labor [14]. The authors of this review concluded that "there is insufficient evidence to evaluate the effect of nipple stimulation for reducing PPH during the third stage of labor and more evidence from high-quality studies is needed."

23.4 What Did Dr. Google Say?

A health survey from the Pew Research Center revealed that 59% of US adults use the Internet and other digital technologies to find health and healthcare information about symptoms, treatments, and medical conditions. The medical information found in search engines such as Google, Yahoo, or Bing comes from various sources across the web. It is available and accessible from every phone or computer with a Wi-Fi connection. Unfortunately, unlike professional search engines and other reliable medical information sources, the medical information retrieved from the web comes from diverse sources that may be unverified and unreliable.

A study by Starman et al. from 2010 [15] showed that the quality and content of health information on the Internet is highly variable across websites. They assessed the reliability and credibility of health-related information using the Health On the Net Foundation (HON) criteria and discovered a consistent relationship between the type of website and the quality of information presented. The highest quality of content was found in nonprofit, academic, and commercial websites with HONcode seal. In contrast, the lowest quality of content was found in news-related and personal websites. Thus, patients seeking health-related information on the Internet should be encouraged to exercise caution and utilize only well-known sites with transparency and accountability practices.

With the abundance of health and medical information on the web, the problem is no longer finding the information but assessing the quality and credibility of the publisher (see Chapter 8 for more details on grading internet information). Readers should always ask about the source of information, who is writing the article, and why. Many online medical articles are written by anonymous journalists who may or may not be physicians, health professionals, or even experts in the field. Therefore, it is better to seek health information from nonprofit websites that end in .org or .gov, from organizations operating from donation or government funding (www.wikipedia.org, www.nih.gov), or from academic websites that end in .ac or .edu, including those affiliated with universities, medical journals, or medical societies.

Google search engine was selected for this review, based on its popularity and availability. Current data show that the Google search engine is the most common method of searching health information on the Internet used by patients, with over 60% of all internet searches in the USA. A Google search was performed in April 2021 via Chrome browser using incognito mode to avoid predisposed personal browsing history, cookies, site data, or current location to influence search results. The Google top-ten hits search results for "nipple stimulation and induction of labor" and "nipple stimulation and postpartum hemorrhage" were collected, reviewed, and analyzed as discussed in the following sections.

23.4.1 Nipple Stimulation and Induction of Labor

Of the top-ten Google search results for "nipple stimulation and induction of labor," two were academic sites and eight were commercial sites. The two academic websites present published peer-reviewed articles on a nonprofit government-funded website (www.pubmed.gov) and will not be discussed in this section. The remaining results were from commercial websites and represent healthcare information articles for pregnant women discussing nipple stimulation for labor induction. The titles of these articles are "Nipple stimulation to induce labor: how does it work?," "Can you use a breast pump to induce labor?," "Does nipple stimulation help to induce labor?," "Nipple stimulation for natural labor induction," "The science behind pumping to induce labor," and so on. The vast majority of the articles from commercial websites have been written or reviewed by physicians in the past four years, include a list of references, and have HONcode seal indicating compliance with transparency and accountability practices. All articles include general information and consultation for parturients who are considering nipple stimulation for labor induction. The articles often include a description of nipple stimulation and other methods of natural induction of labor, a brief review of the literature, and a step-by-step guide of how to perform nipple stimulation. While all articles instruct readers to consult their physician before performing nipple stimulation, only one of them mentions possible adverse outcomes, namely uterine hyperstimulation, fetal distress, and fetal demise following the procedure.

23.4.2 Nipple Stimulation and Postpartum Hemorrhage

All top-ten Google search results for "nipple stimulation and postpartum hemorrhage" led to nonprofit and academic sites. Even after expanding the search for the first 20 results, no commercial, news-related, or personal websites were found. Six results linked to peer-reviewed scientific articles published on governmental nonprofit websites (www.pubmed.gov) or websites affiliated with medical journals (e.g. BMC, ScienceDirect), one book chapter, and two guidelines from websites affiliated with medical societies (e.g. WHO, US-Aid), and one content description linked to the nonprofit website Wikipedia (www.wikipedia.org). The titles of the scientific contents areas follows: "Breastfeeding or nipple stimulation for reducing postpartum haemorrhage in the third stage of labour," "Comparison of the effect of breast pump stimulation and oxytocin administration on the length of the third stage of labor, postpartum hemorrhage, and anemia: a randomized controlled trial," "Active management of the third stage of labor," "Prevention of postpartum hemorrhage: implementing active management of the third stage of labor," "WHO recommendations for the prevention and treatment of postpartum haemorrhage," and so on. All these results have been written by health professionals, physicians, or group experts and provide structured information with sufficient references and supplementary material for, but not only, healthcare personnel.

23.4.3 Summary of Internet Information

The quality of information on the Internet relating to nipple stimulation in pregnancy is highly variable. We analyzed Google's top-ten hits and found great variation in web-related information regarding nipple stimulation for induction of labor and nipple stimulation for postpartum hemorrhage. Of the information on nipple stimulation for induction of labor, 80% comes from commercial websites and includes general information for women contemplating labor induction, whereas all of the information on nipple stimulation and PPH is mainly professional, scientifically structured, and comes from nonprofit and educational websites with high accountability and credibility. Healthcare professionals should be aware of the quality of the information available on the Internet and direct their patients to appropriate high-quality information sources.

23.5 Conclusions

Evidence shows that in low-risk populations, antepartum nipple stimulation seems to be efficient and relatively safe in promoting the onset of labor. However, caution is advised in high-risk pregnancies, especially after previous cesarean delivery or mild placental abruption as uterine tachysystole may increase the risk for fetal distress, placental abruption and, in extreme cases, even fetal loss. The use of nipple stimulation in the third stage of labor is safe and may serve as an additive measure for the prevention of PPH.

References

1. J. Kavanagh, A. J. Kelly, J. Thomas. Breast stimulation for cervical ripening and induction of labour. *Cochrane Database Syst Rev* 2005;(3):CD003392.

2. N. Singh, R. Tripathi, Y. M. Mala, N. Yedla. Breast stimulation in low-risk primigravidas at term: does it aid in spontaneous onset of labour and vaginal delivery? A pilot study. *Biomed Res Int* 2014;2014:695037.

3. G. Demirel, H. Guler. The effect of uterine and nipple stimulation on induction with oxytocin and the labor process. *Worldviews Evid Based Nurs* 2015;12:273–80.

4. K. Takahata, S. Horiuchi, Y. Tadokoro, E. Sawano, K. Shinohara. Oxytocin levels in low-risk primiparas following breast stimulation for spontaneous onset of labor: a quasi-experimental study. *BMC Pregnancy Childbirth* 2019;19:351.

5. O. A. Viegas, S. Arulkumaran, D. M. Gibb, S. S. Ratnam. Nipple stimulation in late pregnancy causing uterine hyperstimulation and profound fetal bradycardia. *Br J Obstet Gynaecol* 1984;91:364–6.

6. M. A. Schellpfeffer, D. Hoyle, J. W. Johnson. Antepartal uterine hypercontractility secondary to nipple stimulation. *Obstet Gynecol* 1985;65:588–91.

7. D. M. Narasimhulu, L. Zhu. Uterine tachysystole with prolonged deceleration following nipple stimulation for labor augmentation. *Kathmandu Univ Med J* 2015;13:268–70.

8. S. D. Eckford, J. Westgate. Breastfeeding and placental abruption. *J Obstet Gynaecol* 1997;17:164–5.

9. M. A. Belfort. Overview of postpartum hemorrhage. UpToDate, 2022. www.uptodate.com/contents/overview-of-postpartum-hemorrhage. (accessed April 11, 2021).

10. T. M. Raams, J. L. Browne, V. J. M. M. Festen-Schrier, K. Klipstein-Grobusch, M. J. Rijken. Task shifting in active management of the third stage of labor: a systematic review. *BMC Pregnancy Childbirth* 2018;18:47.

11. D. W. Irons, P. Sriskandabalan, C. H. Bullough. A simple alternative to parenteral oxytocics for the third stage of labor. *Int J Gynaecol Obstet* 1994;46:15–18.

12. C. H. Bullough, R. S. Msuku, L. Karonde. Early suckling and postpartum haemorrhage: controlled trial in deliveries by traditional birth attendants. *Lancet* 1989;334:522–5.

13. Y. M. Kim, N. Tejani, B. Chayen, U. L. Verma. Management of the third stage of labor with nipple stimulation. *J Reprod Med* 1986;31:1033–4.

14. P. Abedi, S. Jahanfar, F. Namvar, J. Lee. Breastfeeding or nipple stimulation for reducing postpartum haemorrhage in the third stage of labour. *Cochrane Database Syst Rev* 2016;(1):CD010845.

15. J. S. Starman, F. K. Gettys, J. A. Capo, et al. Quality and content of Internet-based information for ten common orthopaedic sports medicine diagnoses. *J Bone Joint Surg Am* 2010;92:1612–18.

Chapter

Sex during the Postpartum
Why the Six-Week Break?

E. Shirin Dason, Abi Kirubarajan, and Mara Sobel

24.1 Introduction

Postpartum resumption of sexual intercourse is an important contributor to a woman's general health and quality of life. Lower sexual function has been linked to increased health service utilization, postpartum depression, relational conflict, and impacts on parenting [1]. Up to 89% of first-time mothers report distressing concerns regarding the impact of body image, physical recovery, and fatigue on sexual function [1]. This is likely related to inadequate counseling regarding expectations for normal postpartum sexual function and inadequate treatment or recommendations for sexual dysfunction. Though separate guidelines on postpartum sexual health exist, most international guidelines on appropriate postpartum care do not address the optimization of sexual function but rather focus on appropriate contraception. Though important, contraception is only one of many aspects of sexual health in the postpartum period [2–4].

24.2 Resumption of Intercourse

Vaginal intercourse is resumed by 52% of women by 5–6 weeks postpartum and by 90% of women by 3 months postpartum [4,5]. Women are often concerned about the risk to their physical health, including the impact of intercourse on their healing, pain, and the chance of conception. Therefore, most women seek the advice of their physician prior to resuming intercourse [6]. Most physicians recommend resuming sexual intercourse after 4–6 weeks; however, there is no specific evidence to support this recommendation. The World Health Organization recommends that providers should discuss the resumption of sexual activity 2–6 weeks after delivery [7]. The biological context for this advice may be influenced by the higher risk of venous thromboembolism with the first 3–6 weeks postpartum, which impacts available contraceptive options and the higher risk of infection and/or hemorrhage in the first 2 weeks postpartum [8]. Rare complications reported by case reports of early resumption of sexual intercourse include delayed uterine rupture after cesarean section (CS) and air embolism [9,10] (see Chapter 19 for more details on air embolism). Ultimately, the underlying basis for this recommendation is likely anecdotal, as this may be when most women have felt physically and mentally ready to engage in intercourse. Sharing this with women as an observation rather than as a medically based recommendation in the context of the discussion of normal postpartum sexual function may be appropriate.

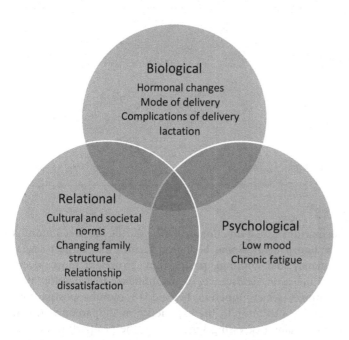

Figure 24.1 Postpartum sexual function.

24.3 Normal Postpartum Sexual Function

While there are many studies that have reported on postpartum sexual dysfunction, it is important to realize that postpartum sexual function is an entity that has yet to be fully described and normalized. Therefore, some of what women consider dysfunctional may actually be functionally normal. Current evidence detailing the presence of sexual dysfunction in the postpartum period is also flawed due to the lack of standardized measurement techniques. It is apparent from the current literature that most women are dissatisfied with their sexual function, whether or not this constitutes true sexual dysfunction. A focus on improving counseling and the provision of treatment recommendations may mitigate this distress.

Postpartum sexual function is a complex entity influenced by biological, psychological, and relational factors (Figure 24.1). Biological factors include the hormonal changes during pregnancy and the postpartum, mode of delivery, complications of delivery, and lactation. Psychological factors include low mood and chronic fatigue. Relational factors may include navigating cultural and societal norms, changing family structure, and relationship dissatisfaction that may reduce feelings of intimacy [1,4].

It is generally well accepted that normal sexual postpartum changes include a reduction in the frequency of sexual intercourse, the presence of vaginal dryness leading to dyspareunia, as well as an overall decline in libido, sexual desire, and orgasm (Table 24.1) [11,12]. Other changes more specifically associated with breastfeeding include the potential for sexual arousal during feeding and ejection of milk.

Table 24.1. Expected postpartum sexual changes

- Reduction in frequency of intercourse
- Decline in libido
- Decline in sexual desire
- Decline in orgasm
- Vaginal dryness
- Sexual arousal with breastfeeding

24.3.1 Biological Factors

Biological factors impact postpartum sexual function primarily during the first 3 months and then begin to gradually improve [4]. Some biological factors that impact sexual function begin during pregnancy and continue postpartum. However, more severe complications such as wound infection, dehiscence, or incontinence that develop after delivery may continue to impact sexual function beyond 18 months postpartum. Biological factors are a primary contributor to the experience of dyspareunia, which represents the most common sexually distressing symptom in the postpartum period. Painful penetration is present in up to 55% of women upon postpartum resumption of intercourse; perineal pain significantly reduces to 10% by 12 weeks postpartum [13,14].

24.3.1.1 Physiology

Most physiological changes and physical symptoms during pregnancy that impact sexual function persist for the first 3–6 months postpartum. These include fatigue, back pain, dyspareunia, infections such as urinary tract infections (UTIs) or vulvovaginitis, and vulvar varicose veins. Pregnant women may also experience diminished clitoral sensation, lack of libido, and orgasmic disorder. Dyspareunia may arise due to multiple physiological mechanisms, including the decrease in connective tissue, increase in muscular fibers of the vaginal wall, and vasocongestion resulting in decreased lubrication. Vasocongestion and resulting edema begin to subside by 3 weeks postpartum when vaginal rugae return [11].

Hormonal changes, such as an increase in estrogen, progesterone, and prolactin, can impact sexual desire and arousal through experienced symptoms such as nausea, vomiting, weight gain, fatigue, and breast tenderness. If a woman is not breastfeeding, levels of prolactin decline allowing levels of luteinizing hormone and follicle-stimulating hormone to increase, leading to the restoration of menstrual cycles in approximately 30 days following delivery [8]. The mean time of first ovulation in nonlactating women has been reported to be between 45 and 94 days postpartum [8]. In a breastfeeding woman, ovulation is typically suppressed until breastfeeding frequency declines with, for example, the introduction of solids [8]. Breastfeeding women may have irregular menstruation leading to a fear of undesired pregnancy, which can impact sexual life negatively [6].

After delivery, the superficial layer of the endometrial decidua sheds, resulting in vaginal bleeding referred to as lochia. Lochia may be present for 24 hours up to 12 weeks postpartum [15]. Some women are counseled to wait until their lochia subsides before resuming intercourse. However, there is no evidence of complications, such as increased ascending infection, during this time. Therefore, lochia should not be used as a gauge for safe resumption of sexual activity.

24.3.1.2 Breastfeeding

While some studies have demonstrated that lactation causes several physiological, contextual, and relationship changes that can lead to lower sexual function, other studies have found that breastfeeding may improve sexual function [1]. Overall, though it may or may not impact sexual satisfaction, breastfeeding has been shown to lead to a delay in the resumption of intercourse [5].

Lactation is facilitated by an elevation in prolactin levels, which decrease ovarian production of androgen and estrogen. Lower androgen levels may result in lower sexual desire. Low estrogen and progesterone levels result in decreased vaginal lubrication, vasocongestion, and atrophy of the vaginal epithelium that may contribute to dyspareunia [14]. The prevalence and degree of dyspareunia has been found to be higher in breastfeeding women during the first 6 months postpartum [14]. Lactation may increase sexual desire and eroticism due to the increased sensitivity and direct stimulation of the breasts [4]. The release of oxytocin during breastfeeding leads to feelings of eroticism during nursing in up to 40% of women. Some patients may be uncomfortable with this experience [4]. Orgasm may also lead to the release of oxytocin, thus causing milk ejection that may also be uncomfortable for women; nursing prior to sex may mitigate this effect [4].

Women who are breastfeeding may also notice psychological effects on sexual function. Breastfeeding can make women feel less sexually attractive, contribute to heightened levels of fatigue due to frequent nursing, and cause feelings of envy in a woman's partner due to the closeness between mother and child [1,4,6].

24.3.1.3 Mode of Delivery

Evidence on the effect of mode of delivery on postpartum sexual function is controversial. While forms of delivery that cause more perineal trauma, such as assisted vaginal delivery or episiotomy, have been associated with an increase in pain with penetration, this effect is largely nonsignificant by 6 months. Factors contributing to persistent dyspareunia past 6 months postpartum include breastfeeding and presence of prepregnancy dyspareunia [13].

The classically proposed protective effect of CS on sexual function has largely been debunked [12]. The only available randomized controlled trial comparing sexual function between women undergoing CS or vaginal delivery (Term Breech Trial) did not demonstrate a difference in sexual function between the two groups. However, this was not measured based on validated questionnaires [4]. Cohort studies assessing the impact of delivery mode on sexual function have produced inconsistent results. This is a challenging research question because women who undergo CS are a heterogeneous group; some may undergo labor prior to CS and others may have an elective CS prior to the onset of labor. Potential mechanisms for the improved sexual function in women undergoing CS include less pelvic floor trauma through minimal pudendal nerve injury and absence of lacerations and perineal pain in the postpartum period. Nevertheless, if a woman also undergoes labor, these effects would not necessarily be mitigated by intrapartum CS. Similarly, while these factors may confer higher sexual function in the first 3 months postpartum, the difference between the effect of modes of delivery on sexual function seems to equalize by 1 year [4].

Operative delivery tends to be associated with a higher rate of sexual dysfunction, although the exact mechanism is difficult to ascertain. It may be due to the increased perineal trauma, the psychological impact of an operative birth, or the presence of anatomical factors that led to the need for operative delivery [4]. A large prospective cohort study of 1507 nulliparous women in Australia demonstrated that women who had a birth assisted with forceps and those who had an episiotomy or laceration were less likely to have resumed vaginal sex by 6 weeks compared to women with a spontaneous vaginal birth and an intact perineum [16].

Up to 85% of women will sustain some form of perineal trauma with vaginal delivery, with at least one-third requiring repair, and up to 20% of women who sustain perineal trauma will continue to experience some pain at 8 weeks postpartum [17] (see Chapter 25 for more details on pelvic floor injuries). The degree of both vaginal laceration and episiotomy has been associated with increased perineal pain and lower sexual function [13]. Obstetric anal sphincter injuries are an independent risk factor for sexual dysfunction and postpone resumption of vaginal intercourse [18]. Signorello et al. [19] demonstrated that compared to patients with an intact perineum or a first-degree laceration, women with a second-degree perineal laceration and those with a third- or fourth-degree laceration were 80% and 270%, respectively, more likely to report dyspareunia at 3 months postpartum. Several other studies have corroborated these effects [4]. Routine use of episiotomy, purported as a potential mitigator to worse perineal trauma, was not found to lower pain with sexual intercourse 6 months or longer after delivery [20].

Complications of obstetric lacerations may include infection and/or dehiscence. It has been suggested that early resumption of sexual intercourse may contribute to these complications, but there have been no studies assessing this. Significant risk factors for wound infection include mediolateral episiotomy, operative vaginal delivery, third- and fourth-degree lacerations, and presence of meconium [21]. The majority of perineal wound infections occur in the first 3 weeks after hospital discharge. Dehiscence may be managed by allowing secondary intention to occur or by resuturing the wound within the first 2 weeks, although evidence suggests that resuturing the laceration reduces dyspareunia and increases satisfaction [21].

24.3.1.4 Delivery Complications

The impact of intrapartum complications such as postpartum hemorrhage, genital tract infections, or obstructed labor on sexual function has not been adequately studied. Following delivery, women may have either short-term or long-term complications. Up to 10.9% of women may have perineal wound complications such as infection or dehiscence following vaginal delivery [17,22]. Long-term consequences of perineal trauma include urinary and fecal incontinence, pelvic organ prolapse, or pain. Early pelvic floor muscle training beginning in early pregnancy may prevent the onset of urinary incontinence in late pregnancy and the postpartum, especially in patients with an elevated body mass index [23].

24.3.2 Psychological Factors

Psychosocial factors are associated with increased sexual dysfunction past 3 months postpartum and contribute to heightened sexual distress [1]. Psychogenic changes such as the anxiety of delivery and motherhood, lack of self-esteem, and sexual guilt can all lead to changed sexual function. Extreme exhaustion due to chronic sleep deprivation, exacerbated by breastfeeding, also impacts sexual function [24].

Sexual dysfunction is commonly associated with postpartum depression (PPD). PPD has been associated with decreased frequency and interest in sexual intercourse at 8–12 weeks and in sexual desire at 6 months [25]. These effects may persist even after depression resolves. Sexual dysfunction can also lead to PPD. In addition, the treatment of depression with selective serotonin reuptake inhibitors or serotonin/norepinephrine reuptake inhibitors can also result in sexual dysfunction. Sexual side effects should be discussed with patients and consideration of agents that have a lower impact on sexual function and are safe in breastfeeding (if applicable) is warranted (i.e. bupropion) [4].

24.3.3 Relational Factors

Sexual distress contributing to sexual dysfunction is also influenced by one's interpersonal relationships. The postpartum period is associated with a decline in relationship satisfaction [1]. Developing a parental relationship, the changes in family structure, and whether this was a planned/unplanned or desired/undesired pregnancy all influence a patient's self-image, mood stability, difficulty, and discomfort with vaginal intercourse [11]. Women can also experience the impact of changing views of intimacy and sexuality [24]. Women have reported engaging in sexual intercourse due to concerns regarding their partner's satisfaction despite not being ready physically or psychologically to engage; this can further impact sexual distress and lead to dysfunction [1].

Societal influences, such as poor sex education, general role traditionality and cultural values, can also contribute to sexual function as it can shape first-time mothers' expectations [1]. Parity also affects sexual function, as primiparous women tend to be less secure in their sexual function due to lack of experience and suffer from more dyspareunia due to the higher trauma associated with first births [5].

24.4 Evaluation and Management Principles

It is important to initiate sexual health discussions during pregnancy in order to build rapport and normalize the conversation. Starting the conversation early and revisiting the subject as a component of general health is important in normalizing sexual health for both patient and provider.

24.4.1 Measurement of Sexual Function

It is important to begin by determining prepregnancy sexual function. Important historical points include relationship assessment, presence of support networks, planned/unplanned pregnancy, outcomes of pregnancies, previous deliveries, current children's health, and contraception. An assessment for the presence of mood symptoms should be undertaken. There are standardized screening questionnaires available to assist providers in specifically assessing postpartum sexual problems. Patients may feel more

Table 24.2. Plouffe: three sexual health screening questions

- Are you sexually active?
- Do you have any sexual problems?
- Do you experience sexual pain?

comfortable with a standardized questionnaire rather than a clinical interview. A screening questionnaire published by Plouffe describes three questions: whether the patient is sexually active, whether there are any sexual problems, and whether there is any sexual pain (Table 24.2). These questions can be asked during a postpartum history or included in a postpartum historical questionnaire. Other screening questionnaire options include the Female Sexual Function Index, the McCoy Female Sexual Function Questionnaire, the Brief Sexual Symptom checklist, the Female Distress Scale, and the Pelvic Organ Prolapse/Urinary Incontinence Sexual Questionnaire [4]. After determining baseline sexual function, providers should initiate a discussion of the expected changes with pregnancy.

24.4.2 Intrapartum Prevention of Perineal Pain

Given the likely impact of perineal trauma on sexual function, efforts to limit the degree of trauma and subsequent complications have been found to reduce penetrative pain. Evidence-based mechanisms for the reduction of postpartum perineal pain include continuous suturing rather than the use of interrupted sutures, use of absorbable sutures, a single dose of aspirin, a single dose of paracetamol, and/or a single dose of a nonsteroidal anti-inflammatory drug (NSAID) [17,26–29]. Antibiotic prophylaxis with intravenous antibiotics for women with operative vaginal deliveries, regardless of type of laceration, reduces infectious puerperal morbidity and improves perineal pain [30]. However, antibiotic prophylaxis does not reduce wound infection after episiotomy in uncomplicated vaginal birth [31]. Routine episiotomy does not result in a lower incidence of dyspareunia at 6 months [20]. One trial demonstrated a reduction in perineal wound complications following a single dose of second-generation cephalosporin administered intravenously at the time of third- or fourth-degree perineal tears [32].

24.4.3 Postpartum Sexual Health Management Principles

An early discussion of expectations surrounding perineal pain, dyspareunia, and initiation of postpartum sexual activity should take place, ideally before a patient leaves the hospital or within the first 1–2 weeks postpartum (Table 24.3). Patients who know what to expect may experience less sexual distress overall. At the 6-week postpartum follow-up, specific efforts should be made to assess sexual function and concerns (using a questionnaire) and assessing the presence of dyspareunia and/or other physical symptoms and performing an appropriate examination [4]. Women should be counseled to expect a reduction in frequency of sexual intercourse, libido, desire, and orgasm. if vaginal dryness or dyspareunia is a primary concern, use of vaginal lubricants should be

Table 24.3. Three important management principles to improve postpartum sexual health

- Normalize the conversation: ask your patient about their sexual function and discuss expected sexual changes in the postpartum period

- Dyspareunia is the most commonly experienced distressing symptom: offer vaginal lubricants, alternative sexual positions, vaginal estrogen, or pelvic floor physiotherapy

- Psychological or relational factors: encourage alone time, ask about childcare support, offer individual or couple-based therapy

encouraged and vaginal estrogen considered. In addition, more frequent intercourse and sexual positions that allow women more control over the depth of penetration may be helpful. Alternatives to intercourse such as genital stimulation may allow partners to discover new ways to express their sexuality and maintain sexual health [11]. Relationship partners should be counseled to work on communication, teamwork, time together as a couple, and agreement on priorities [24]. Optimization of sleep is an important factor, which may be improved by childcare support [24]. In addition, referral for postpartum pelvic floor muscle training may provide some benefit, especially in women experiencing dyspareunia or urinary and/or anal incontinence [5]. Psychological and relational factors may be better addressed by individual or family counseling; however, this has yet to be specifically studied in this population.

24.5 What Did Dr. Google Say?

There is a multitude of information readily available on searching the question "How to have sex after having a baby?" As with most topics, recommendations available on popular websites frequented by women have varying levels of evidence-based information. Most of the recommendations readily available on the Internet are reasonable. Most popular websites recommend discussing the resumption of intercourse with a healthcare provider, although they acknowledge that there is no set timeline. One website, Today's Parent, in their article "A low-key guide to sex for new parents," explains that the 6-week visit is not always required, provided a woman's incision or tear looks sufficiently healed [33]. The major risk associated with the resumption of intercourse "too soon" is often cited to be infection; some websites even go on to recommend that women should wait until lochia has resolved [34].

Normal postpartum changes that may impact sexual function described by popular websites include vaginal dryness, loss of libido, fatigue, low mood, low body image, possibility of leaking milk during intercourse, and potential for dyspareunia. Advice usually given to women includes performing Kegel exercises, ensuring appropriate birth control, using lubricants or a supportive pillow, trying top or side-to-side positions to control the depth of penetration, pumping prior to intercourse to avoid milk leakage, encouraging intimacy with their partner through communication and other nonsexual or nonpenetrative experiences, and seeking out a pelvic physiotherapist [35–38]. One website, What to Expect, advises women to try acetaminophen and ibuprofen prior to sexual intercourse [35].

References

1. S. J. Dawson, M.-P. Vaillancourt-Morel, M. Pierce, N. O. Rosen. Biopsychosocial predictors of trajectories of postpartum sexual function in first-time mothers. *Health Psychol* 2020;**39**:700–10.

2. C. Haran, M. van Driel, B. L. Mitchell, W. E. Brodribb. Clinical guidelines for postpartum women and infants in primary care: a systematic review. *BMC Pregnancy Childbirth* 2014;**14**:51.

3. J. Lamont, K. Bajzak, C. Bouchard, et al. Female sexual health consensus clinical guidelines. *J Obstet Gynaecol Can* 2012;**34**:769–75.

.4. L. M. Leeman, R. G. Rogers. Sex after childbirth: postpartum sexual function. *Obstet Gynecol* 2012;**119**:647–55.

5. O. Gutzeit, G. Levy, L. Lowenstein. Postpartum female sexual function: risk factors for postpartum sexual dysfunction. *Sex Med* 2020;**8**:8–13.

6. F. Alp Yılmaz, A. Şener Taplak, S. Polat. Breastfeeding and sexual activity and sexual quality in postpartum women. *Breastfeeding Med* 2019;**14**:587–91.

7. World Health Organization. *WHO Recommendations on Postnatal Care of the Mother and Newborn.* Geneva: World Health Organization, 2013.

8. A. Glasier, S. Bhattacharya, H. Evers, et al. Contraception after pregnancy. *Acta Obstet Gynecol Scand* 2019;**98**:1378–85.

9. H.-F. Tsai. Delayed uterine rupture occurred 4 weeks after cesarean section following sexual intercourse: a case report and literature review. *Taiwan J Obstet Gynecol* 2013;**52**:411–14.

10. P. A. Batman, J. Thomlinson, V. C. Moore, R. Sykes. Death due to air embolism during sexual intercourse in the puerperium. *Postgrad Med J* 1998;**74**:612–13.

11. C. E. Johnson. Sexual health during pregnancy and the postpartum. *J Sex Med* 2011;**8**:1267–84.

12. S. Lurie, M. Aizenberg, V. Sulema, et al. Sexual function after childbirth by the mode of delivery: a prospective study. *Arch Gynecol Obstet* 2013;**288**:785–92.

13. Z. Abdool, R. Thakar, A. H. Sultan. Postpartum female sexual function. *Eur J Obstet Gynecol Reprod Biol* 2009;**145**:133–7.

14. L. Lagaert, S. Weyers, H. V. Kerrebroeck, E. Elaut. Postpartum dyspareunia and sexual functioning: a prospective cohort study. *Eur J Contracept Reprod Health Care* 2017;**22**:200–6.

15. S. Fletcher, C. A. Grotegut, A. H. James. Lochia patterns among normal women: a systematic review. *J Womens Health* 2012;**21**:1290–4.

16. E. McDonald, S. Brown. Does method of birth make a difference to when women resume sex after childbirth? *BJOG* 2013;**120**:823–30.

17. S. Webb, M. Sherburn, K. M. K. Ismail. Managing perineal trauma after childbirth. *BMJ* 2014;**349**:g6829.

18. S. Anglès-Acedo, C. Ros-Cerro, S. Escura-Sancho, et al. Coital resumption after delivery among OASIS patients: differences between instrumental and spontaneous delivery. *BMC Womens Health* 2019;**19**:154.

19. L. B. Signorello, B. L. Harlow, A. K. Chekos, J. T. Repke. Postpartum sexual functioning and its relationship to perineal trauma: a retrospective cohort study of primiparous women. *Am J Obstet Gynecol* 2001;**184**:881–90.

20. H. Jiang, X. Qian, G. Carroli, P. Garner. Selective versus routine use of episiotomy for vaginal birth. *Cochrane Database Syst Rev* 2017;(2):CD000081.

21. A. Kamel, M. Khaled. Episiotomy and obstetric perineal wound dehiscence: beyond soreness. *J Obstet Gynaecol* 2014;**34**:215–17.

22. S. L. Woodd, A. Montoya, M. Barreix, et al. Incidence of maternal peripartum

infection: a systematic review and meta-analysis. *PLoS Med* 2019;**16**:e1002984.

23. S. J. Woodley, P. Lawrenson, R. Boyle, et al. Pelvic floor muscle training for preventing and treating urinary and faecal incontinence in antenatal and postnatal women. *Cochrane Database Syst Rev* 2020;(5):CD007471.

24. H. Woolhouse, E. McDonald, S. Brown. Women's experiences of sex and intimacy after childbirth: making the adjustment to motherhood. *J Psychosom Obstet Gynaecol* 2012;**33**:185–90.

25. S.-R. Chang, W.-A. Lin, H.-H. Lin, M.-K. Shyu, M.-I. Lin. Sexual dysfunction predicts depressive symptoms during the first 2 years postpartum. *Women Birth* 2018;**31**:e403–11.

26. C. Kettle, T. Dowswell, K. M. Ismail. Continuous and interrupted suturing techniques for repair of episiotomy or second-degree tears. *Cochrane Database Syst Rev* 2012;(11):CD000947.

27. E. Abalos, Y. Sguassero, G. Gyte. Paracetamol/acetaminophen (single administration) for perineal pain in the early postpartum period. *Cochrane Database Syst Rev* 2021;(1):CD008407.

28. F. Wuytack, V. Smith, B. Cleary. Oral non-steroidal anti-inflammatory drugs (single dose) for perineal pain in the early postpartum period. *Cochrane Database Syst Rev* 2021;(1):CD011352.

29. E. Shepherd, R. Grivell. Aspirin (single dose) for perineal pain in the early postpartum period. *Cochrane Database Syst Rev* 2020;(7):CD012129.

30. T. Liabsuetrakul, T. Choobun, K. Peeyananjarassri, Q. Islam. Antibiotic prophylaxis for operative vaginal delivery. *Cochrane Database Syst Rev* 2020;(3): CD004455.

31. M. Bonet, E. Ota, C. E. Chibueze, O. T. Oladapo. Routine antibiotic prophylaxis after normal vaginal birth for reducing maternal infectious morbidity. *Cochrane Database Syst Rev* 2017;(11): CD012137.

32. P. Buppasiri, P. Lumbiganon, J. Thinkhamrop, B. Thinkhamrop. Antibiotic prophylaxis for third- and fourth-degree perineal tear during vaginal birth. *Cochrane Database Syst Rev* 2014; (10):CD005125.

33. K. Rope. A low-key guide to sex for new parents. Today's Parent, 2018. www.todaysparent.com/family/parenting/a-low-key-guide-to-sex-for-new-parents/ (accessed April 29, 2021).

34. Sex and childbirth. Women's Health Matters. www.womenshealthmatters.ca/health-centres/sexual-health/pregnancy/sex-and-childbirth.html (accessed April 29, 2021).

35. K. Weiss. Your guide to sex after giving birth. What to Expect, 2021. www.whattoexpect.com/first-year/postpartum-health-and-care/sex-after-birth/ (accessed April 29, 2021).

36. E. Z. Ruddy. 8 Surprising truths about postpartum sex after birth. Parents, 2021. www.parents.com/parenting/relationships/sex-and-marriage-after-baby/how-to-have-great-postpartum-sex/ (accessed April 29, 2021).

37. E. Moore. I had sex 4 weeks after giving birth. Today's Parent, 2020. www.todaysparent.com/baby/postpartum-care/i-had-sex-4-weeks-after-giving-birth/ (accessed April 29, 2021).

38. Mayo Clinic. Sex after pregnancy: set your own timeline. www.mayoclinic.org/healthy-lifestyle/labor-and-delivery/in-depth/sex-after-pregnancy/art-20045669#:~:text=While%20there's%20no%20required%20waiting,first%20two%20weeks%20after%20deliver (accessed April 29, 2021).

Sex after Pelvic Floor Injuries

María del Mar Muñoz Muñiz, Sara Serrano Velayos, and Ángeles Leal García

25.1 Introduction

Sexuality, for both men and women, varies throughout life and is influenced by a number of factors or events such as health, personal relationships, and sociocultural variables. For women, circumstances may also influence their reproduction.

During pregnancy and the postnatal period a woman undergoes a series of physiological changes that affect the entire body. In general, women return to their prepregnancy condition after the birth, although in some cases this process can take up to 6 months.

25.2 Intrapartum Perineal Lacerations

The descent and engagement of the fetal head in the birth canal causes compression of the nerves and the elevator ani muscles with a certain degree of ischemia. Also, vaginal delivery can produce lacerations and tears to the vagina, bladder and urethra, as well as the endopelvic fascia. Expulsion of the fetus produces significant strain on the pubococcygeus muscle, with deformation of the perineum during crowning and elongation of the pudendal nerves.

Because of these consequences, vaginal delivery represents a direct trauma to the pelvic floor, potentially damaging its functionality. This perineal trauma can be divided anatomically into anterior, affecting the labia, urethra, anterior vagina, and clitoris and which carries less morbidity, and posterior. In the latter, there is higher morbidity and possible pelvic floor dysfunction, as the damage affects the vagina, perineal muscles, and anal sphincter and mucosa. All these injuries can occur independently of an episiotomy or vaginal tear.

Obstetric anal sphincter injuries (OASIS) constitute a clear risk factor for posterior pelvic floor dysfunction, mainly fecal incontinence. Their prevalence is variable, comprising up to 1% of all vaginal deliveries, and their prevention constitutes the primary objective of today's obstetric practices. The most important risk factors have been widely described (Table 25.1) and different societies have published specific guidelines [1,2].

The levator ani muscle, most prominently its puborectal part, frequently suffers injuries during delivery, although these are not included in perineal tear classification. Nevertheless, they are relevant as they can occur in up to 13–36% of vaginal deliveries. A meta-analysis by Friedman et al. [3] showed that the relative risk of levator ani avulsion was similar between eutocic and vacuum-assisted deliveries, while it was seven times higher with forceps-assisted deliveries. This muscle injury, whether partial or complete, over time causes the signs and symptoms of pelvic floor dysfunction, mainly pelvic organ prolapse (POP) due to enlargement of the genital hiatus.

Table 25.1. OASIS risk factors

Nulliparity	RR 6.97
Fetal weight >4 kg	OR 2.27
Shoulder dystocia	OR 1.90
Occiput posterior presentation	RR 2.44
Prolonged second stage of labor	2–3 hours: RR 1.47 3–4 hours: RR 1.79 >4 hours: RR 2.02
Instrumental delivery	Vacuum without episiotomy: OR 1.89 Vacuum with episiotomy: OR 0.57 Forceps without episiotomy: OR 6.53 Forceps with episiotomy: OR 1.34
Previous OASIS	OR 5.51

OASIS, obstetric anal sphincter injuries; OR, odds ratio; RR, relative risk.

25.3 Postpartum Sexual Dysfunction

Resuming sexual intercourse after childbirth should be delayed until the perineum, vagina, and uterus have healed properly. It must also be remembered that the postnatal hormonal changes involve a decrease in sex hormones due to the release of prolactin for breastfeeding. This can have a negative influence on libido and emotional state in general, but within the genital region causes atrophy of the vaginal epithelium, which is thinner and more fragile, with less lubrication capacity.

This decrease in sexual desire is compounded by other factors, such as fatigue, lack of sleep, attention focused on the newborn, body image, stress, and sometimes depression.

There is also a fear of pain after the experience of pain during childbirth and in the immediate postnatal period, and the common belief that early postpartum intercourse will be painful. There can be pain during intercourse after an episiotomy or tearing, and some vaginal dryness, although this is not always the case [5].

The postpartum period brings numerous vital changes that, depending on the couple and their environment, can lead to an improvement in their intimacy and sexuality, or conversely create a sexual dysfunction. Health workers play a key role in support, guidance, and prevention at this time. Their work should focus on talking about difficulties and fears, clarifying that they are normal and temporary; explaining that it is good to resume sexual activity as soon as possible but gradually and without pressure; guiding and explaining the importance of dialogue, patience, and mutual exploration; and looking for ways to approach sex that are satisfactory for both partners.

Anglés-Acedo et al. [6] published a retrospective study that examined when intercourse with vaginal penetration was resumed and analyzed the variables that influenced resumption at 6 months postpartum in patients with and without OASIS depending on the mode of delivery. Globally, 73% of patients had resumed intercourse, with a significantly lower proportion in the OASIS group. When comparing between the different modes of delivery using the PISQ-12 questionnaire, the authors observed that women with an instrumental delivery resumed coital activity later and had worse sexual function than patients with a eutocic delivery.

The prevalence of postpartum sexual dysfunction ranges from 41– 83% at 2–3 months postpartum to 64% at 6 months postpartum. Although many women experience sexual problems during this period, the number of consultations for this issue is relatively low, estimated at less than 15%. This may be partly due to prioritizing care for the newborn, but also to embarrassment about discussing sexual problems with health professionals. Lack of time and, in many cases, of specific training in handling sex-related issues can also contribute to the infrequency with which the issue is addressed [7].

Pain disorder is the most common type of sexual dysfunction during the postpartum period. Perineal pain and pain during intercourse are often the result of perineal trauma from episiotomy, spontaneous tearing, or tearing secondary to instrumental delivery. It can affect up to 42% of women immediately after delivery, dropping to 22% and 10% at 8 and 12 weeks postpartum, respectively [8].

With regard to the impact of episiotomy on sexual function, the data in the available literature vary considerably. While some studies find higher rates of dyspareunia compared to women with an intact perineum or a spontaneous perineal tear, the Cochrane review published in 2017 concluded that there was no difference in dyspareunia rates, from 6 months postpartum, in women with a vaginal birth with or without episiotomy. According to most studies, perineal pain and dyspareunia are directly related to the degree of any perineal tear, with pain being more intense and longer-lasting in third- and fourth-degree tears than in first- and second-degree tears [7,9].

In a retrospective study of 626 first-time mothers assessed over a 6-month period postpartum, Signorello et al. [10] found that, compared with women who gave birth with an intact perineum, women with second-degree perineal trauma were 80% more likely to have dyspareunia at 3 months postpartum (confidence interval [CI] 1.2–2.8), while those with third- or fourth-degree perineal trauma were up to 270% more likely to suffer dyspareunia (CI 1.7–7.7). Similar results were found in a Swedish population-based study in which it was observed that the relative risk of not having resumed sexual activity at 6 months postpartum was directly proportional to the degree of perineal injury, doubling in women with high-degree tears compared to women without perineal injury [11].

One of the possible benefits perceived by patients with cesarean delivery is the lack of mechanical damage to the pelvic floor and consequently the absence of sexual function problems. In fact, there is a dearth of good scientific evidence that either route of delivery is better than the other in terms of subsequent sexual function. The only randomized controlled trial assessing postpartum sexual function outcomes after elective cesarean section versus vaginal delivery was the Term Breech Trial, which found no difference in sexual function at 2-year follow-up. However, this study had several limitations: including a heterogeneous sample of both nulliparous and multiparous women, the use of nonvalidated questionnaires to evaluate sexual function, the use of different measurements at different follow-up visits, and problems in generalizing the results given that postpartum sexual function after vaginal breech delivery could be different from a vaginal cephalic delivery [12].

In a survey by Abdool et al. [8] of 484 primiparous women at 6 months postpartum no significant difference was observed in the resumption of sexual intercourse after birth regardless of the form of delivery, whereas the study by Griffiths et al. [13] observed a significant reduction in sexual satisfaction scores among women who had a vaginal delivery versus those who had an elective cesarean section at 2 years follow-up. Finally, a 2017 meta-analysis of 2851 Chinese primiparous women found that the route of delivery did not affect sexual satisfaction at 3 and 6 months postpartum, although significant differences were found in the areas of resumption of sexual intercourse and dyspareunia at both 3 and 6 months [14].

Although the correlation between dyspareunia and sexual dysfunction with perineal trauma seems to be proven, since prevalence is higher in the group of vaginal births compared with that in cesarean births, both groups are highly heterogeneous in terms of the effects on the pelvic floor. This is because a scheduled cesarean section has little in common with an intrapartum cesarean section after a prolonged expulsion time, a complicated instrumental delivery with some degree of tearing, or with a eutocic delivery with an intact perineum. Consequently, although cesarean section appears to result in a lower incidence of dyspareunia at 3–6 months postpartum, this advantage does not persist over time.

Vaginal delivery is a well-recognized risk factor of pelvic floor dysfunction due to the perineal trauma it causes, with a direct relationship to a woman's parity. Also, the mode of delivery increases the likelihood of having urinary incontinence and/or POP, mainly after a forceps-assisted delivery but to a lesser extent in a vacuum-assisted delivery as well.

We must not overlook that there are other factors that can increase pelvic floor trauma and consequently the incidence of future pelvic floor dysfunction, such as episiotomy, fetal head size and birthweight, and the elasticity of maternal tissue. The grade of the injury as well as its recovery will be fundamental in the development or not of those dysfunctions [15].

Depending on the pelvic floor's basal function it is possible that these lesions will not produce immediate symptoms, but with age-related deterioration symptoms will arise. In some cases, the degree of damage can cause immediate symptoms [16]. When POP or urinary or anal incontinence appear early in the postpartum period, they also contribute to sexual dysfunction due to worsening of body self-image.

In women with pelvic floor dysfunction, sexual activity is not routinely evaluated in usual clinical practice, hence the lack of solid data on the impact of these dysfunctions on sexual function and the influence of the different possible treatments. With regard to postpartum sexual dysfunction, the available information is even scarcer, with most of the studies focusing exclusively on resuming coital activity and evaluating the presence of dyspareunia, without evaluating sexual function globally with validated questionnaires.

25.4 Postpartum Recovery

During the first 6–8 weeks of the postpartum period the tissues and the uterus slowly involute. In general, it is not recommended to resume intercourse with penetration until vaginal and/or perineal wounds have healed and bleeding has ceased. Massage of the perineal scar tissues is recommended to promote early recovery of tissue elasticity, minimizing discomfort with coital activity.

After those first weeks it is convenient to carry out an individualized assessment for the presence of symptoms, as well as a perineopelvic exam to determine if it is necessary to use any specific technique for pelvic floor rehabilitation. In this way, healthcare professionals will help prevent the development of pelvic floor dysfunctions such as sexual dysfunction.

During this phase Kegel exercises are also recommended in order to restore pelvic floor muscle function, which has been damaged during delivery, although they should be postponed until there is adequate perineal healing. It is paramount that during this period the woman avoids performing classical abdominal exercises, as these could worsen pelvic floor distension when exercising with a distended perineum and a lax vagina.

Diaphragmatic aspiration exercises are also useful during this period. They are performed in respiratory apnea using certain positions that facilitate diaphragmatic relaxation. These exercises achieve a decrease in intra-abdominal pressure, provoking reflex contraction of the abdominal muscles, which are flaccid, as well as toning perineal muscles due to reflex contraction of the pelvic floor during the aspiration exercise.

According to a systematic review in 2019 [17], pelvic floor exercises performed in the postpartum period have a positive impact on sexual function, although these data must be interpreted with caution because of the risk of bias, small sample sizes, and the heterogeneity of evaluation tools used in the studies reviewed. The need for further well-designed studies in this area is warranted.

Often little attention is paid to sexuality during pregnancy. Medical care during pregnancy and childbirth are aimed at the prevention of possible complications, frequently excluding sexual issues, partly due to poor specific training of professionals on this subject. Moreover, occasionally the information the patient receives is imprecise and susceptible to misinterpretation due to the presence of many cultural prejudices that have been passed on for generations. It is therefore essential to encourage research and the training of health professionals who attend women so that they can convey clear ideas to couples, helping to alleviate anxiety and improve adaptation to their new situation and preventing potential dysfunctions from appearing over time. The allows the opportunity to provide precise information and dissipate myths and, despite initial reservations, women will probably express gratitude for the sensitive recognition of the topic.

In the case of a pelvic floor injury during delivery, such as OASIS or a levator ani muscle avulsion, with clear risk factors for pelvic floor dysfunction, we should offer the patient an individualized care plan and follow-up that takes into account not only her present situation but her future well being too.

25.5 What Did Dr. Google Say?

There is much information on the Internet openly available for patients that addresses the topics presented in this chapter. In 2008, the Global Library of Women's Medicine (GLOWM), an educational platform of the International Federation of Gynaecology and Obstetrics (FIGO), published a comprehensive article reviewing the physical and psychological aspects of sexuality during pregnancy, childbirth, and the postpartum. The authors aimed to provide information to healthcare professionals so that they can help and advise women and their partners on this issue, providing scientific data on the topic [18].

The websites of health institutions such as the National Health Service (UK) or the American College of Obstetricians and Gynecologists (ACOG) also provide similar information about the changes that women may experience in terms of sexuality during pregnancy as well as when to resume sexual relations after childbirth in a safe and satisfactory way, with advice about contraception at this stage. In addition, the NHS website specifically addresses particular myths about sex and pregnancy and the postnatal period [19,20].

Many nonmedical sites have articles about resuming sexual activity after a vaginal tear suffered during a vaginal delivery [21–23]. The physiological changes that occur during the postpartum are reviewed, as well as the changes on libido. No specific timeline for resuming intercourse is given. Recommendations include Kegel exercises, discussing the topic with the partner, or using lubricants.

When looking for OASIS on an internet search engine, the classification and risk factors for it are described on some sites [22,24]. Perineal massage from weeks 32–34 is recommended by some sites as a means to reduce the possibility of suffering significant vaginal tears during delivery [22]. Some of the sites with specific information are actually rehabilitation clinics that offer pelvic floor rehabilitation. Kegel exercises can be easily found on many sites, with explanatory videos.

25.6 Conclusions

- Resumption of penetrative sexual intercourse after childbirth should be delayed until the perineum, vagina, and uterus have healed adequately. It should be remembered that hormone levels in the puerperal period have a negative influence on a woman's desire and emotional state, and can also cause trophic changes in the genitals and decreased lubrication.

- The prevalence of sexual dysfunction after childbirth is high, although few couples consult a doctor. Pain is the most frequent symptom, together with low libido. Other negative factors are fatigue, lack of sleep, changes in body image, and stress. Sexual function usually returns to prepregnancy levels by 6 months postpartum.

- Individualized assessments of women must be done at 6–8 weeks postpartum, allowing the implementation of specific techniques for pelvic floor recovery, and thus contributing to the prevention of future pelvic floor dysfunction.

References

1. Royal College of Obstetricians and Gynaecologists. *The Management of Third- and Fourth-Degree Perineal Tears.* Green-top Guideline No. 29. London: RCOG, 2015. www.rcog.org.uk/globalassets/documents/guidelines/gtg-29 .pdf (accessed July 22, 2021).

2. Committee on Practice Bulletins – Obstetrics. ACOG Practice Bulletin no. 198: prevention and management of obstetric lacerations at vaginal delivery. *Obstet Gynecol* 2018;**132**:e87–102.

3. T. Friedman, G. D. Eslick, H. P. Dietz. Delivery mode and the risk of levator muscle avulsion: a meta-analysis. *Int Urogynecol J* 2019;**30**:901–7.

4. K. Van Delft, A. H. Sultan, R. Thakar, et al. The relationship between postpartum levator ani muscle avulsion and signs and symptoms of pelvic floor dysfunction. *BJOG* 2014;**121**:1164–71.

5. L. M. Leeman, R. G. Rogers. Sex after childbirth: postpartum sexual function. *Obstet Gynecol* 2012;**119**:647–55.

6. S. Anglés-Acedo, C. Ros-Cerro, S. Escura-Sancho, et al. Coital resumption aflter delivery among OASIS patients: differences between instrumental and spontaneous delivery. *BMC Womens Health* 2019;**19**:154–60.

7. O. Gutzeit, G. Levy, L. Lowenstein. Postpartum female sexual function: risk factors for postpartum sexual dysfunction. *Sex Med* 2020;**8**:8–13.

8. Z. Abdool, R. Thakar, A. H. Sultan. Postpartum female sexual function. *Eur J Obstet Gynecol Reprod Biol* 2009;**145**:133–7.

9. H. Jiang, X. Qian, G. Carroli, P. Garner. Selective versus routine use of episiotomy for vaginal birth. *Cochrane Database Syst Rev* 2017;(2):CD000081.

10. L. B. Signorello, B. L. Harlow, A. K. Chekos, J. T. Repke. Postpartum sexual functioning and its relationship to perineal trauma: a retrospective cohort study of primiparous women. *Am J Obstet Gynecol* 2001;**184**:881–8.

11. R. Radestad, A. Olsson, E. Nissen, C. Rubertsson. Tears in the vagina, perineum, sphincter ani, and rectum and first sexual intercourse after childbirth: a nationwide follow-up. *Birth* 2008;**35**:98–106.

12. M. E. Hannah, H. Whyte, W. J. Hannah, et al. Maternal outcomes at 2 years after planned cesarean section versus planned vaginal birth for breech presentation at term: the international randomized Term Breech Trial. *Am J Obstet Gynecol* 2004;**191**:917–27.

13. A. Griffiths, S. Watermeyer, K. Sidhu, N. N. Amso, B. Nix. Female genital tract morbidity and sexual function following vaginal delivery or lower segment caesarean section. *J Obstet Gynaecol* 2006;**26**:645–9.

14. D. Fan, S. Li, W. Wang, et al. Sexual dysfunction and mode of delivery in Chinese primiparous women: a systematic review and meta-analysis. *BMC Pregnancy Childbirth* 2017;**17**:408.

15. E. S. Lukacz, J. M. Lawrence, R. Contreras, C. W. Nager, K. M. Luber. Parity, mode of delivery and pelvic floor disorders. *Obstet Gynecol* 2006;**107**:1253–60.

16. J. O. L. Delancey, L. K. Low, J. M. Miller, D. A. Patel, J. A. Tumbarello. Graphic integration of causal factors of pelvic floor disorders: an integrated lifespan model. *Am J Obstet Gynecol* 2008;**199**:610.e1–5.

17. S. S. Sobhgol, H. Priddis, C. A. Smith, H. G. Dahlen. The effect of pelvic floor muscle exercise on female sexual function during pregnancy and postpartum: a systematic review. *Sex Med Rev* 2019;**7**:13–28.

18. C. S. Brown, J. B. Bradford, F. W. Ling. Sex and sexuality in pregnancy. Global Library of Women's Medicine. www.glowm.com/section-view/heading/Sex%20and%20Sexuality%20in%20Pregnancy/item/111# (accessed July 22, 2021).

19. National Health Service. Sex in pregnancy. www.nhs.uk/pregnancy/keeping-well/sex (accessed July 22, 2021).

20. American College of Obstetricians and Gynecologists. Is it safe to have sex during pregnancy? www.acog.org/womens-health/experts-and-stories/ask-acog/is-it-safe-to-have-sex-during-pregnancy (accessed July 22, 2021).

21. How to deal with vaginal tearing while having sex. Enkimd, 2018. www.enkimd.com/vaginal-tearing-during-intercourse.html (accessed September 26, 2021).

22. L. Hickman. Tears during a vaginal delivery: what you need to know. 2020. https://femalehealthawareness.org/en/tears-during-a-vaginal-delivery-what-you-need-to-know/ (accessed September 26, 2021).

23. K. Holland. What to expect from sex after giving birth. 2019. www.healthline.com/health/pregnancy/sex-after-birth (accessed September 26, 2021).

24. What to expect when you have a 2nd degree tear. Mamamend, 2019. www.mamamend.com/postpartum-health/second-degree-tear (accessed September 26, 2021).

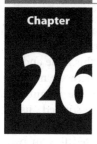

Miscarriages, Spontaneous Abortions, Stillbirths, and Sex

Orli Silverberg and Dan Farine

26.1 Introduction

Losing a pregnancy is undoubtedly an awful outcome that pregnant women dread. In this chapter we look at this issue from a number of different perspectives:

- Can having sex result in miscarriage or stillbirth?
- Should women refrain from having sex in order to prevent pregnancy loss?
- When can sexual intercourse be resumed after a miscarriage?
- Should sex be avoided or postponed after a miscarriage?
- Should a miscarriage in the past be a reason to avoid sex in the current pregnancy.

As outlined, this topic comprises completely unrelated issues and therefore we have divided this chapter into four separate sections:

1. Can sex result in a stillbirth or miscarriage?
2. Does violent sex cause such results?
3. When can intercourse be resumed after a pregnancy loss?
4. Is loss in a previous pregnancy a reason to refrain from sex in the current one?

26.2 Terminology

The definitions vary in different jurisdictions but the following are generally accepted:

- Spontaneous abortion (SA): loss of the pregnancy in the first trimester (up to 20 weeks as defined by some authorities).
- Miscarriage: usually same as above.
- Missed abortion: a dead fetus in utero without any maternal symptoms.
- Threatened abortion: bleeding in the first trimester.
- Stillbirth: death of the baby in utero after 20 weeks.

The management of these conditions is different. In all but threatened abortion the baby has died. In the past we used to believe that the psychological trauma to the pregnant woman was significant late in pregnancy and minimal in early pregnancy, but we now know that it is the event itself and less its timing.

26.3 Methodology

In medicine there is a hierarchy to the quality of evidence. We consider the best evidence to be derived from randomized controlled trials (RCTs). The second best is from meta-analysis where such RCTs are lumped together in a careful way. Then come very large cohort studies (e.g. data of a whole country) and last come smaller observational studies and case reports.

This creates a problem in trying to research the issues at hand. This is illustrated by a paper published by Gordon Smith from Cambridge [1]. He performed a meta-analysis of all the RCTs comparing the outcomes of jumping from an airplane with or without a parachute. To his surprise, he could not find a single study addressing this issue and his meta-analysis had therefore no papers at all. His conclusion was that "there are no good studies showing the superiority of jumping with a parachute." What he meant and succeeded in doing was to show that not all issues can be studied using such methodologies.

Another phenomenon is that many years ago some studies suggested that in twin pregnancies preterm birth could be associated with having sex. Interestingly, in studies that examined only sex there was higher chance of finding it was a risk factor than in studies that examined several risks. The study by Langer and Hod [2] provides an answer by finding that women lied 80% of the time (and in 90% of those), claiming that the glucometer readings they charted manually were lower than the readings on the glucometer memory.

These issues imply that most papers on these topics have a problematic methodology. In addition, many have selection biases and a small number of subjects. The result is that the suggestions provided in this chapter are most likely to be expert opinion at best.

26.4 Sections of This Chapter

1. **One mechanism for sex to result in stillbirth is bleeding**: Bleeding in either early or late pregnancy is associated with pregnancy loss. Bleeding usually implies placental separation; a massive bleed may result in total abruption and fetal death. These issues are covered in other chapters (see Chapter 13 for more details on bleeding in the first trimester and Chapter 14 on bleeding in the second and third trimesters). Therefore, the issue of stillbirth following bleeding as the result of sex is not discussed in this chapter.
2. **Violence in pregnancy**: Violence in pregnancy is unfortunately very common. In the last few years it has finally gained the attention it deserves. Such violence is often also sexual in nature. Violent sex is quite different from the nonviolent sex that is the topic of this book. For the sake of completeness, we refer briefly to this topic.
3. **Resuming sex following a pregnancy loss**: Technically, it is not a pregnancy issue as the pregnancy is over. However, it is an important question, as it signifies in a way that life is back to normal and sex could be important not only on its own but as part of a support system.
4. **Sex in a subsequent pregnancy**: In a woman who has experienced a pregnancy loss there is a major concern that this may reoccur in a subsequent pregnancy. The question that most of these women have is whether pregnancy is safe and will not trigger another pregnancy loss. This is discussed in detail.

Each of these topics was selected to shed light on subjects that we think are important and distinct.

26.5 Can Sex Result in a Stillbirth or Miscarriage?

Whether sexual intercourse can cause pregnancy loss is a controversial and poorly studied topic. Pregnant patients often seek out guidance from healthcare providers about a healthy lifestyle during the antenatal period, including avoidance of alcohol and unpasteurized dairy. There is little evidence that coitus can cause stillbirth and most of it concerns bleeding. As discussed earlier in the book, placental separation and abruption increase the likelihood of fetal demise in utero.

Over time societal norms evolve and the taboos surrounding sexual health have begun to dissipate. As recently as 40 years ago, sexual intercourse was described in textbooks as a risk factor and precipitant for pregnancy loss. Later revisions then suggested that coitus did not have any impact on pregnancy. Nevertheless, if a patient has recurrent miscarriages or the pregnancy is at risk, sexual activity in pregnancy is "unwise." There have been very few peer-reviewed and evidence-based articles examining whether coitus can increase the risk of pregnancy loss. It seems that the default advice to avoid the act is rooted in our paternalistic society and culture. Without previous evidence to support these statements, they were derived from a lack of knowledge and support for sexuality in pregnancy. There have been minimal advances in the field and current practitioners remain divided on counseling and instructing on this topic [3].

As mentioned above, coitus used to be discouraged by practitioners on the basis of minimal evidence, and the few papers that supported this opinion were of low quality and neglected to control for relevant contributing factors. However, a large collaborative study published in *The Lancet* from the 1980s found no association between any adverse outcome in pregnancy and sexual activity [4]. Almost 40 000 pregnancies were included and intercourse during the third trimester of pregnancy did not have an impact on the outcome of these pregnancies. Vaginitis and urinary tract infection, which are known to follow sexual activity, did not influence the results whether included in the statistical analyses or not. To date, this is still the largest study of its kind conducted in the USA and should be used as a guideline for counseling with regard to sexual activity during pregnancy.

In 1981, a study by Mills et al. [5] disputed the previously well-accepted notion that coitus may precipitate stillbirth and miscarriage. Premature rupture of membranes, preterm birth, and chorioamnionitis were all proposed methods of the alleged risk imposed by sexual activity. The authors described the shortcomings of the previous literature and demonstrated, with a large sample size and effective blinding techniques, no association between intercourse and demise of a pregnancy.

It seems that this topic is one that has been historically neglected by clinicians and researchers and the previously proposed risk was made on the basis of poor-quality studies and historical societal norms. To date, there is no good evidence that sexual activity imposes any increased risk of pregnancy loss. However, it is also clear that there is a need for further high-quality evidence on the topic.

26.5.1 What Did Dr. Google Say?

Doctor Google agrees with the literature. Many of the articles reference the historical advice to sexual abstinence during pregnancy (Verywell family website). This site thoughtfully acknowledges the well-being of individual patients and recognizes that intercourse is a healthy and normal part of life. The risks associated with sexual intercourse and pregnancy are centered around specific situations, such as high-risk sexual behaviors with nonmonogamous partners in which the chances of contracting a sexually transmitted infection (STI) are increased. There is also mention that placenta previa and bleeding may be special circumstances in which coitus should be avoided.

Another article on the National Health Service site normalizes the increased or decreased desire to engage in sexual activity while pregnant. Either way, it becomes a personal decision and one that is not about the risk to the pregnancy, so much as the well-being of an individual. The article also mentions that there are instances where coitus should be avoided, including multiple gestation, rupture of membranes, and placenta previa. The article also emphasizes the importance of protection against STIs since they may affect pregnancy outcomes.

It seems that the information available to lay people as well as the evidence-based articles explains that in general coitus does not precipitate pregnancy loss. There is a history of conflicting evidence, but with the evolution of medicine and a new emphasis on sexual health, this myth will hopefully be debunked.

26.6 Does Violent Sex Result in Stillbirths?

Violence in pregnancy is an underrecognized and devastating global health pandemic that contributes to poor health outcomes. For individuals who normally endure intimate partner violence (IPV), pregnancy serves as a protective factor or, paradoxically, exacerbates the ongoing abuse [6,7]. We define IPV here as abuse in any form – sexual, physical, emotional – that may be carried out by any person. Although this topic is seemingly unrelated to the rest of this book, which focuses on sexual intercourse and how it affects pregnancy, sexual violence does unfortunately occur in the context of pregnancy. Sex in pregnancy is distinct from violence in pregnancy, and although sex may be a presentation of violence it is in reality a disgusting demonstration of aggressive dominance. It is a topic that has been historically neglected, but greatly affects health outcomes. In the following, we discuss what the literature reveals about violence of a sexual nature in pregnancy as well as how it relates to loss of pregnancy.

Social determinants of health play a central role in global health; notably, one in five women in low-income areas experience physical IPV [8]. Other risk factors for violence include low education level and socioeconomic status, young maternal age, increasing parity, and substance abuse in the partner [6,9,10]. The World Health Organization (WHO) estimates that a staggering 30% of women internationally are subject to IPV, whether sexual, emotional, physical, or otherwise [11]. A study encompassing various regions of Africa determined that 2.3–57.1% of pregnant women may experience IPV [7]. The likely underreported estimated prevalence of IPV in pregnancy in various countries is quoted at 30% in Tanzania, 33% in Vietnam, 23% in Ethiopia, and up to 20% in the USA [7,10]. A study by Tiruye et al. [9] stated that above 40% of women during pregnancy experience partner-incited violence. From the above it is very clear that abuse in pregnancy is not infrequent and must not be neglected by healthcare professionals.

Individuals who experience IPV are significantly more likely to report premature rupture of membranes, preterm birth, low birthweight, and admission to the neonatal intensive care unit [6,7,9–13]. More sinister outcomes associated with IPV include pregnancy loss in any trimester, stillbirth, and perinatal death. As outlined by another study, these patients are also three times more likely to experience fetal death [14]. Sexual abuse, specifically, escalates the risk of perinatal death, as well as additional adverse pregnancy outcomes [6,10]. Individuals who reported stillbirth as the outcome of their pregnancy were also more likely to have endured domestic abuse in the previous year [15].

These devastating consequences may be partly due to the confounding factors that often accompany abuse; these include psychological stress, low socioeconomic status, and unemployment. However, one study notes that employed individuals and middle to upper class women are not immune to this detrimental abuse during pregnancy [10]. Additionally, a study by Tiruye et al. [9] described an association between IPV and pregnancy loss after controlling for the confounding variables listed above. The risk may also be associated with hazardous unwanted sexual encounters resulting in infection (e.g. HIV), as well as stress and psychosocial illness following sexual assault [7–9]. Stress may also incite or exacerbate medical illness such as hypertension of pregnancy, which is known to induce adverse outcomes through alterations in the hypothalamic–pituitary–adrenal axis. The psychological impact of violence may lead to the demise of a pregnancy through behavioral changes and increase in substance abuse [6]. This coping mechanism adopted by victims of trauma is well known to be harmful to pregnancies and likely furthers the association of IPV with negative outcomes [10]. Physical violence in any form, including sexual, may jeopardize a pregnancy [10,11]. As evidenced by the above, there are numerous well-understood pathways by which physical and sexual violence in pregnancy may precipitate stillbirth.

In a study from sub-Saharan Africa, physical IPV was linked with higher risk of miscarriage and stillbirth [8,11]. This was a direct consequence of abdominal trauma precipitating uterine rupture, placental abruption, or antepartum hemorrhage [6,8,9,12]. The uterus is very thin in the third trimester of pregnancy, leaving women particularly vulnerable to rupture following violence [12]. Similar patterns are described in Asia, Africa, Latin America, Colombia, South Carolina, and California [7,16].

Heazell et al. [15] noted that pregnant women who suffer from abuse may have difficulty with access to, or experience a delay in seeking, antenatal care, increasing the risk of complication and stillbirth in this population. In the same study, it was identified that women who preferred not to answer questions about domestic abuse were also at higher risk of stillbirth. This signifies the importance and underreporting of abuse.

IPV may be more prevalent than other commonly diagnosed issues, such as pre-eclampsia or gestational diabetes [16]. It is a statistically underrepresented problem due to the hesitation and shame many victims feel when deciding to disclose information [9]. Healthcare providers are generally not well equipped to approach situations regarding sexual abuse and do so less than recommended [12]. Although the American College of Obstetrics and Gynecology (ACOG) recommends screening for IPV at the first antenatal visit, once per trimester and postpartum, many providers hesitate to do so [12]. Universal screening is imperative to avoid missing cases that go undetected due to a lack of red flags or other typical physical exam findings [17]. Tiruye et al. [9] suggests implementing an IPV prevention and screening program for pregnant women, in addition to reinforcing confidentiality at each encounter. Another possibility for change is the integration of education about relationships and coping mechanisms into school programs for young adolescents [12]. Early detection and intervention has the potential to improve outcomes of pregnancies in patients experiencing IPV as well as improve health outcomes overall [6,7].

For this section, Dr. Google was not consulted because it is inconceivable to imagine that any website would condone domestic violence against pregnant individuals.

26.7 When Can Intercourse Be Resumed after Pregnancy Loss?

The complex and devastating experience of pregnancy loss is known to provoke grief, anxiety, and guilt in parents, damaging their well-being and quality of relationships. Following a period of grieving, parents may feel that their relationship and own quality of life has changed. Many of these factors contribute to the decision to resume sexual activity following a pregnancy loss.

Reduced sexual intimacy is common following stillbirth and Lang et al. [18] observed that 60% of postpartum patients were aware of sexual distress as well as a loss of interest following stillbirth or loss of a child. Feelings of guilt and blame that emerge from enduring this loss greatly contributes to patients reporting decreased libido [19]. Patients exhibit a wide range of individual variation in baseline libido, personal coping skills, and relationships that will contribute to their view on resuming sexual intercourse. Some patients feel that intercourse may provide comfort by achieving physical closeness to their partner. However, others may find it to be triggering and a burdensome reminder of the tragedy that has occurred [20]. It is important to adopt a person-centered approach and uncover how each individual patient may view the situation.

Campbell-Jackson et al. [21] noted that following stillbirth or death of a child, male patients had the tendency to desire sexual intimacy earlier than female patients. Depending on the desires and values of their partners, this may put strain on their relationship. In general, sexual intimacy was an accurate indicator of how adequately men were managing grief a few years after the loss of an infant or fetus [18].

Aside from the emotional and interpersonal aspects, there is the question of when to resume intercourse in an attempt to conceive again after stillbirth. In 2019, the WHO recommended postponing family planning for at least 6 months. This statement is based on evidence that a decreased interval between pregnancies is associated with increased adverse pregnancy outcomes. Paradoxically, a meta-analysis from Dyer et al. [22] did not support the recommendation of the WHO. Following the loss of a pregnancy, many women experience an urge to become pregnant again, and 80% become pregnant within the subsequent 18 months [22]. Involving a health professional in future family planning is encouraged regardless of the individual patient decision surrounding timing. Thus, the interpregnancy opportunity to attenuate modifiable risk factors for subsequent pregnancies, such as diabetes, obesity, or smoking, may be the most important and effective way of lowering risk [23].

In the literature, there is also an expressed concern that if women become pregnant immediately after the miscarriage, without time to properly grieve and cope, they may attempt to psychologically replace the fetus with another child. In this case, it may be harmful to the emotional grieving process and mothers should be counseled to understand that another child should not, and cannot, be a replacement child [20].

The decision to resume sexual activity following stillbirth is both a medical and deeply personal matter. The recommendation as to when depends on individual, psychological, and emotional circumstances; there is no simple answer. The best way to support patients through this difficult time without clear answers is to be present and available to provide advice and answer questions. In a study by Dyer et al. [22], the decision about, and the planning of, a subsequent pregnancy was based on individual and social factors rather than on advice from medical professionals. As health advocates, the role of physicians should be to broach the topic if appropriate and provide information accordingly. Dyregrov and Gjestad [19] found that only 11% of patients had the subject of satisfaction in sexuality broached by their care providers following a stillbirth. It is worth noting that in that same study, close to 80% of couples had resumed sexual intercourse within 3 months of child loss or stillbirth. It may therefore be useful to encourage normalization of this emotional expression, need for physical comfort, and potential escape from the tragedy that has befallen them. Conveying the necessary medical information regarding the stillbirth is still imperative, but acknowledgment of their sexuality may help with some of the guilt many individuals feel following stillbirth [19]. On the other hand, some women who did not receive any advice about planning subsequent pregnancies felt that they were given time and space to do so when they felt ready. This demonstrates that assessing when to provide advice appropriately may have a more significant positive impact than the content of what is being conveyed. Overall, advice about timing may be most useful rather than specific recommendations [23]. All factors must be considered to give a specific ideal time to resume sexual activity following a stillbirth or miscarriage.

26.7.1 What Did Dr. Google Say?

The Society of Obstetricians and Gynecologists of Canada (SOGC) publishes guidelines that are available on the Internet regarding when to resume sexual activity following the demise of a pregnancy. However, the site does state that there is currently no precise recommendation regarding when to resume sexual intercourse during subsequent pregnancies.

On the BC Women's Hospital and Health Centre website, in an article on how to cope with a stillbirth, there is a section on sexuality. It details that individuals may either desire or stray away from sexual intercourse after this traumatic event. The article encourages communication between partners about the topic and suggests other physical maneuvers that may aid in feeling comfort from physical closeness, such as cuddling. There are a few strategies to reduce sexual dysfunction, such as lubrication, expressing breast milk prior to intercourse, and exploration of intimacy through means other than intercourse. The recommendation is that once any vaginal lacerations have healed and vaginal bleeding has decreased, it is medically safe to resume sexual activity.

A blog called Scary Mommy (2019) emphasizes that curiosity about sexuality following a miscarriage is very common. The loss of a pregnancy comes with the loaded question of whether fertility is affected, and when it will be safe to reengage in intimate behaviors with partners. There is mention of an infection risk immediately after miscarriage and a recommendation to arrange a physical exam with an obstetrician prior to recommencing sexual activity. In addition to the physical safety check, the importance of emotional readiness is emphasized. Communicating with your partner is suggested to enable effective decision-making when both parties feel prepared. If individuals do decide to resume sexual intercourse, they should explore methods to reduce the risk of STI as well as contraception if desired. Unprotected intercourse can still result in an unwanted pregnancy and patients should be counseled that they are likely fertile following a pregnancy loss. For patients that would like to conceive, the article recommends waiting for one menstrual cycle, but does note that there is controversy surrounding this time interval.

Another article (Meredith Shur, VeryWell Family, 2020) advises waiting 6 weeks, until the postpartum visit, to resume sexual activity; however, ensuring physical and emotional readiness is the most important factor. As with the previous resources, the article emphasizes the importance of contraception if a subsequent pregnancy is not desired.

Six months is the suggested waiting time on the Tommy's website, to ensure physical and emotional recovery prior to initiating intercourse. Discussion centers on planning to conceive and provides recommendations on folic acid supplementation and lifestyle factors such as halting smoking and alcohol consumption. Fertility may return as quickly as 2 weeks following a stillbirth, but the advice is to wait until the cervical os has closed and episiotomy scars have healed before resuming sexual activity.

In summary, the advice from Dr. Google generally incorporates the various factors that surround the personal decision to resume sexual activity following a pregnancy loss. There is advice about emotional processing, relationship factors, physical and medical indications, and future family planning. Generally, the recommendation for the correct amount of time varies from article to article and these do note the controversy in the medical community as well.

26.8 Is a Loss in a Previous Pregnancy a Reason to Refrain from Having Sex in the Current One?

The most common etiology of stillbirth is idiopathic, and 50% of women conceive less than 1 year following their loss [21]. Guilt, shame, and blame often accompany this devastating loss and impact the actions of mothers in subsequent pregnancies. Many feel an overwhelming sense of duty to protect the unborn fetus by whatever means possible, which addresses the question at hand: Does sexual intercourse in a pregnancy following stillbirth impact outcome?

As explored in the previous sections, sexual intercourse was historically thought to be a factor in precipitating fetal demise. In a previous edition of *Gynecology by Ten Teachers*, coitus was deemed to be safe in a healthy pregnancy, but viewed as "unwise" in a subsequent pregnancy following a stillbirth. This was not supported by sound evidence and in a later edition of the same text the statement was removed. However, if there is no current evidence demonstrating that sexual intercourse can cause misfortune in pregnancy, a recommendation of abstinence in the future antepartum period would not be sound [3].

The SOGC statement on stillbirth details that after such tragic outcomes, subsequent pregnancies are at a twofold to tenfold increased risk; however, the absolute risk of pregnancy loss remains low. It is important to include the etiology of loss in the assessment of subsequent risk; however, there is no recommendation or guideline regarding sexuality in future pregnancies.

26.8.1 What Did Dr. Google Say?

Dr. Google takes a more haphazard approach, with one site (Grow by WebMD) recommending that individuals with a history of previous miscarriage avoid sexual intercourse during pregnancy. No reasoning or evidence is provided for this statement. However, consulting a healthcare provider to determine the risk at hand is recommended.

Sexuality during pregnancy has historically been a taboo, controversial, and understudied topic that has caused confusion among providers and patients alike. The subject of sex and stillbirth is one that must be further explored. However, there is currently no recommendation for how to approach a subsequent pregnancy. Personal, medical, and situational factors must be considered on an individual basis to make a decision for each patient.

References

1. G. C. Smith, J. P. Pell. Parachute use to prevent death and major trauma related to gravitational challenge: systematic review of randomised controlled trials. *BMJ* 2003;**327**:1459–61.

2. O. Langer, M. Hod. Management of gestational diabetes mellitus. *Obstet Gynecol Clin North Am* 1996;**23**:137–59.

3. A. Moscrop. Can sex during pregnancy cause a miscarriage? A concise history of not knowing. *Br J Gen Pract* 2012;**62**: e308–10.

4. M. A. Klebanoff, R. P. Nugent, G. G. Rhoads. Coitus during pregnancy: is it safe? *Lancet* 1984;**324**:914–17.

5. J. L. Mills, S. Harlap, E. E. Harley. Should coitus late in pregnancy be discouraged? *Lancet* 1981;**318**:136–8.

6. J. L. Alhusen, E. Ray, P. Sharps, L. Bullock. Intimate partner violence during pregnancy: maternal and neonatal outcomes. *J Womens Health (Larchmt)* 2015;**24**:100–6.

7. K. Z. Gebreslasie, S. Weldemariam, G. Gebre, M.-A. Mehari. Intimate partner violence during pregnancy and risk of stillbirth in hospitals of Tigray region Ethiopia. *Ital J Pediatr* 2020;**46**:107.

8. N. Rao, A. N. Turner, B. Harrington, et al. Correlations between intimate partner violence and spontaneous abortion, stillbirth, and neonatal death in rural Malawi. *Int J Gynaecol Obstet* 2017;**138**:74–8.

9. T. T. Tiruye, C. Chojenta, M. L. Harris, E. Holliday, D. Loxton. Intimate partner violence against women and its association with pregnancy loss in Ethiopia: evidence from a national survey. *BMC Womens Health* 2020;**20**:192.

10. A. L. Coker, M. Sanderson, B. Dong. Partner violence during pregnancy and risk of adverse pregnancy outcomes. *Paediatr Perinat Epidemiol* 2004;**18**:260–9.

11. A. Afiaz, R. K. Biswas, R. Shamma, N. Ananna. Intimate partner violence (IPV) with miscarriages, stillbirths and abortions: identifying vulnerable households for women in Bangladesh. *PLoS ONE* 2020;**15**:e0236670.

12. N. Auger, N. Low, G. E. Lee, A. Ayoub, T. M. Luu. Pregnancy outcomes of women hospitalized for physical assault, sexual assault, and intimate partner violence. *J Interpers Violence* 2021; DOI: https://doi .org/10.1177/0886260520985496.

13. R. M. Román-Gálvez, S. Martín-Peláez, J. M. Martínez-Galiano, K. S. Khan, A. Bueno-Cavanillas. Prevalence of intimate partner violence in pregnancy: an umbrella review. *Int J Environ Res Public Health* 2021;**18**:707.

14. G. Pastor-Moreno, I. Ruiz-Pérez, J. Henares-Montiel, D. Petrova. Intimate partner violence during pregnancy and risk of fetal and neonatal death: a meta-analysis with socioeconomic context indicators. *Am J Obstet Gynecol* 2020;**222**:123–33.e5.

15. A. Heazell, J. Budd, L. K. Smith, et al. Associations between social and behavioural factors and the risk of late stillbirth: findings from the Midland and North of England Stillbirth case–control study. *BJOG* 2021;**128**:704–13.

16. G. Pastor-Moreno, I. Ruiz-Pérez, J. Henares-Montiel, et al. Intimate partner violence and perinatal health: a systematic review. *BJOG* 2020;**127**:537–47.

17. N. A. Deshpande, A. Lewis-O'Connor. Screening for intimate partner violence during pregnancy. *Rev Obstet Gynecol* 2013;**6**:141–8.

18. A. Lang, L. N. Gottlieb, R. Amsel. Predictors of husbands' and wives' grief reactions following infant death: the role of marital intimacy. *Death Stud* 1996;**20**:33–57.

19. A. Dyregrov, R. Gjestad. Sexuality following the loss of a child. *Death Stud* 2011;**35**:289–315.

20. J. Thomas. The effects on the family of miscarriage, termination for abnormality, stillbirth and neonatal death. *Child Care Health Dev* 1995;**21**:413–24.

21. L. Campbell-Jackson, J. Bezance, A. Horsch. "A renewed sense of purpose": mothers' and fathers' experience of having a child following a recent stillbirth. *BMC Pregnancy Childbirth* 2014;**14**:423.

22. E. Dyer, R. Bell, R. Graham, J. Rankin. Pregnancy decisions after fetal or perinatal death: systematic review of qualitative research. *BMJ Open* 2019;**9**: e029930.

23. K. Joronen , M. Kaunonen, A. L. Aho. Parental relationship satisfaction after the death of a child. *Scand J Caring Sci.* 2016;**30**:499–506.

Index

Printed in the United States
by Baker & Taylor Publisher Services